Repair and Regeneration of Ligaments, Tendons, and Joint Capsule

Orthopedic Biology and Medicine

SERIES EDITOR: ***Yuehuei H. An and A. U. Daniels***
Orthopaedic Research Laboratory
Medical University of South Carolina, Charleston, SC

Repair and Regeneration of Ligaments, Tendons, and Joint Capsule, edited by ***William R. Walsh,*** 2005

Repair and Regeneration of Ligaments, Tendons, and Joint Capsule

Edited by

William R. Walsh, PhD

Orthopaedic Research Laboratory, University of New South Wales
Sydney, Australia

HUMANA PRESS ✱ TOTOWA, NEW JERSEY

999 Riverview Drive, Suite 208
Totowa, New Jersey 07512

www.humanapress.com

This publication is printed on acid-free paper. ∞

ANSI Z39.48-1984 (American Standards Institute) Permanence of Paper for Printed Library Materials.

Cover design by Patricia F. Cleary.

Cover illustrations: *Background*: Figure 11, Chapter 12. *Foreground (from left to right)*: Figure 13, Chapter 12; Figure 3, Chapter 2; Figure 9B, Chapter 11; Figure 5, Chapter 12.

For additional copies, pricing for bulk purchases, and/or information about other Humana titles, contact Humana at the above address or at any of the following numbers: Tel: 973-256-1699; Fax: 973-256-8341; E-mail: humana@humanapr.com, or visit our Website: http://humanapress.com

Printed in the United States of America. 10 9 8 7 6 5 4 3 2 1

Library of Congress Cataloging in Publication Data

Repair and regeneration of ligaments, tendons, and joint capsule / edited by William R. Walsh.
p. cm. — (Orthopedic biology and medicine)
Includes bibliographical references and index.
ISBN 1-58829-174-X (alk. paper) eISBN 1-59259-942-7
1. Ligaments—Wounds and injuries. 2. Tendons—Wounds and injuries. 3. Joints—Wounds and injuries. 4. Joints—Regeneration. 5. Orthopedic surgery. I. Walsh, William R. II. Series.
RD688.R47 2005
617.4'74044—dc22 2004030489

Preface

The molecular biology and mechanical properties of tendon and ligament healing and soft tissue (i.e., tendon, ligament, capsular tissues) to bone are a vital aspect of many surgical disciplines. Recent advances, both surgical and experimental, have provided great insight into new techniques, mechanisms of healing, and strategies for augmentation and repair.

Repair and Regeneration of Ligaments, Tendons, and Joint Capsule provides a comprehensive review of some of the most important scientific and clinically relevant topics in biology, biomechanics, and surgical reconstruction today. It is hoped that this book will set the standard of excellence in these fields and become a valuable resource for clinical understanding, postgraduate research, and resident training. In addition, chapters on the shoulder, hand, and knee should be valuable to those involved in the research and practice of sports medicine. The book is written by distinguished contributors who have graciously provided new techniques and experimental findings in their respective fields.

***William R. Walsh,* PhD**

Contents

Contributors

Scott D. Allen, MD • *Department of Orthopaedic Surgery, Brown University School of Medicine, Providence, Rhode Island*

Andrew A. Amis, DSc • *Departments of Mechanical Engineering and Musculoskeletal Surgery, Imperial College of Science, Technology, & Medicine, London, UK*

Yuehuei H. An, MD • *Orthopaedic Research Laboratory, Medical University of South Carolina, Charleston, SC*

Maria Apreleva, PhD • *Center for Musculoskeletal Surgery, Sports Traumatology and Arthroscopy Service, Charité, Campus Virchow Klinikum, Berlin, Germany*

Randip R. Bindra, MD, FRCS • *Center for Hand and Upper Extremity Surgery, Orthopaedic Surgery Department, University of Arkansas for Medical Sciences, Little Rock, AR*

Eric M. Bluman, MD, PhD • *Department of Orthopaedic Surgery, Brown University School of Medicine, Providence, Rhode Island*

Gino Bradica, PhD • *Department of Pathology and Laboratory Medicine, UMDNJ-Robert Wood Johnson Medical School, Piscataway, NJ*

Warwick J. Bruce, MD • *Orthopaedic Department, Concord Hospital, Concord, New South Wales, Australia*

Adam M. Butler, PhD • *Orthopaedic Research Laboratories, Prince of Wales Hospital, University of New South Wales, Sydney, Australia*

Jeffrey S. Cartmell, PhD • *Departments of Orthopaedic Surgery and Bioengineering, McKay Orthopaedic Research Laboratory, University of Pennsylvania, Philadelphia, PA*

Tracey Clarke, MSc, CHT, MAPA, MAHTA • *Hand Therapist, Hand & Upper Limb Therapy, Castle Hill, NSW, Australia*

Eddy Dona, MBBS • *Orthopaedic Research Laboratories, Prince of Wales Hospital, University of New South Wales, Sydney, Australia*

Michael G. Dunn, PhD • *Orthopaedic Research Laboratory, Department of Orthopaedic Surgery, UMDNJ-Robert Wood Johnson Medical School, New Brunswick, NJ*

Richard O. Evans, MSc, FRCS(Tr&Orth) • *Consultant Orthopaedic Surgeon, University Hospital of Wales, Cardiff, Wales, UK*

Paul D. Fadale, MD • *Department of Orthopaedic Surgery, Brown University School of Medicine, Providence, RI*

Joseph W. Freeman, PhD • *Department of Pathology and Laboratory Medicine, UMDNJ-Robert Wood Johnson Medical School, Piscataway, NJ*

Mark P. Gianoutsos, MBBS, MD, FRACS (Plast) • *Head of the Department of Paediatric Plastic Surgery, Sydney Children's Hospital, and Adjunct Associate Professor, University of New South Wales, Sydney, Australia*

R. Mark Gillies, PhD • *Orthopaedic Research Laboratories, Prince of Wales Hospital, University of New South Wales, Sydney, Australia*

Jerome Goldberg, MBBS, FRACS • *Orthopaedic Research Laboratories, Prince of Wales Hospital, University of New South Wales, Sydney, Australia*

David Hartright, MD • *Orthopaedic Research Laboratories, Prince of Wales Hospital, University of New South Wales, Sydney, Australia*

Christopher M. Hill, VMD • *Orthopaedic Research Laboratory, Medical University of South Carolina, Charleston, SC*

Peter J. Hughes, BSc(HONS), MBChB, FRCS(Tr&Orth) • *Department of Orthopaedics, Lancashire Teaching Hospitals NHS Trust, Preston, United Kingdom*

Jon Karlsson, MD, PhD • *Department of Orthopaedics, Sahlgrenska University Hospital, Göteborg, Sweden*

Norimasa Nakamura, MD, PhD • *Department of Orthopaedics, Osaka University Graduate School of Medicine, Osaka, Japan*

Beata Niechoda, MBBS • *Orthopaedic Research Laboratories, Prince of Wales Hospital, University of New South Wales, Sydney, Australia*

Sven Scheffler, MD • *Center for Musculoskeletal Surgery, Sports Traumatology and Arthroscopy Service, Charité, Campus Virchow Klinikum, Berlin, Germany*

Frederick H. Silver, PhD • *Department of Pathology and Laboratory Medicine, UMDNJ-Robert Wood Johnson Medical School, Piscataway, NJ*

Louis J. Soslowsky, PhD • *Departments of Orthopaedic Surgery and Bioengineering, McKay Orthopaedic Research Laboratory, University of Pennsylvania, Philadelphia, PA*

David H. Sonnabend, MBBS, FRACS • *Orthopaedic Department, Royal North Shore Hospital, Sydney, Australia*

Paul C. Stephens, MB ChB, MRCS (Glas) • *Orthopaedic Research Laboratories, Prince of Wales Hospital, University of New South Wales, Sydney, Australia*

Andrew L. Wallace, PhD, FRACS • *Department of Orthopaedic Surgery, St. Mary's Hospital, Imperial College, London, UK*

William R. Walsh, PhD • *Orthopaedic Research Laboratories, University of New South Wales, Sydney, Australia*

Andreas Weiler, MD, PhD • *Center for Musculoskeletal Surgery, Sports Traumatology and Arthroscopy Service, Charité, Campus Virchow Klinikum, Berlin, Germany*

Frank A. Young, DS • *Orthopaedic Research Laboratory, Department of Materials Science, Medical University of South Carolina, Charleston, SC*

Part I
Introduction

1

Tendon Repair and Regeneration

An Overview

Eric M. Bluman, Scott D. Allen, and Paul D. Fadale

INTRODUCTON

To fully understand the healing and regeneration of tendons, the relevant anatomy of each of these structures must be first understood. Each tendon is made up of a hierarchical arrangement of collagen bundles. These bundles—organized in parallel—are responsible for the tendon's tensile strength. Tendons are primarily composed of type I collagen, but they also contain small amounts of types III, IV, V, and VI collagen. Proteoglycans are also present with decorin predominating, but biglycan, lumican, and fibromodulin have been detected as well. Proteoglycans are thought to regulate the diameter of collagen fibers, separate individual fiber bundles, and minimize the shear stresses that fibers experience as they move relative to each other during normal function. Although tendons function primarily under tensile loads, they do experience compressive loads passing around skeletal prominences. Some pressures in these regions are substantial, with measurements reported in the range of 700 mmHg. Glycosaminoglycan content in these areas is elevated relative to the rest of the tendon. This is probably a functional adaptation, which allows for greater water content and secondary structural resiliency under compressive conditions.

Adaptive changes in tendons are also observed in the flexor and extensor tendons of the hand. At birth, both groups have identical mechanical properties, but as the flexor tendons encounter a greater load (as a consequence of the biomechanical arrangement of the hand), they become stronger and stiffer relative to their extensor counterparts.

The blood supply to tendons is paramount in their healing and maintenance. This supply is from three sources: the perimesium, the periosteal insertion of the tendon, and the paratenon. The paratenon derives its blood supply from the surrounding tissues. Flexor tendons of the hand and wrist also have an additional blood supply—the mesotenon that is condensed into the vincula. Avascular regions are believed to be supplied by diffusion.

INFLAMMATORY AND TRAUMATIC PATHOLOGIES

The conditions that affect the tendons, as well as the manifestations of each, are diverse. The mechanisms and pathogenesis of these injuries are also quite different.

From: *Orthopedic Biology and Medicine: Repair and Regeneration of Ligaments, Tendons, and Joint Capsule*
Edited by: W. R. Walsh © Humana Press Inc., Totowa, NJ

Tendinopathies may involve the tenosynovium, the peritenon, the tendon itself, or a combination of these structures. One current view espouses that the initial condition is inflammation of the peritenon secondary to overuse. If this inflammation becomes chronic, the tendon proper may become inflamed or hypovascular as a result of reduced perfusion through the peritenon. The resultant ischemia induces degenerative changes in the tendon. This discussion is limited to those conditions affecting the tendon proper.

Before reviewing the healing of ligaments and tendons, the mechanisms of injury must be discussed because they have a direct impact on how these structures heal. There are three main mechanisms of tendon and ligament injury: laceration, contusion, and tensile overload. Tensile overload may result in midsubstance tears, tears at the musculotendinous junction, avulsion from bone, or avulsion fracture of the bone at the insertion site.

One way in which these pathologies may be cognitively organized is by the acuity of their onset. Lacerations, contusions, tears, and avulsion from bone are the most sudden in their acuity. Although the treatment of these injuries may be similar, the reasons for their occurrence are quite different. Because most tendons can handle tensile forces greater than their accompanying muscles can generate and forces greater than the sheer forces able to be withstood by the bones into which they anchor, midsubstance tears are uncommon. For this reason, musculotendinous junction tears or avulsion fractures are more typical. Midsubstance tears of tendons require pre-existing tendonopathy at, or near the site, of the tear.

Paratenonitis, tendinosis, and enthesopathies are less acute in their onset. Paratenonitis most commonly occurs as a result of overuse and is characterized by macroscopic or microscopic injury to superficial collagen fibrils, tendon matrix, and the supporting microvasculature that causes inflammation and, secondarily, pain. Overuse injuries account for almost half of all occupational injuries in the United States, as well as half of all sports injuries. The histologic appearance of paratenonitis has been described as angiofibroblastic hyperplasia. The inflammatory cells present are not characteristic of other acute inflammatory conditions. It is not believed to be strictly an inflammation of the tendon proper; for this reason, the descriptor paratenonitis is more accurate than the term tendonitis. Enthesopathies are defined as diseases that occur at the insertion site of muscle tendons and ligaments into bone or joint capsules. Enthesopathies are not reviewed as these are beyond the scope of this chapter.

Tendinoses are chronic degenerative conditions of tendons. More specifically, tendinosis refers to intrasubstance degeneration without histologic or clinical signs of inflammation within the tendon. The morphologic changes evident in tendinosis include proliferation of fibroblasts, appearance of new capillary tufts, a decrease in collagen fibril diameter, and a more wavy orientation of the collagen fibers. Matrix components also show histologic changes. At the gross level, tendinosis shows thickened, condensed, and dessicated-appearing regions. Histologically, tendinosis is characterized by interstitial microscopic failure of the tendon substance or central tissue necrosis with mucoid degeneration *(1)*. Because inflammation may or may not be a part of this process, it is unclear whether paratenonitis is associated with symptoms.

At the biochemical level, degenerative tendons demonstrate an increase in type III collagen and proteoglycan content. The type III isoform is generally perceived as linked to regeneration of collagenous tissues. The tensile strength of collagenous tissues is inversely correlated with type III collagen content, as is an increased level of proteoglycan relative to collagen.

Although paratenonitis and tendonoses may be secondary to systemic disease, most cases result from overuse syndromes, which all have some component of chronic inflammatory response that occurs in or around the tissue. A "tendinosis cycle" has been described in which tendinosis is caused by changes in the load experienced by tendons that are not compensated by adaptations of the cell matrix. Microtears happen through pathologic tendinous tissue and eventually result in tissue failure if there is not an adequate healing, reparative, or hypertrophic response *(2)*.

Fluoroquinolones and Tendinopathy

Over the past decade, the increased use of fluoroquinolones as antimicrobial chemotherapeutic agents has resulted in numerous reported cases of fluoroquinolone-induced tendinopathies. Some frank ruptures were reported to occur. Undoubtedly, hundreds of other cases have occurred whose association with the use of these drugs went unrecognized or were just not reported. An increased relative risk of Achilles tendon disorders with the standard use of these drugs has been epidemiologically demonstrated, and it is estimated at 3.2 times that of a control population. It appears that this increased risk is limited to those patients who are over 60 yr of age. Concomitant use of these antibiotics with corticosteroids in those over age 60 further increases the risk to 6.7 times that of a control population. The risk of tendinopathy increased in those currently using the drugs, not in those who have used them in the past *(3)*.

Shakibaei et al. demonstrated that even limited doses in a rat model of fluoroquinolone-induced Achilles tendonitis resulted in degenerative alterations of the tenocytes. Electron microscopic findings included multiple vacuoles and vesicles in the cytoplasm that had developed from swellings and dilatations of cell organelles. Cells not only lost normal cell–matrix interactions but also detached from the extracellular matrix as well *(4)*.

The pathophysiologic effects that these drugs have on tendons is not fully characterized, but it is believed that the adverse effects are because of altered tendon fibroblast metabolism. Culture of tendon fibroblasts with ciprofloxacin resulted in a 66% reduction in cell proliferation in comparison to controls cultures. Collagen synthesis was decreased by up to half of control values, and proteoglycan synthesis was also diminished. These studies also suggested that fluoroquinolones stimulate tendon matrix degradation with the upregulation of protease activity. At this point, it seems likely that fluoroquinolones not only decrease the synthesis of tendon structural components, but also accelerate the degradation of these components *(5)*.

NORMAL HEALING RESPONSES

Tendons pass through three phases in their healing process that have characteristic cellular, temporal and biomechanical patterns. The first phase is considered the inflammatory phase and occurs in the first week following injury. It starts with the migration of macrophages from tissues surrounding the injury. During this phase, the macrophages remove necrotic tissue and hematoma from the area of the injury thereby preparing the tissue bed for reconstruction. Collagenases and matrix metalloproteinases have a key role in removing not only collagen debris, but also matrix components from the site of injury *(6)*.

The second phase of the healing response is the fibroblastic phase. Fibroblasts proliferate and begin to synthesize collagen and other proteins required for extracellular matrix construction at this time. The fibroblastic phase is initiated approx 1 wk following injury, but collagen synthesis reaches a maximum 3–4 wk after injury. The fibroblasts that drive this phase are believed to originate from locally resident cells of the perivascular tissues *(7)*. Revascularization at the injury site is also initiated during the fibroblastic phase.

The last phase has been termed the remodeling phase. At approx 8 wk after injury, the recently laid down collagen fibers are brought into orientation along the axis of the tendon. The collagen fibers are originally oriented perpendicular to the long axis of the tendon. It is during this period that adhesions may become more numerous and tenacious. Older individuals have a lower metabolic activity within these structures that may be responsible for the diminished age-related tendon-healing capacity observed.

Throughout tendon healing, there is a dynamic balance between collagen breakdown and synthesis. Initially, collagenase activity and collagen breakdown predominate, but these levels diminish and become equal to the rising synthesis levels by 4–6 wk postinjury. After this time, synthesis and remodeling occur at a much greater rate than breakdown.

In the middle of last century, Mason and Allen demonstrated that the biomechanical strength of surgical tendon repairs closely matches the histologic phases through which tendons pass when healing. During the inflammatory phase, there is a decrease in the tensile strength of the repair likely secondary to edema and tendon degradation. In the fibroblastic phase, there is an increase in strength, which is further elevated during the remodeling phase *(8)*.

Investigations into the pathogenesis and normal healing responses of these conditions is both reliant on, and severely hampered by, the animal models used to study them. Most tendon, ligament, and capsular injuries result from either acute trauma to the tissues or overuse syndromes. With the exception of lacerations, recreating either acute or chronic soft tissue injuries in laboratory animals is difficult to perform and standardize. Unlike the exquisite knock-out or knock-in recombinant techniques that have resulted in transgenic animals to model single molecular defect diseases, no elegant models for most tendon, ligament, and capsular disease amenable to repair are available.

In the past, there was debate regarding whether healing of tendon injury was predominantly an intrinsic or extrinsic phenomenon. The extrinsic mechanism depends on fibroblasts and inflammatory cells entering from the periphery of the injury to effect repair of the tendon. The intrinsic mechanism involves migration of fibroblasts and inflammatory cells from within the tendon and epitenon. It is now believed that tendon healing involves both intrinsic and extrinsic mechanisms, with the latter predominating in the early phases and the intrinsic predominating in a more delayed fashion. Some hypothesize that an imbalance favoring the extrinsic mechanism leads to increased collagen content at the repair site, as well as a suboptimal level of collagen organization and, hence, material properties of the reparative tissue. Consequently, predominance of the extrinsic mechanism may cause scar formation and adhesions between the tendon and surrounding tissues.

CONTRIBUTION OF THE NERVOUS SYSTEM IN TENDON HEALING

Until very recently, tendons were believed to be without direct innervation. Ackermann et al. have demonstrated that nerve fibers are present in healing tendon, suggesting that the neuropeptides associated with these fibers may have a central role in cell proliferation and angiogenic patterns observed in this process *(9)*.

Using immunohistochemical techniques, this group showed that abundant neuronal ingrowth was present in the early phases of healing rat tendon. Interestingly, there was effective, complete regression of these neurons by 12–16 wk after the start of healing. Furthermore, a temporal pattern of specific neuropeptide expression was observed that correlated with the nociceptive responses of experimental animals. They hypothesized that the peripheral nervous system may modulate neuropeptide expression in relation to the phase of tendon healing *(10)*. These findings seem to raise the question of whether coupling of nociceptive and healing responses in animals may provide a protective function by optimizing the physical environment in which tendons undergo healing.

REGENERATION OF TENDONS AFTER HARVESTING

Numerous investigators have reported the regeneration of the semitendinosis tendon after harvesting for anterior cruciate ligament (ACL) reconstructive procedures. This regeneration has been looked at clinically (using imaging modalities) and histologically. Feretti et al. looked at the regenerated tissue histologically in a limited number of patients after they noted regrowth clinically. Six months after the procedure, they noted fibroblastic proliferation surrounded by a few vessels and a sheath of fibrous tissue. In those specimens looked at 2 yr postharvesting, there was a central thickened portion with well-oriented tendon-like fibers and cells that appeared to be mature tenocytes *(11)*. These results were similar to those of Eriksson et al. *(12)*.

PHYSICAL MODIFIERS OF TENDON HEALING

Effects of Ultrasound and Shock Wave Therapy on Healing

The effect of ultrasound on tendon healing has been researched in both rat and canine models. Using a canine tenotomy-tenorrhaphy model, Saini et al. demonstrated that ultrasound-treated animals had less lameness in the early postoperative period, fewer adhesions, histologically better union patterns, and earlier initiation of collagen bundle formation than control animals *(13)*. The ultrasound-treated animal also showed earlier improved ultrasonographic appearance of repaired tendon, but this difference diminished after longer term evaluation. deCunha et al. investigated the optimal ultrasound mode for tendon healing. Utilizing both continuous and pulsed treatment regimens, they evaluated healing parameters in a rat tenotomy repair model. Histologic examination of the tendons showed that animals treated with the pulsed mode showed better aggregation and organization of collagen bundles. Using the pulsed mode decreased the time to healing relative to control animals that received mock ultrasound treatments. Interestingly, treatment with the continuous mode did not show the same shortened time to healing that the pulsed mode demonstrated *(14)*.

Utilizing a rat model of surgical Achilles tenotomy, Orhan et al. *(15)* observed the effect of low-energy extracorporreal shock wave therapy on the healing of surgically created tenotomy sites. After transsection followed by either suture repair or sham operation, 500 shock waves were applied to the surgical site under ultrasound guidance. Hydroxyproline levels were elevated in the tenotomized animal compared with control groups, indicating that healing occurred at an accelerated rate in animals treated with the shock wave therapy. Extracorporeal shock wave application has also been shown to induce neovascularization at the bone tendon interface *(16)*.

BIOLOGIC MODIFIERS TO HEALING

At a gross level, physical stabilization (and some degree of approximation) of injured tendons, ligament, and capsular tissue is required for proper healing. Modulation at the molecular environment with biologic response modifiers may be required to more closely approximate a native state once healing is complete. Gelberman and colleagues believe that the limit is being reached of improving the healing of flexor tendon injuries by manipulating repair techniques and rehabilitation variables alone. They suggest that to improve tendon healing further, the focus must be more closely and critically on the biologic response modifiers that affect tendon healing *(17)*. Several systemic and local treatments have been applied to injured tendons toward this goal. Experimental gene therapy of tendon and ligament healing is in its infancy but holds promise as a therapeutic modality *(18)*.

Hyperbaric Oxygen Therapy

Because vascular ingrowth is a normal part of the inflammatory and healing process seen after tendon injury, researchers have tried to augment the availability of oxygen to the healing tendon. Hyperbaric oxygen allows a greater concentration of oxygen to be delivered to tissues during intermittent treatments. Using a rat ligament laceration model, Ishii et al. demonstrated that there was better gross and histologic healing in animals exposed to hyperbaric treatments. A significant increase in the amount of collagen synthesis was observed in animals exposed to oxygen at two atmospheres for 1 h/d for a duration of 14 d *(19)*. The systemic nature of hyperbaric oxygen therapy precludes the determination of whether a purely local phenomenon is being observed at the site of ligament injury or whether systemic effects are also exerting an impact on healing.

Topical treatments seek to modify the local environment to promote better healing at the injury site. Researchers have approached the use of such treatments from several angles: creation of a physical scaffold onto which the body can base its reparative processes, application of growth factors at the site of injury, and a combination of both that allows the augmentation of scaffolds with growth factors. Modalities that have been investigated include autografting, application of biologic response modifiers, and local physical treatments.

Fibrin

The scaffold that is formed by a fibrin clot has been shown to have both chemotactic and mitogenic properties. Attempts to exploit these properties have used both purified fibrin glues and fibrin clots.

Recent investigations that compared fibrin glue to suture repair and conservative treatment in a rabbit model of Achilles tendon healing demonstrated that application of this glue to the injured site at the time of surgery resulted in better stiffness, maximum force to rupture, and tensile stress to rupture compared to suture repair alone or conservative therapy. However, these differences were not evident at later time points *(20)*. Other researchers have reported that the addition of a fibrin clot to a rat rotator cuff model caused a decrease in material properties *(21)*.

BIOLOGIC RESPONSE MODIFIERS

The Bone Morphogenentic Protein (BMP) Family of Growth Factors

BMPs and CDMPs are members of the transforming growth factor-β (TGF-β) superfamily that have been shown to enhance the formation of bone and cartilage formation at fracture sites. BMP-12 is a recently discovered member of the BMP family. It is the human homolog of mouse GDF-7. BMP-12 has been shown to induce some cells to form tendon. Recent in vitro studies have shown that rhBMP12 could increase the proliferation of tendon fibroblasts and increase the gene expression of procollagen type I and type III while decreasing the gene expression of decorin. It has been suggested that BMP-12 has a role in early phases of regeneration of tendons *(22)*.

BMPs and CDMPs can induce bone, cartilage, or tendon-like tissue depending on the conditions in which they are applied. OP-1 (BMP-7) has been shown to be ineffective in the augmentation of tendon healing. Animals that received this factor after the creation of surgically created tendon defects developed bony rests within the tendon that compromised mechanical strength of the tendon. However, for those that received CDMP-1 or -2, the area of healing tendon became bigger and stronger *(23)*.

Rodeo's group has used a combination of BMPs, as well as other growth factors, in a rabbit model of autograft hamstring ACL reconstruction in an attempt to improve tendon-to-bone tunnel healing. Histologic analysis demonstrated that animals treated with a growth factor–impregnated collagen sponge at the bone tunnel site had more consistent interface between the tendon and bone with closer apposition of new bone to the graft. The experimental grafts also had higher load to failure rates than the controls *(24)*.

Gene transfer of BMP-12 expression constructs into tenocytes of an in vivo tendon laceration chicken model resulted in a twofold increase in the tensile strength and stiffness of the repaired tendons *(26)*.

Local injections of CDMP-2 into surgically created rat Achilles tendon defects resulted in tendons that were 39% stronger than uninjected control animals at 8 wk postinjury *(25)*.

These growth factors show promise in augmenting the healing process of ligaments and tendons. More work needs to be done to optimize the conditions for their use and investigate the initiation of induction of tendon outgrowth from pluripotential tissues. At present, fully matured tendon has not been formed *de novo* through the use of these substances, but continuing work may prove that these substances are a key link in either in vitro or in vivo growth of graft material.

Growth and Differentiation Factor-5

GDF-5 is essential for normal skeletal development and induces tendon- and ligament-like structures at ectopic sites. GDF-5 was tested using a surgically created and repaired rat model of Achilles tendon healing. Although histological tests positive for type II collagen were present in the areas of the coated suture material used in this study, experiments demonstrated thicker and stiffer tendons than controls *(27)*.

Modulation of Adhesion Formation

Strong repair of a deficient tendon unit alone will not suffice. In most cases, a repaired tendon must maintain a substantial amount of its excursive ability to maintain function. This ability is dependent on the ability to achieve a strong repair at the injury site and to prevent adhesions from forming during the healing process. Adhesions can severely restrict tendon gliding after tendon healing has occurred. As mentioned earlier, it is thought that an overaggressive extrinsic healing response results in the formation of these adhesions. Physical, pharmacologic, and biologic approaches have been used to combat this problem.

5-Fluorouracil (5-FU) is a pyrimidine analog that exerts its effects by causing thymidine depletion and disrupting RNA processing. The use of this pharmacologic agent as a topical applicant to prevent tendon adhesions has been reviewed by a number of investigators. Recently, groups have observed the molecular, cellular, histologic, and functional outcomes in preventing adhesions after application of 5-FU to repaired tendons. Khan et al. applied 5-FU to the sites of tendon repair in a rabbit model. In addition to a less vigorous cellular response, they demonstrated a decrease in the local levels of TGF-β, which is a known potentiator of the fibrotic response *(28)*. Another group using a similar protocol in a chicken model of tendon repair looked at the microscopic and functional outcome of 5-FU as an inhibitor of tendon adhesion formation. After suture repair of the flexor digitorum profundus 5-FU was applied at four different concentrations to the tendon sheath for 5 min. Fewer adhesions were observed histologically, and lower forces were needed for digit contraction relative to controls in animals that had concentrations of 25 mg/mL applied to their repair sites *(29)*.

Other groups have applied human amniotic fluid *(30)* or hyaluronic acid membranes *(31)* to the sites of suture-repaired tendons and found that these treatments resulted in fewer adhesions compared to control groups. Although further work needs to be done to identify and isolate the factors responsible for the inhibitory properties of human amniotic fluid, the latter treatment may provide an available, cost-effective, and convenient physiochemical barrier by which peritendinous adhesions can be minimized or prevented at repair sites.

Recently, application of supraphysiologic temperatures to areas of tendon repair has been shown to decrease the amount of peritendinous adhesions without adverse affect on gliding or strength of the treated tendons *(32)*. The authors hypothesized that induction of heat shock proteins limited the local inflammatory response and subsequent adhesion formation.

CONCLUSION

Tendon injuries continue to be costly and debilitating conditions. Although there is a good understanding of the normal healing processes of these structures, how we, as physicians, can augment the body's natural healing and regenerative properties remains a challenge. Recent advances in the surgical treatment and rehabilitation of these diseases have not been met by advances in the biological augmentation of tendon healing. As the physical treatment of these conditions is perfected, we must redouble our efforts and investigations into maximizing the biology of tendon repair and regenerative processes.

REFERENCES

1. Jones D. Tendon disorders of the foot and ankle. *J Am Acad Orth Surg* 1993;1:87–94.
2. Leadbetter WB. Cell-matrix response in tendon injury. *Clin Sports Med* 1992;11:533–578.
3. van der Linden PD, Sturkenboom MC, Herings RM, Leufkens HG, Stricker BH. Fluoroquinolones and risk of Achilles tendon disorders: Case-control study. *BMJ* 2002;324: 1306–1307.
4. Shakibaei M, Pfister K, Schwabe R, Vormann J, Stahlmann R. Ultrastructure of achilles tendons of rats treated with ofloxacin and fed a normal or magnesium-deficient diet. *Antimicrob Agents Chemother* 2000;44:261–266.
5. Williams RJ, III, Attia E, Wickiewicz TL, Hannafin JA. The effect of ciprofloxacin on tendon, paratenon, and capsular fibroblast metabolism. *Am J Sports Med* 2000;28:364–369.
6. Creemers LB, Jansen ID, Docherty AJ, Reynolds JJ, Beertsen W, Everts V. Gelatinase a (mmp-2) and cysteine proteinases are essential for the degradation of collagen in soft connective tissue. *Matrix Biol* 1998;17:35–46.
7. Grillo HC. Origin of fibroblasts in wound healing: An autoradiographic study of inhibition of cellular proliferation by local X-irradiation. *Ann Surg* 1963;157:453–467.
8. Mason M, Allen H. The rate of healing of tendons: An experimental study of tensile strenth. *Ann Surg* 1941;113:424–459.
9. Ackermann PW, Ahmed M, Kreicbergs A. Early nerve regeneration after achilles tendon rupture—a prerequisite for healing? A study in the rat. *J Orthop Res* 2002;20:849–856.
10. Ackermann PW, Li J, Lundeberg T, Kreicbergs A. Neuronal plasticity in relation to nociception and healing of rat achilles tendon. *J Orthop Res* 2003;21:432–441.
11. Ferretti A, Conteduca F, Morelli F, Masi V. Regeneration of the semitendinosus tendon after its use in anterior cruciate ligament reconstruction: A histologic study of three cases. *Am J Sports Med* 2002;30:204–207.
12. Eriksson K, Kindblom LG, Hamberg P, Larsson H, Wredmark T. The semitendinosus tendon regenerates after resection: A morphologic and MRI analysis in 6 patients after resection for anterior cruciate ligament reconstruction. *Acta Orthop Scand* 2001;72:379–384.
13. Saini NS, Roy KS, Bansal PS, Singh B, Simran PS. A preliminary study on the effect of ultrasound therapy on the healing of surgically severed Achilles tendons in five dogs. *J Vet Med A Physiol Pathol Clin Med* 2002;49:321–328.
14. da Cunha A, Parizotto NA, Vidal Bde C. The effect of therapeutic ultrasound on repair of the Achilles tendon (tendo calcaneus) of the rat. *Ultrasound Med Biol* 2001;27:1691–1696.
15. Orhan Z, Alper M, Akman Y, Yavuz O, Yalciner A. An experimental study on the application of extracorporeal shock waves in the treatment of tendon injuries: Preliminary report. *J Orthop Sci* 2001;6:566–570.
16. Wang CJ, Huang HY, Pai CH. Shock wave-enhanced neovascularization at the tendon-bone junction: An experiment in dogs. *J Foot Ankle Surg* 2002;41:16–22.
17. Silva MJ, Boyer MI, Gelberman RH. Recent progress in flexor tendon healing. *J Orthop Sci* 2002;7:508–514.
18. Hoeller D, Petrie N, Yao F, Eriksson E. Gene therapy in soft tissue reconstruction. *Cells Tissues Organs* 2002;172:118–125.
19. Ishii Y, Ushida T, Tateishi T, Shimojo H, Miyanaga Y. Effects of different exposures of hyperbaric oxygen on ligament healing in rats. *J Orthop Res* 2002;20:353–356.
20. Thermann H, Frerichs O, Biewener A, Krettek C. Healing of the Achilles tendon: An experimental study. *Foot Ankle Int* 2001;22:478–483.
21. Thomopoulos S, Soslowsky LJ, Flanagan CL, Tun S, Keefer CC, Mastaw J, Carpenter JE. The effect of fibrin clot on healing rat supraspinatus tendon defects. *J Shoulder Elbow Surg* 2002;11:239–247.

22. Fu SC, Wong YP, Chan BP, Pau HM, Cheuk YC, Lee KM, Chan KM. The roles of bone morphogenetic protein (BMP) 12 in stimulating the proliferation and matrix production of human patellar tendon fibroblasts. *Life Sci* 2003;72:2965–2974.
23. Aspenberg P, Forslund C. Bone morphogenetic proteins and tendon repair. *Scand J Med Sci Sports* 2000;10:372–375.
24. Anderson K, Seneviratne AM, Izawa K, Atkinson BL, Potter HG, Rodeo SA. Augmentation of tendon healing in an intraarticular bone tunnel with use of a bone growth factor. *Am J Sports Med* 2001;29:689–698.
25. McAuliffe JA. Flexor tendon repair, healing and rehabilitation: A brief commentary. *Hand Surg* 2002;7:29–31.
26. Lou J, Tu Y, Burns M, Silva MJ, Manske P. BMP-12 gene transfer augmentation of lacerated tendon repair. *J Orthop Res* 2001;19:1199–1202.
27. Rickert M, Jung M, Adiyaman M, Richter W, Simank HG. A growth and differentiation factor-5 (GDF-5)-coated suture stimulates tendon healing in an Achilles tendon model in rats. *Growth Factors* 2001;19:115–126.
28. Khan U, Kakar S, Akali A, Bentley G, McGrouther DA. Modulation of the formation of adhesions during the healing of injured tendons. *J Bone Joint Surg Br* 2000;82:1054–1058.
29. Moran SL, Ryan CK, Orlando GS, Pratt CE, Michalko KB. Effects of 5-fluorouracil on flexor tendon repair. *J Hand Surg [Am]* 2000;25:242–251.
30. Ozgenel GY, Samli B, Ozcan M. Effects of human amniotic fluid on peritendinous adhesion formation and tendon healing after flexor tendon surgery in rabbits. *J Hand Surg [Am]* 2001;26:332–339.
31. Isik S, Ozturk S, Gurses S, Yetmez M, Guler MM, Selmanpakoglu N, Gunhan O. Prevention of restrictive adhesions in primary tendon repair by ha-membrane: Experimental research in chickens. *Br J Plast Surg* 1999;52:373–379.
32. Mulhall KJ, McLaughlin R, Kay E, Kiely P, Bouchier-Hayes D, Murray P. Thermal preconditioning prevents peritendinous adhesions and inflammation. *Clin Orthop* 2002; 405:258–266.

Part II

Basic Science

2

Structure and Function of Ligaments, Tendons, and Joint Capsule

Frederick H. Silver, Joseph W. Freeman, and Gino Bradica

INTRODUCTION

For vertebrates to achieve locomotion and to hurl objects efficiently, they must be able to develop muscular forces, store elastic energy in tendon, and then transfer this energy to the attached joints. After joint movement has been achieved, excess energy dissipates by reverse transmission from the joint to the muscle–tendon unit, where it is dissipated in the muscle. Locomotion and joint movement are the result of the coordinated development of muscle forces that are transmitted to bone using the tendon. However, although muscle can generate force, the tendon stores most of the muscular force as work *(1)*. The tendon not only transmits the developed muscular force to the bone, but it also acts as an energy storage device *(2,3)*. Elastic energy is stored in the tendon through reversible stretching of collagen molecules *(3)*. Consequently, the muscle–tendon unit produces energy that is transferred to the joint. Energy stored in the joint is used for movement, and also leads to joint deformation. Ligaments and the capsule attached to the joint function to seal the joint space and to provide passive stability by limiting movement. Thus, energy generated by the muscle–tendon unit is used for movement, and it is stored during ligament and capsule deformation. The energy stored during ligament and capsule deformation is then transferred back to the muscle through the tendon, where it dissipates as heat.

BACKGROUND

Elastic energy storage in tendons in the legs and feet of many animals is an important mechanism that saves substantial quantities of muscular energy during locomotion *(4,5)*. During normal gait, potential energy is stored as strain energy in the muscles and tendons that are stretched upon impact with the ground *(4,5)*. Elastic recoil, primarily by the tendons, converts most of the stored energy back to kinetic energy. Elastic energy storage in tendons has been studied in several animal models. In the pig, the digital flexor tendons are involved in the elastic storage of strain energy *(6)*; the amount of elastic energy stored in the digital flexor tendons decreases with age after the animal reaches maturity. In the turkey, direct measurement of force and fiber length in the lateral gastrocnemius muscle reveals that the active muscle produces high force but

From: *Orthopedic Biology and Medicine: Repair and Regeneration of Ligaments, Tendons, and Joint Capsule*
Edited by: W. R. Walsh © Humana Press Inc., Totowa, NJ

little work, while the tendon produces most of the work because of elastic deformation and recovery *(1)*. A recent study in horses suggests that the muscle–tendon unit not only stores energy during extension, but it also dissipates the energy after extension is complete *(7)*.

Although tendons are involved in energy storage and transmission in the musculoskeleton, ligaments and joint capsule (*see* Fig. 1A) function to stabilize synovial joints by limiting movement (ligaments and capsule) and preventing loss of synovial fluid that lubricates the joint (capsule). In accomplishing either energy storage or force transmission, the tendon, ligament, and capsule must cyclically undergo reversible deformation with limited structural reorganization. This chapter examines the structures of these tissues and how energy is stored and transmitted at the molecular level. Structurally, the tissues are made up of dense fibrous connective tissue with aligned collagen fibers that are separated by rows of cells. Each tissue contains regions with specialized structures and functions, such as the connections to muscle, cartilage, and bone. This chapter only reviews the regions that make up the midsubstance of these tissues to simplify the analysis. The composition and structure of these dense fibrous tissues is now considered.

Dense Regular Connective Tissue: Structure and Development

Dense regular fibrous connective tissue, also termed the extracellular matrix (ECM), consists of cells, aligned collagen and elastic fibers, proteoglycans, and water. Although elastic fibers are present in the ligament and capsule, they are only minor components of these tissues. Collagen is the most abundant protein in dense fibrous connective tissue and forms essential mechanical building blocks in the musculoskeletal system. It can be found in both fibril and nonfibril forms. The fibril-forming collagens provide the structural framework of tissues and include types I, II, III, V, and XI collagens *(8)*. All fibril-forming collagens self-assemble into cross-striated fibrils with a characteristic 67-nm repeat; they all share a triple helical region that is roughly 1000 amino acid residues long with a length of about 300 nm *(8)*. These collagens are synthesized within cells in a precursor form termed procollagen, which has amino and carboxyl terminal nonhelical ends that are approx 15.0 and 10.0 nm long, respectively (Fig. 1B). In addition, fibril-associated collagens with interrupted triple helical sequences, e.g., type XII collagen, are found on the surface of collagen fibrils and may connect fibrillar collagens to other components of the ECM *(9)*.

The tendon, ligament, and joint capsule are composed primarily of type I collagen, but they contain small amounts of types III and V *(10–14)*. The type III collagen content has been reported to be 10% for ligament as opposed to 5% for tendon *(15)*. Collagen types II, VI, XII, and XIV have also been reported to be in the ligament and capsule *(12,16,17)*. However, these collagens appear to be associated with fibrocartilage that is found at the junction with bone, not in the midsubstance. The high content of type I collagen in these joint tissues not only leads to mechanical stability, but it also promotes elastic energy storage.

The mechanical stability of dense fibrous connective tissue and type I collagen in the tendon, ligament, and capsule is related to the rod-like structure of type I collagen and its inherent flexibility *(18,19)*. The rod-like behavior of type I collagen was first established based on the measurement of the translational diffusion coefficient *(20–*

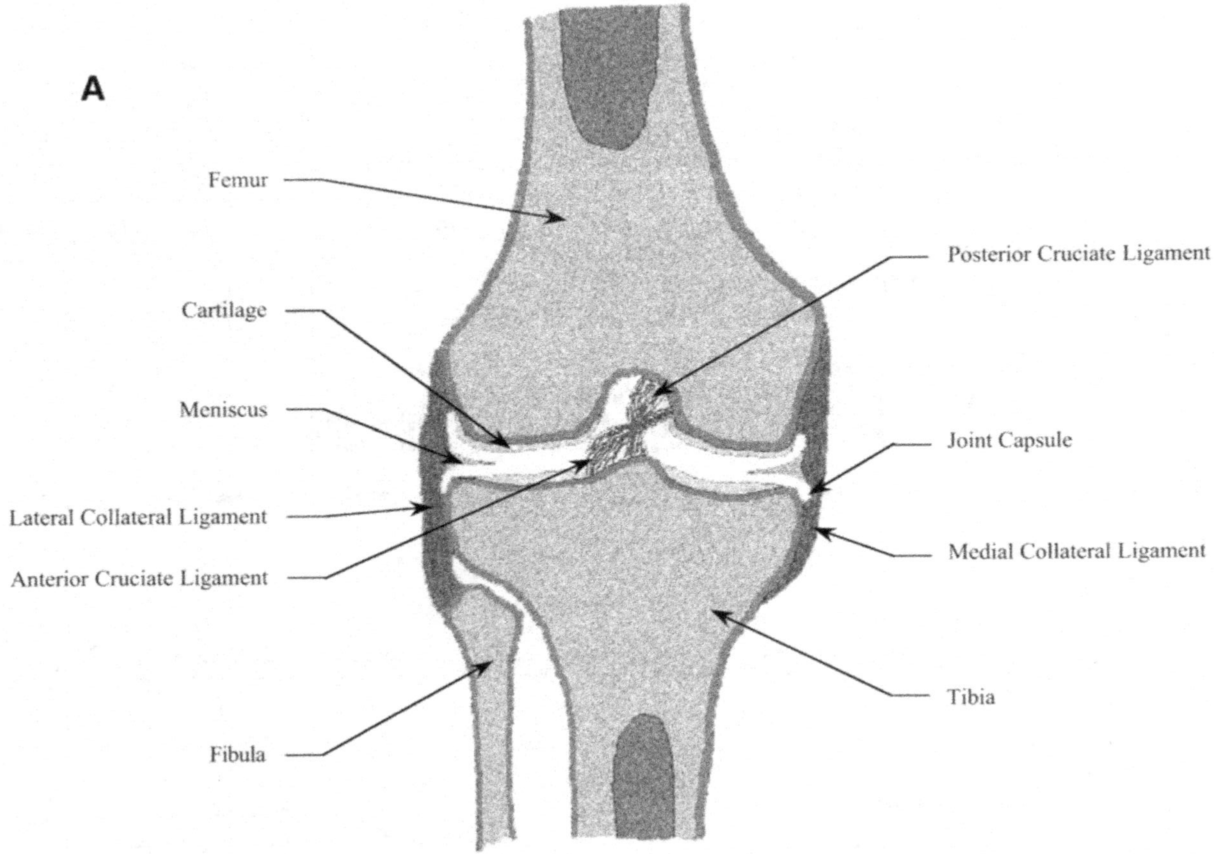

Fig. 1. Diagram of the knee joint. **(A)** Frontal view of the knee and the location of dense connective tissue, including the anterior and posterior cruciate ligaments, medial and lateral collateral ligaments, and joint capsule in the knee. The patellar tendon (not shown) is found in front of the cruciate ligaments. All these structures contained aligned collagen fibrils composed of collagen molecules in a quarter-staggered packing pattern shown in Fig. 2.

(Continued on next page.)

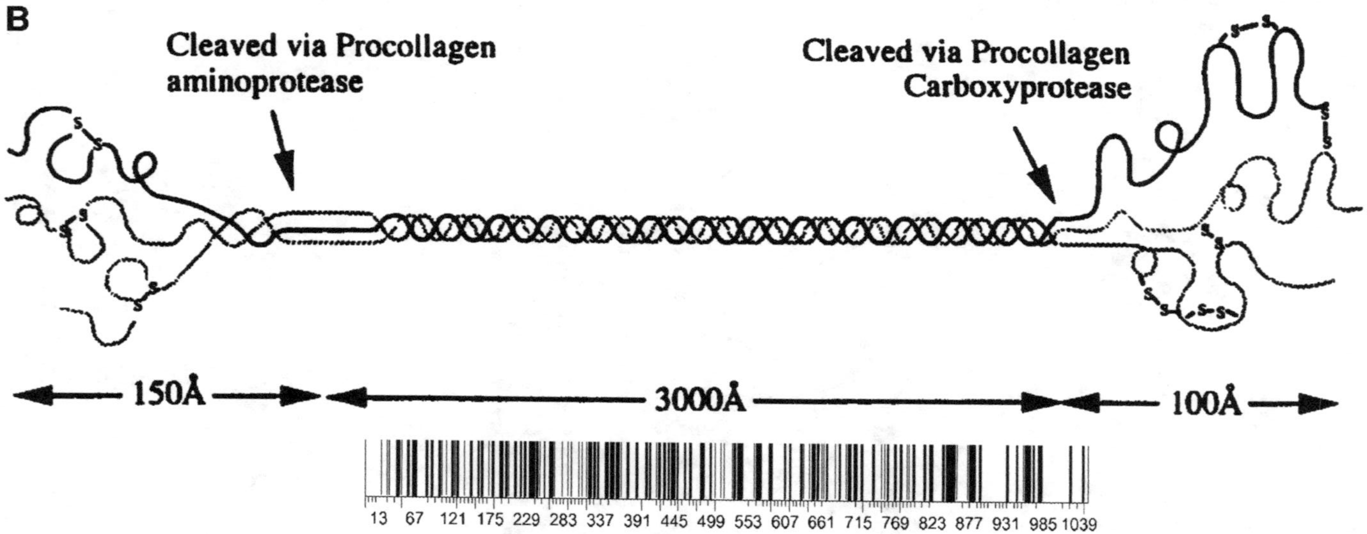

Fig. 1. *(Continued)* **(B)** The structure of procollagen type I, the precursor of collagen molecules found in the tendon, ligament, and joint capsule. The procollagen molecule shown consists of aminopropeptides (large left-hand portion of molecule), a triple-helical region (3000 Å long), and a carboxylic propeptide (right-hand end of molecule). The amino (N–) and carboxylic (C–) propeptides are cleaved by specific proteinases during collagen self-assembly and aid in regulating linear and lateral fibril growth (*see* Fig. 4). The circles in the triple helix represent major sequences devoid of proline and hydroxyproline that are the likely sites of folds where flexibility is introduced into a normally rigid helix. The striated pattern shown below the helical portion of the molecule is a diagrammatic representation of the flexible (dark bands) and rigid regions (light bands) found in the triple helix. Note the ends of the triple helix are rigid, whereas sequences toward the center of the molecule are more flexible.

22). Yet, later measurements indicated that the type I collagen molecule had numerous bends and was not completely rigid *(23)*. Type II and III collagen molecules have slightly higher translational diffusion coefficients and slightly shorter end-to-end distances *(23)*, suggesting that the later collagen molecules are more flexible than type I collagen. Results of recent modeling studies suggest that the types I–III collagen molecules are made up of alternating rigid and flexible domains that are conserved within the collagen fibril with types II and III collagen molecules being more flexible than type I *(19)*. The flexible domains at first approximation coincide with the positively stained bands in the collagen D period observed in the electron microscope after staining with heavy metals *(19,24)*.

The molecular basis for the flexibility of type I collagen derives from sequences that lack the amino acids proline and hydroxyproline (Fig. 1B). These sequences are the sites where bends can occur in the triple helix. Five sites have been identified by Hofmann et al. *(25)* based on electron microscopic images; these sites occur at characteristic distances of 30–45, 90–105, 150–157.5, 210–217.5, and 270–277.5 nm from the C-terminus of the molecule. However, recent modeling studies suggest that additional flexible sites are present *(19)*. Results of another modeling study indicate that sequences without the amino acid residues, proline and hydroxyproline, are able to form internal loops *(26)* that give these regions more flexibility than the other regions of the triple helix. Stereochemical maps constructed for dipeptides with amino and imino acid residues also imply that the number of available conformations and, consequently, the flexibility are increased in the absence of proline and hydroxyproline *(8,27)*. A flexibility profile as a function of axial displacement for the type I collagen triple helix is shown in Fig. 2. This diagram suggests that the collagen triple helix can be considered a composite of regions with varying degrees of stiffness. Regions of the molecule that are devoid of proline and hydroxyproline appear to have the highest flexibility, whereas regions with the sequence Gly-Pro-Hyp or sequences containing lysine or hydroxylysine are very rigid. This variation in molecular flexibility affects collagen self-assembly, as well as the resulting mechanical properties of tendons, ligaments, and joint capsule.

Research suggests that fibril diameters appear to be inversely related to collagen molecular flexibility *(19)* and that the application of external mechanical loading appears to be consistent with stretching of the flexible regions *(19)*. Energy storage during stretching is thought to be linked with an increase in steric energies owing to van der Waals and electrostatic interactions that occur with the stretching of oppositely charged pairs of amino acid side chains on collagen (*see* Fig. 2; *24*). Modeling studies on a five-molecule-wide subfibrillar structure composed of quarter-staggered collagen molecules suggest that the most flexible regions are bands a3, a4, a2, b1, b2, and d and regions between bands b1 and b2 and between bands c1 and c2 (*see* Fig. 2). These areas are consistent with the flexible sites identified by Hofmann et al. *(27)* and are consistent with Ramachandran plots constructed based on peptide sequences observed in collagen *(27)*.

Small amounts of types III and V collagen are found in mixtures with type I in the tendon, ligament, and capsule in a single fibril, indicating that tissue-specific differences in mechanical properties may reflect different mixtures of these collagen types *(28,29)*. The recent belief that the type III collagen molecule is more flexible than the

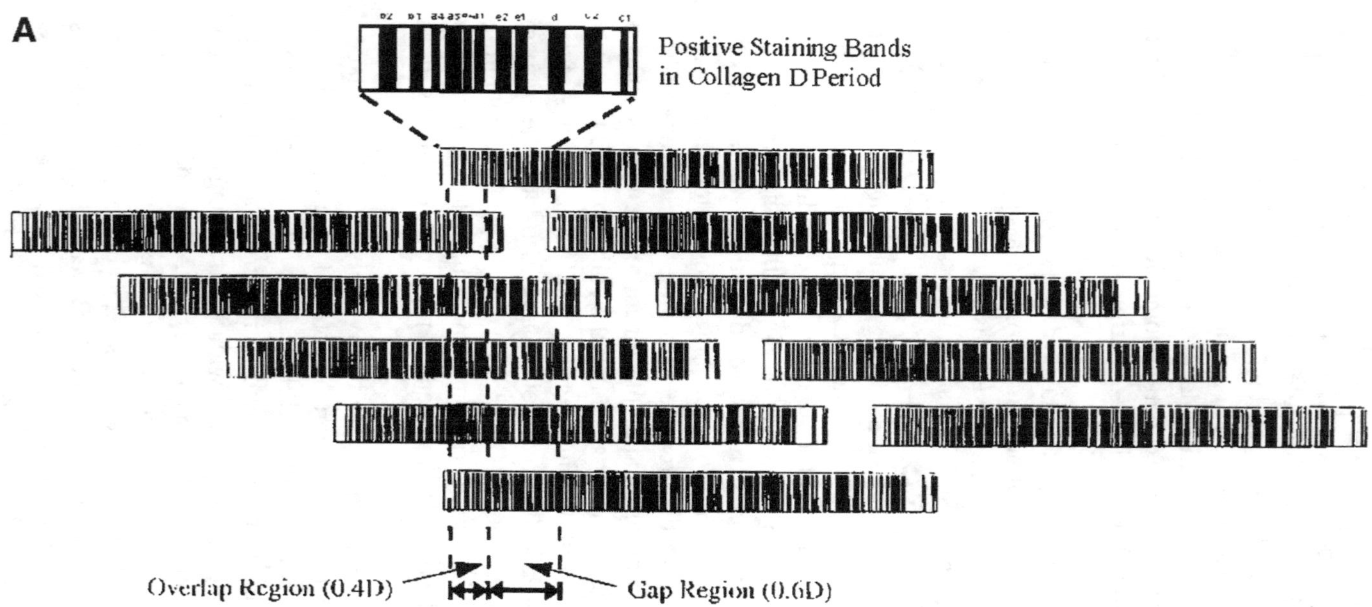

Fig. 2. Quarter-stagger packing pattern of type I collagen molecules in collagen fibrils. **(A)** In the quarter-stagger packing pattern, neighboring collagen molecules (4.4 D long) are staggered relative to their nearest neighbors. In the tendon, ligament, and joint capsule, the collagen molecules are shifted by a distance D (equal to 67 nm) with respect to their nearest neighbors after they are self-assembled into fibrils in tissues. When collagen molecules are stained with metal ions, then viewed in the electron microscope, a series of light and dark bands are observed across the axis of the fibril and are designated b2, b1, a4, a3, a2, a1, e2, e1, d, c2, and c1. The distance D is made up of a hole region approx 0.6 D and an overlap region approx 0.4 D. The D period is the characteristic fingerprint of fibrous collagen. Note proteoglycans are observed bound to the d and e bands in the positive-staining pattern. **(B)** *(opposite page, top)* When the collagen fibril is stretched in tension, the energy is stored as potential energy in the flexible regions contained in the positive-staining bands. This diagram illustrates how external mechanical loading increases the separation distance between pairs of oppositely charged amino acid residues in the flexible regions of the collagen molecules that make up the fibrillar elements in tendon. **(C)** *(opposite page, bottom)* This diagram illustrates space-filling molecular models constructed using a SYBYL molecular modeling program of a: (a) d band in a single collagen molecule; (b) model of five D-staggered collagen molecules in the d band of a collagen microfibril; and (c) segment of the d band of a collagen microfibril stretched 5%. The arrows in b illustrate the location of holes in a collagen microfibril, which are closed after a 5% axial stretch. These holes may be the sites for decorin and mineral attachment to type I collagen fibrils.

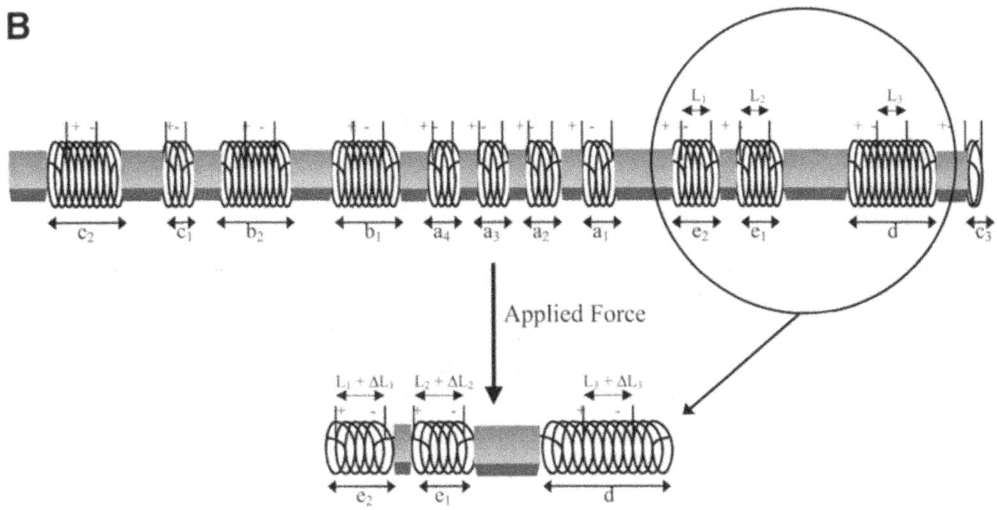
B
L1
L2
L3
c2
c1
b2
b1
a4
a3
a2
a1
e2
e1
d
c3
Applied Force
L1 + ΔL1
L2 + ΔL2
L3 + ΔL3
e2
e1
d

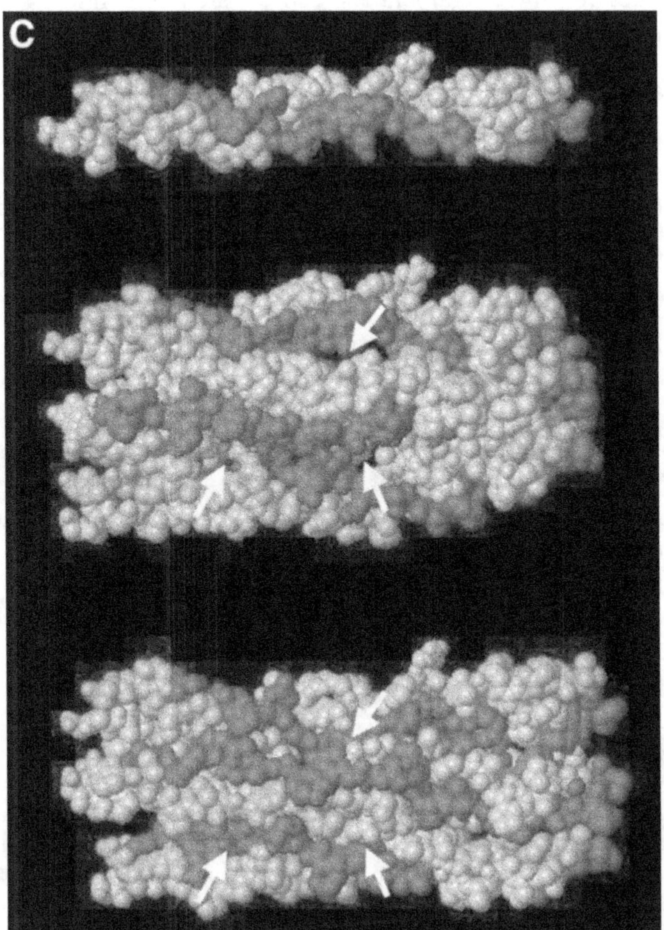
C

type I collagen molecule reports that mixing collagen types would alter the elastic modulus of collagen fibrils *(19)*.

Immunolocalization and/or chemical crosslinking studies have shown that collagen types I and V can be present as heteropolymers *(28)*. Although the type V molecule is somewhat larger than that of type I, owing to the N-terminal domain, type V molecules are assembled into typical quarter-staggered fibrils characteristic of type I collagen. The mixture formation of such heterotrophic or heterotypic fibrils provides a way to modulate self-assembly and modify mechanical properties *(28)*. The presence of a large N-terminal domain is likely to modify fibrillar packing and slippage of collagen molecules during mechanical deformation. Experimental observations on a mouse model with a structurally abnormal α2(V) collagen chain indicate that the resultant collagen fibrils are loosely packed in skin. This is consistent with the hypothesis that the large N-terminus of the type V collagen molecule may regulate the growth of skin fibrils *(30)*.

Knowledge of the relationship between cells and their ECM mostly comes from the analysis of developing tendon. The association between collagen fibril development and changes in mechanical properties has been studied extensively using the chick extensor model *(31,32)*. In addition, mineralization and the related changes in the mechanical properties of turkey leg tendon have also been studied a great deal *(24,32,33)*. Although the structures of the ligament and capsule are not identical to that of tendon, they are similar at first approximation.

Collagen Assembly in Developing Tendon

The ability of collagen molecules to assemble into crosslinked fibrils is an important requirement for the development of tissue strength, as well as for the storage and dissipation of elastic energy during locomotion. The process of collagen fibril formation is under cellular control, possibly through feedback mechanisms associated with mechanochemical transduction processes, but the tendency for collagen molecules to form cross-striated fibrils is a property of the molecular sequence *(34)*.

The tendon has a hierarchical structure, including collagen molecules, fibrils, fibril bundles, fascicles, and tendon units that run parallel to the geometrical axis *(35)* as diagrammed in Fig. 3A. This architecture is important for its ability to transmit large loads efficiently and also to store elastic energy during locomotion. The fundamental structural element is type I collagen in the form of fibrils. Collagen is synthesized in a precursor form, procollagen, which contains amino- (N) and carboxylic terminal (C) extensions *(36,37)*. These extensions have been shown to limit self-assembly of procollagen intracellularly *(38)*, and their removal by specific proteinases occurs prior to final fibril assembly *(39)*. The C-propeptides are essential for both the initiation of procollagen molecular assembly from the constituent chains *(40)* and lateral assembly of procollagen

Fig. 3. *(Opposite page)* Structural hierarchy in the tendon. **(A)** This diagram illustrates the relationship between collagen molecules, fibrils, fibers, fascicles, and tendon units. Although the diagram does not show fibril subunits, collagen fibrils appear to be self-assembled from intermediates integrated within the fibril. The structural hierarchy in the ligament and joint capsule is similar to that of tendon, but other components, such as elastic tissue, are also present in the latter types of connective tissue. **(B)** Scanning electron micrograph of a rat-tail tendon fiber showing the fascicles (*see* asterisks) that make up the tendon unit.

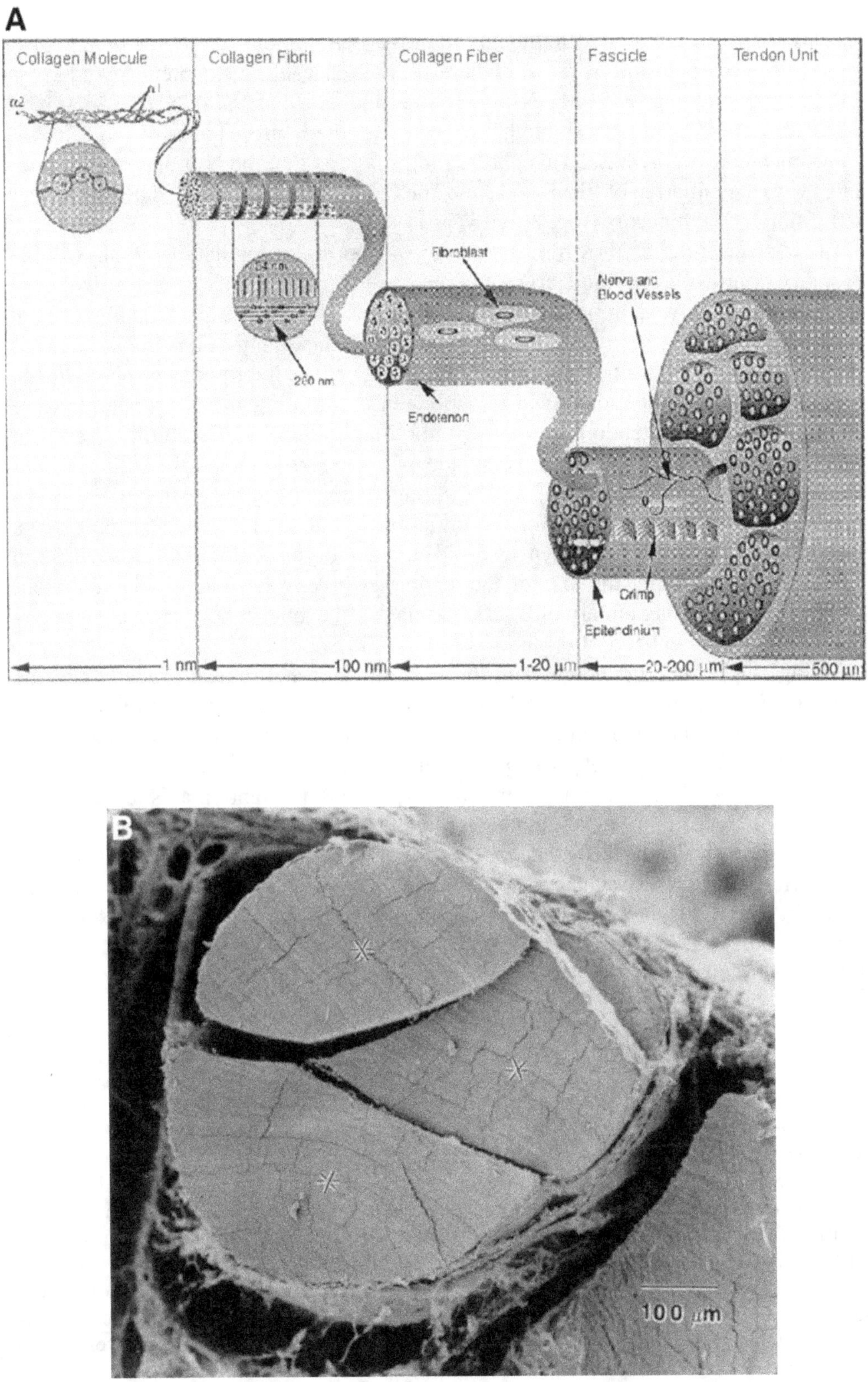
A
Collagen Molecule
Collagen Fibril
Collagen Fiber
Fascicle
Tendon Unit
Fibroblast
Nerve and
Blood Vessels
200 nm
Endotenon
Crimp
Epitendinium
1 nm
100 nm
1-20 μm
20-200 μm
500 μm
B
100 μm

molecules. Procollagen molecular assembly in vivo initiates within intracellular vesicles *(41)*. These vesicles are thought to move from regions within the Golgi apparatus to deep cytoplasmic recesses, where they discharge their contents. Studies on embryonic tissue suggest that the N-propeptides remain attached to fibrils 20–30 nm in diameter after collagen is assembled; however, after the N-propeptide is cleaved, fibril diameters appear to increase. This observation suggests that the N-propeptide is associated with the initiation of fibrillogenesis. The C-propeptide is removed before further lateral fibril growth occurs (Fig. 4; ref. *42*).

The C-propeptide of fibril-forming collagens appears to regulate later steps in the assembly of procollagen into fibrils; it is removed from small-diameter fibrils during growth *(43)* possibly when fibril fusion occurs. The C-propeptide has been observed in fibrils with diameters between 30 and 100 nm *(44)* indicating that it is involved in the initiation and growth of fibrils (Fig. 4). Procollagen and the intermediates, pN-collagen (containing the N-propeptide) and pC-collagen (containing the C-propeptide), are present in developing tendon up to 18-d embryonic *(44,45)*. Collagen oligomers isolated from developing chick tendons include 4-D staggered dimers (the collagen molecule is 4.4 D long, where D is 67 nm) of collagen molecules, suggesting that this is a preferred molecular interaction for the initiation of collagen fibrillogenesis in vivo. About 50% of the fibrils formed in 18-d-old chick embryos are bipolar (molecules run in both directions along the axis of the tendon), whereas the other half is unipolar. Analysis of the staining pattern of fibrils reveals that the axial zone of molecular polarity isto be highly localized *(46)*.

During chick tendon development, the structure and mechanical properties of the tendon change rapidly *(31,32,46–48)*. The morphology of embryonic development of collagen fibrils in the chick tendon has been studied and characterized extensively *(31, 32,35,48–52)*. Two levels of structural organization seem to occur during development of chick hind limb extensor tendons *(31)*. Along the tendon axis, cytoplasmic processes of one or more axial tendon fibroblasts are observed to direct formation of groups of short collagen fibrils that appear to connect cells together (Fig. 5). A second type of fibroblast that forms bundles of collagen fibers encircles groups of axial tendon cells. This type encircles groups of collagen fibrils with a sheath that separates fascicles. Initially, axial tendon cells appear at both ends of growing fibrils (Fig. 5). Once the fibrils begin to elongate, they are then packed closely side to side (Fig. 6).

Fig. 4. *(Opposite page)* Diagram modeling the role of N- and C-propeptides in type I collagen self-assembly. The procollagen molecule is represented by a straight line with bent (N-propeptide) and circular (C-propeptide) regions (*see* Fig. 1B). **(A)** Initial linear and lateral aggregation is promoted by the presence of both the N- and C-propeptides. Linear and lateral aggregation leads to the formation of the quarter-staggered packing pattern (*see* Fig. 2A) that is the characteristic fingerprint of collagen fibrils viewed in the electron microsope. **(B)** *(Continued on page 26)* In the presence of both propeptides, lateral assembly is limited and the fibrils are narrow. Removal of the N-propeptide results in lateral assembly of narrow fibrils; removal of the C-propeptide causes the additional lateral growth of fibrils. As indicated in the diagram, the presence of the N- and C-propeptides physically interferes with fibril formation.

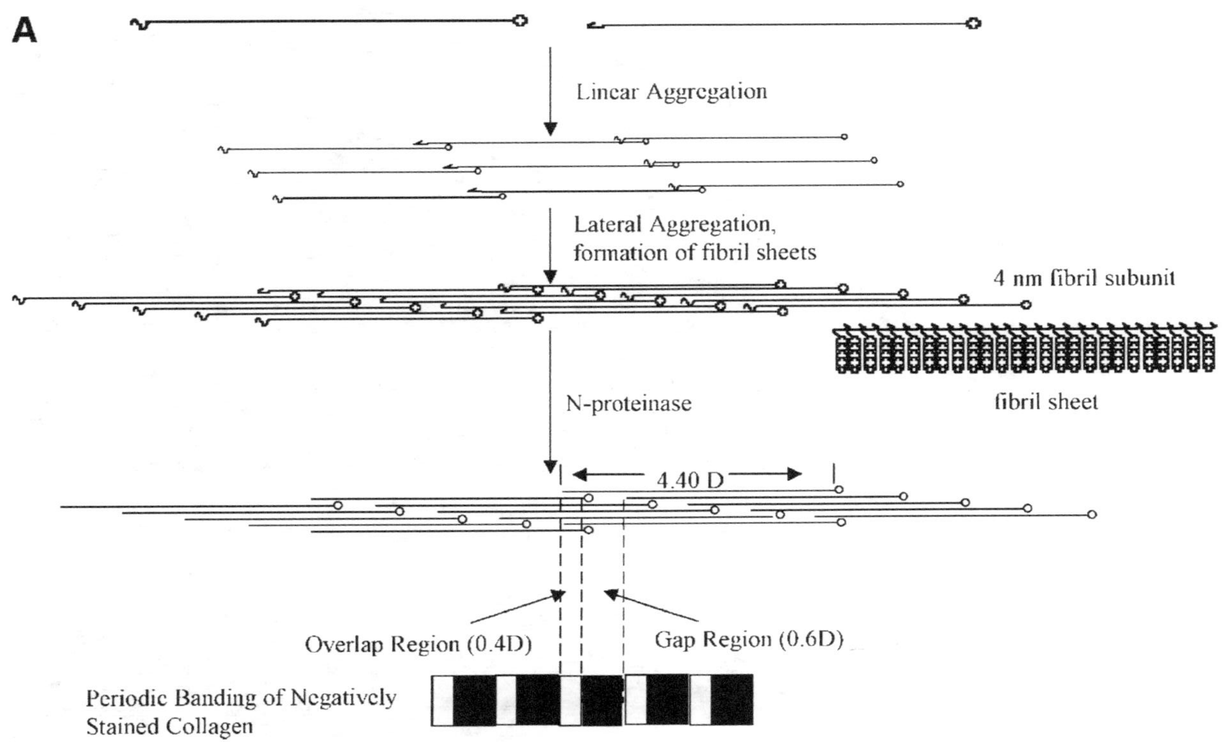

Fig. 4. *(Caption on opposite page)*

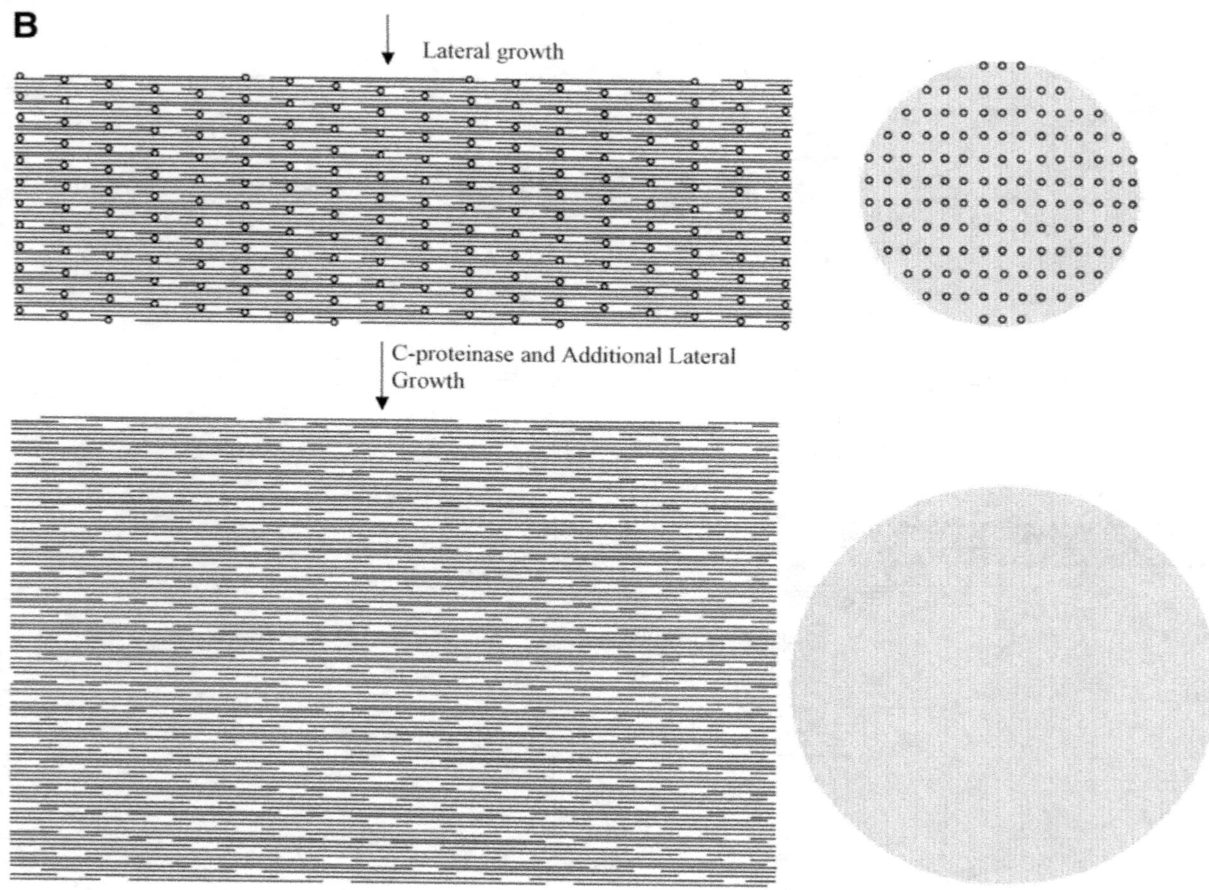

Fig. 4. *(Continued from page 24.)*

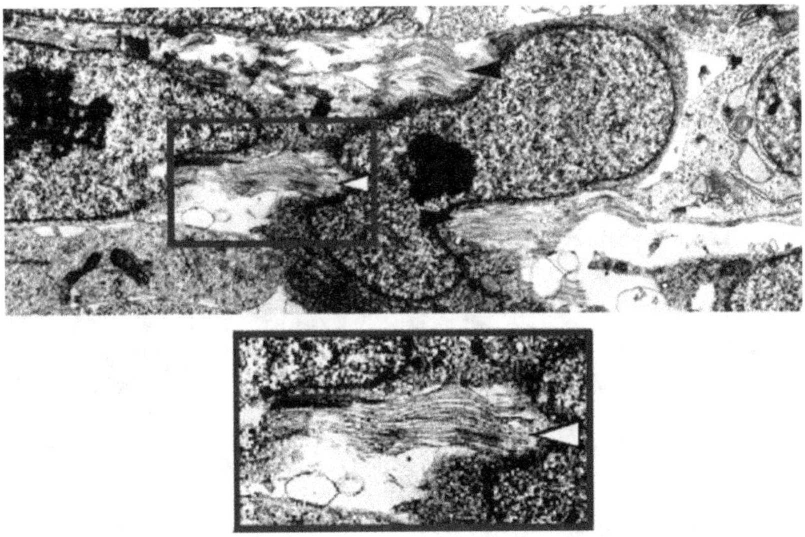

Fig. 5. Directed cellular self-assembly of axial collagen fibrils during chick tendon development. Transmission electron micrograph showing collagen fibrils (*see* arrow in box) from a 7-d-old chick leg extensor tendon that appear to be connecting two fibroblasts during tendon development. Insert shows a high-magnification view of the collagen fibrils that originate from invaginations in the cell membranes on either side of the fibril. The collagen fibrils shown are about 50 nm in diameter. Adapted from ref. *48*.

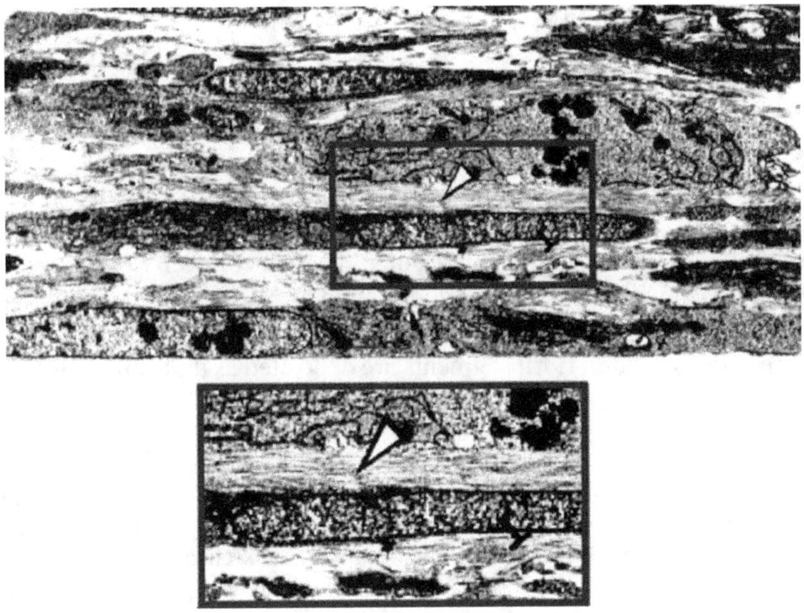

Fig. 6. Lateral condensation of axial collagen fibrils and alignment of tendon fibroblasts. Transmission electron micrograph showing collagen fibrils from a leg extensor tendon of a 10-d-old chick. Note the fibrils (*see* arrow) and fibroblasts appear to be more highly aligned and densely packed compared to the same structures at d 7. Fibrils shown have diameters of approx 50 nm, and the insert shows a high-magnification view of the relationship between the collagen fibrils and the cell surfaces on either side of the collagen fibrils. Adapted from ref. *48*.

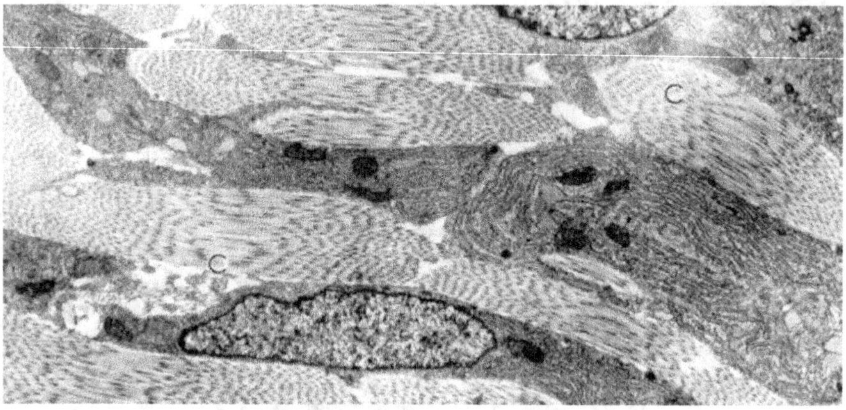

Fig. 7. Formation of crimp in axial collagen fibrils during development of chick extensor tendon. Transmission electron micrograph showing collagen fibrils (C) from a leg extensor tendon of a 17-d-old chick. Note the fibrils appear to be going in and out of the plane of the section consistent with the formation of a crimped planar zig-zag pattern. Fibrils shown have diameters of approx 100 nm. Adapted from ref. *48*.

Later, a planar crimp is introduced into collagen fibrils, possibly from the contraction of cells at the fibril ends or by shear stresses introduced by tendon cells between layers of collagen fibrils (Fig. 7). Recent modeling studies show that the molecule and fibril have many points of flexibility *(19)*, where crimp could develop.

In the cross-section, collagen fibers are made up of individual fibrils that appear to be released from invaginations in the cell membrane (Fig. 8). Further collagen fibril diameter growth occurs by adding materials that appear to originate inside the Golgi apparatus. During lateral growth, these invaginations in the cell membrane disappear, causing lateral fusion of fibrils (Fig. 9). Macroscopically, this results in increased fibril diameter and length.

Birk and coworkers have studied the manner in which collagen fibrils are assembled from fibril "segments" in developing chick tendon *(52)*. During development, fibril segments are assembled in extracytoplasmic channels defined by the fibroblast. In 14-d-old chick embryos, tendon fibril segments are deposited as units 10–30 μm in length.

Fig. 8. *(Opposite page)* Addition of axial collagen fibrils within invaginations in the cell membrane to a growing fibril. **(A)** Transmission electron micrograph showing collagen fibril formation in invaginations within the cell membrane of an extensor tendon from a 14-d-old chick embryo. Collagen fibrils are seen as circular elements within collagen fibril bundles (fibers). The collagen fibril bundle shown for illustration has two letter "x" connected by a line that represents the collagen fibril bundle diameter (2 μm). Arrows are placed in micrograph areas where collagen fibrils appear to be in the ECM and are in close proximity to the cell membrane. **(B)** Higher magnification views of areas shown in boxes labeled A, B, C, and D in part **(A)**, illustrating the close proximity between the collagen fibrils formed within deep cytoplasmic recesses and the growing fibril bundle seen in the ECM (*see* arrow). Adapted from ref. *48*.

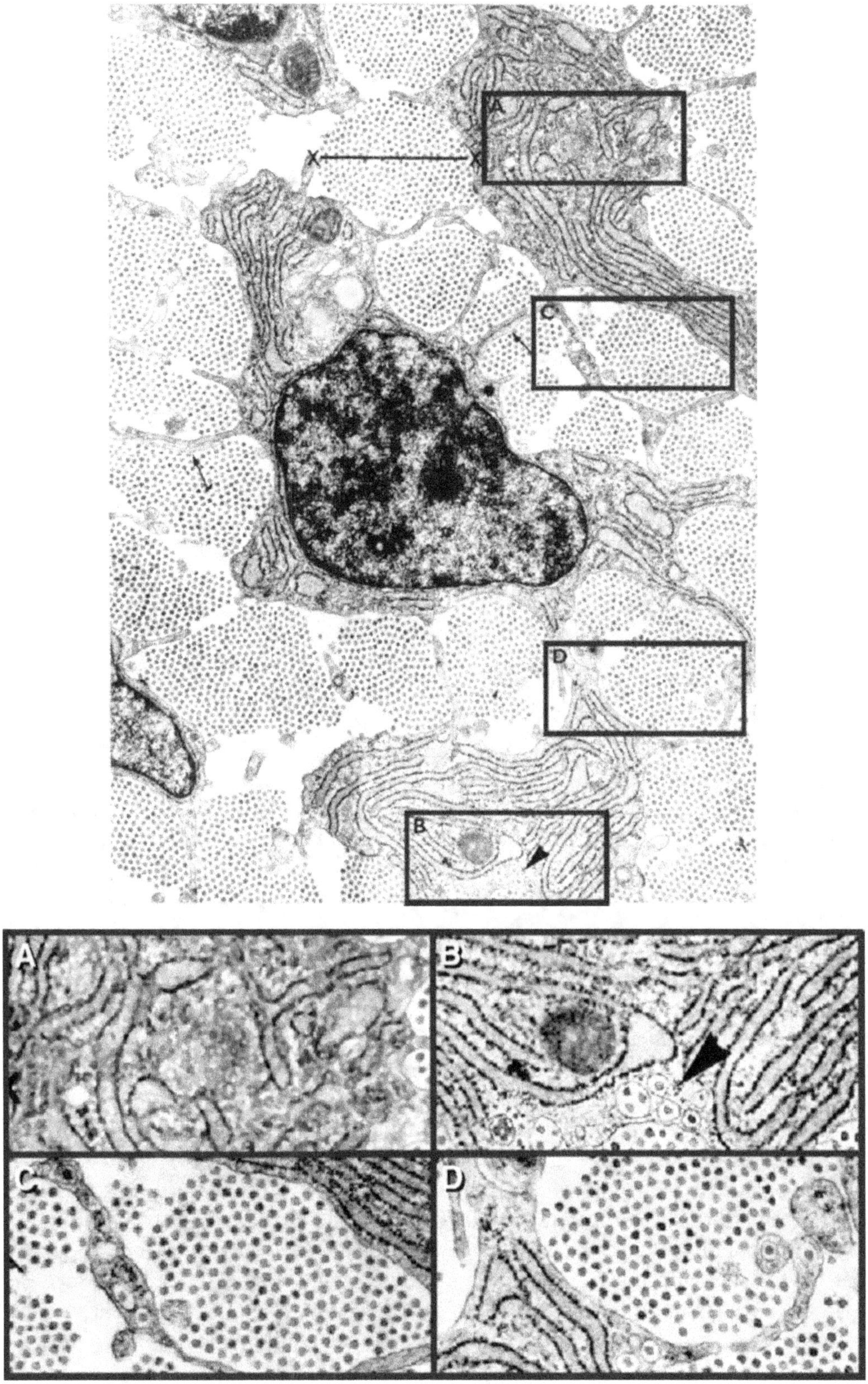
A
B
C
D
A
B
C
D

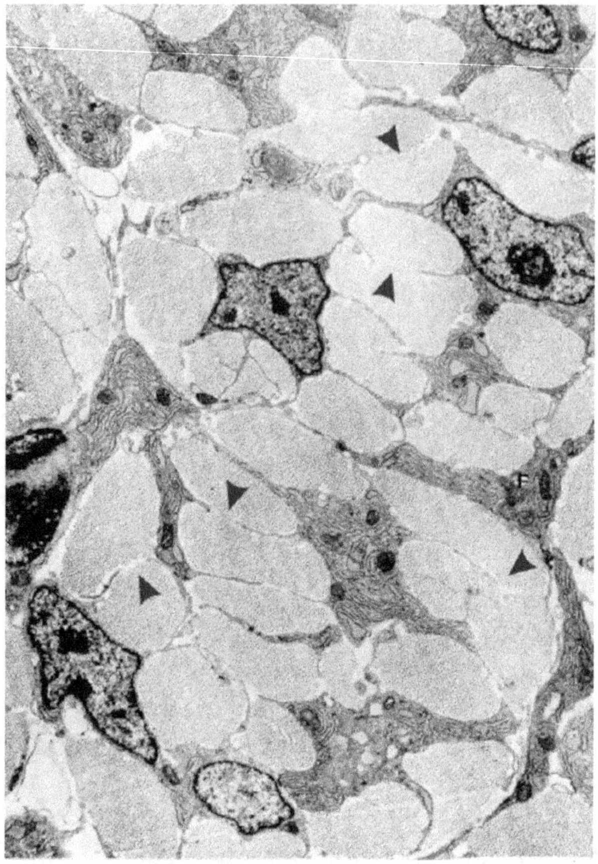

Fig. 9. Transmission electron micrograph showing the lateral fusion of collagen fibrils at d 17 of chick embryogenesis. This transmission electron micrograph shows several collagen fibrils that appear to be in the fusion process (see arrows). Fusion leads to lateral growth and increased collagen fibril diameters. The fibril bundle (fiber) diameter is still approx 2 µm before fusion similar to that observed on d 14. Adapted from ref. *48*.

These segments can be isolated from tendon and studied by electron microscopy *(51)*. Holmes and coworkers have shown that fibrils from 12 d-old chick embryos grow in length at a constant diameter *(46)* and that end-to-end fusion requires the C-terminal end of a unipolar fibril *(53)*. By 18 d, embryonic fibril growth occurs at both fibril ends and is associated with increased diameter *(46)*. Because fibril segments at 18 d cannot be isolated from developing tendon, it is likely that fibril fusion and crosslinking occur simultaneously.

In the mature tendon, collagen fibril bundles (fibers) have diameters between 1 and 300 µm, and fibrils have diameters from 20 to over 280 nm (*11*; Fig. 3). The presence of a crimp pattern in the collagen fibers has been established for rat-tail tendon *(54)* as well as for patellar tendon and anterior cruciate ligament (ACL) *(55)*; the specific geometry of the pattern, however, differs from tissue to tissue. It is not clear that the crimp morphology is actually present in tendons that are under normal resting muscular forces.

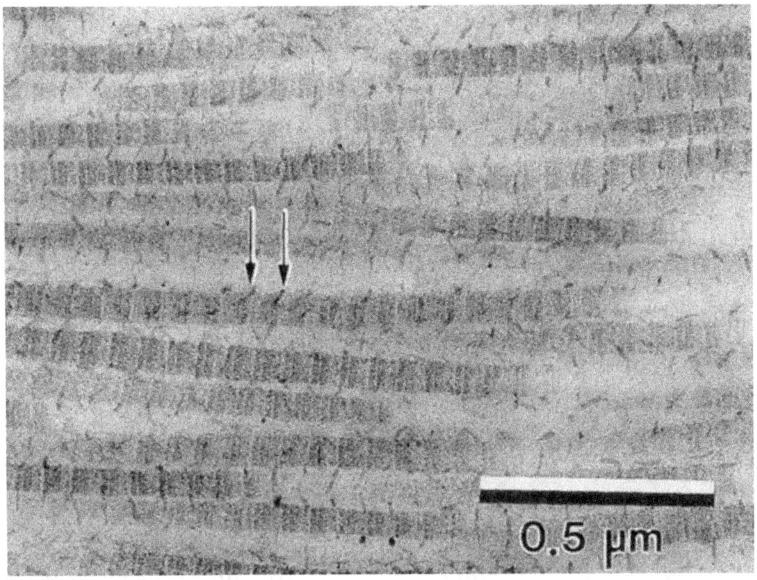

Fig. 10. Relationship between PGs and collagen fibrils in the tendon. Transmission electron micrograph showing positive-staining pattern of type I collagen fribrils from rabbit Achilles tendon stained with quinolinic blue. This stain specifically stains PG filaments (arrows) attached to collagen fibrils at the d and e bands. Adapted from ref. *71*.

Role of Proteoglycans (PGs) in Tendon Development

The tendon contains a variety of PGs, including decorin *(56)*, a small leucine-rich PG that binds specifically to the d band of positively stained type I collagen fibrils *(57)*, as well as hyaluronan, a high-molecular-weight polysaccharide. Other small leucine-rich PGs are biglycan, fibromodulin, lumican, epiphycan, and keratocan. In mature tendon, the PGs are predominantly proteodermochondran sulfates *(56)*. PGs are seen as filaments regularly attached to collagen fibrils in electron micrographs of tendon stained with Cupromeronic blue (Fig. 10; *58*). In relaxed mature tendon, most PG filaments are arranged orthogonally across the collagen fibrils at the gap zone—usually at the d and e positively staining bands *(57)*. In immature tendons, PGs are observed either orthogonal or parallel to the D period *(58)*, and the amount of PGs associated with collagen fibrils in the tendon decreases with increased fibril diameter and age *(59)*.

Animal models employing genetic mutations that lack decorin demonstrate collagen fibrils with irregular diameters and decreased skin strength *(60)*, whereas a model lacking lumican shows abnormally thick collagen fibrils and skin fragility *(61)*. Downregulation of decorin has been shown to cause the development of collagen fibrils with larger diameters and higher ultimate tensile strengths in ligament scar *(62)*. Models without thrombospondin 2—a member of a family of glycoproteins found in ECM—exhibit abnormally large fibril diameters and skin fragility *(63)*. These observations suggest that PGs, e.g., decorin and other glycoproteins found in the ECM, are required for normal collagen fibrillogenesis. Decorin also appears to assist in the alignment of collagen molecules and to facilitate sliding during mechanical deformation *(64,65)*.

Scott and coworkers studied the role of decorin in tendon development *(57,59,64)*, and their results suggest that interactions between collagen and PGs are an important aspect. A specific relationship between PGs and the d band of the positive-staining pattern of collagen fibrils exists *(57)*. They speculated that PGs might (1) inhibit collagen fibril radial growth through the interference with crosslinking and (2) inhibit calcification by occupying the hole in the gap zone *(57)*. Scott and coworkers subsequently demonstrated that the interactions between collagen and PGs could be broken down into three phases during tendon development *(59)*. During the first 40 d after conception, collagen synthesis leads to the formation of thin fibrils in an environment rich in PGs. Between d 40 and 120, when growth of existing collagen fibrils occurs, PG and hyaluronan content decreased to a critical value. After 120 d fibril diameter growth decreased, and the PG content per fibril surface area remained constant. Recently, Scott *(64)* has proposed that small PGs act as tissue organizers, orienting and ordering collagen fibrils.

Comparative Structure of the Tendon, Ligament and Capsule

Many studies exist in the literature on tendon structure; however, there are fewer studies on the structure of the ligament and capsule. Fibril diameters for knee ligaments are reported to be between approx 59 and 85 nm *(66,67)*, and those reported for the capsule average about 45 nm. In ACL, the fascicles containing collagen fibrils are reported to be 1–32 μm in diameter *(67)*. Although the collagen fibrils in the center of the ACL are similar to those found in the tendon and show a parallel alignment with respect to the tendon axis, the fibrils on the surface showed a crossing pattern *(67)*. In contrast, collagen fibrils in the posterior cruciate ligament are predominantly aligned along the ligament axis *(67)*.

Mineralization of Tendon

Although the mineralization of the tendon, ligament, and capsule appear to be pathological responses to trauma or injury, there are examples in nature of tendon mineralization that occur during development. The major leg tendons of the domestic turkey, *Meleagris gallopavo* (including the Achilles or gastrocnemius tendon), begin to naturally calcify when the birds reach about 12 wk of age *(32)*. Whether this is an adaptive response to increased loading or a pathologic response owing to overloading is unclear. This seems to be in response to external forces, but the relationship between skeletal changes and such forces is still not understood *(68)*. The gastrocnemius is a relatively thick tendon at the rear of the turkey leg that passes through a cartilaginous sheath at the tarsometarsal joint and inserts into the muscles at the hip of the bird *(32)*. After passing through the sheath, the tendon divides into two portions, with a decrease in total cross-sectional area relative to the original cross-section. This division results in an alteration of the load borne by the sections after the bifurcation. Initiation of calcification occurs at or near the point of bifurcation, then calcification proceeds along the bifurcated sections *(32)*.

Morphological observations indicate that initiation of calcification occurs on the surface of collagen fibrils close to or at the center of the tendon in 15-wk-old animals *(69)*. This is associated with changes in the collagen fibril structure. The collagen fibrils appear to become straighter and pack into narrower bundles, and to align with their D periods in register. Mineral is laid down within the gap region of the collagen D period *(69)*; the crystal *c* axis is parallel to the long axis of the fibril. Later, mineralization occurs within the fibril. Whether mineralization is linked with changes in PG content is unclear.

In areas away from the mineralization site, tendon cells are spindle-shaped and have cellular processes that extend into the ECM, eventually connecting with processes of neighboring cells *(32)*. The diameters of collagen fibrils in these areas range from 75 to 500 nm. In regions near the site, the tendon cells appear to have increased amounts of endoplasmic reticulum, Golgi apparatus, and thin cellular processes that weave between tightly packed collagen fibrils *(32)*. Vesicles containing calcium and phosphate are also seen within and outside cellular processes and in regions where mineralization is seen *(32)*.

As the turkey gastrocnemius tendon mineralizes, there are associated changes in both the mechanical properties and elastic energy storage. Mineralization appears to increase the elastic modulus as well as increase the elastic energy storage at a fixed strain *(24,33)*. Thus, changes in mechanical properties of developing tendons reflect changes in tendon structure and function.

Mechanical Properties of Developing Tendons

Understanding the relationship between the structure and mechanical properties of dense regular connective tissue generally derives from analysis of the mechanical properties of developing tendon. The properties of developing tendons rapidly change just prior to the onset of locomotion. McBride et al. *(31)* reported that the ultimate tensile strength (UTS) of developing chick extensor tendons increases from about 2 MPa (d 14 embryonic) to 60 MPa 2 d after birth. This rapid increase in UTS is not related to changes in fibril diameter, but is associated with increases in collagen fibril lengths *(31)*, which is linked to the viscoelastic properties of tendons *(2)*.

The relationship between tendon UTS and fibril length is based on an association developed with fibril length and mechanical behavior. Measurements of stress-strain curves and incremental stress-strain curves for tendon and self-assembled collagen fibers suggest that both UTS and the elastic modulus are more dependent on fibril length than diameter *(2,33)*. Application of incremental strains to the tendon, followed by measuring the initial and equilibrium stresses, yields information on the molecular and fibrillar bases for energy storage and transmission in dense regular connective tissue (Fig. 11). From the equilibrium stresses obtained at different strains, an elastic stress-strain curve can be plotted while from the difference between the total and elastic stress, a viscous stress-strain curve can be constructed *(2,19,70)*. The slope of the elastic stress-strain curve is proportional to the elastic modulus of the collagen molecule and fibril; using hydrodynamic theory, the viscous stress is proportional to the fibril length *(2,33)*. Fibril lengths calculated from incremental stress-strain curves for postembryonic rat-tail and turkey tendons are within the range of approx 400–800 μm *(2,33)*. These fibril lengths are much greater than the fibril lengths observed prior to the onset of locomotion, suggesting that increases in fibril length are associated with energy storage and transmission.

When effective fibril lengths (calculated from mechanical measurements) are plotted against reported values of the fibril lengths measured on chick metatarsal tendons

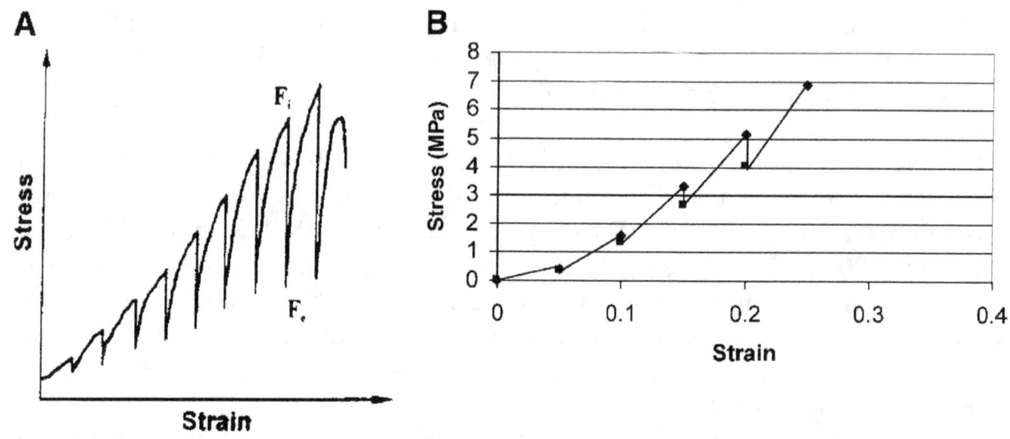

Fig. 11. **(A)** Incremental stress-strain testing of the tendon. This diagram illustrates the construction of an incremental stress-vs-strain curve from initial and equilibrium stress measurements. The sample is loaded in tension by stretching to a predetermined strain increment at a constant strain rate, then allowing the specimen to relax to equilibrium. The initial stress or force is recorded, as well as the equilibrium stress or force. After equilibrium is achieved (i.e., the force does not change by >2% during a 20-min time interval), an additional strain increment is added, and the cycle is repeated until the specimen fails. The total stress is obtained by dividing the total force, Fi, by the cross-sectional area, whereas the elastic stress is obtained by dividing the equilibrium force, Fe, by the cross-sectional area. The viscous stress is defined as the difference between the total stress and elastic stress. **(B)** Total (open boxes), elastic (closed diamonds), and viscous (closed squares) stress-strain curves for rat tail tendon. Error bars represent one standard deviation of the mean. The data were collected at a strain rate of 10%/min, a strain increment of 5%, and a temperature of 22°C. The time required to reach equilibrium ranged from 20 min to several hours for a single strain increment. Reproduced from ref. *2*.

during development *(49,51)*, a linear relationship is observed *(71)*. Elevations in UTS during development appear to be related to increased fibril lengths *(24)* and may be a consequence of fibril fusion and crosslink formation in vivo.

On a molecular basis, the slope of the elastic stress-strain curve (elastic modulus) can be related to the stretching of collagen triple helices within crosslinked collagen fibrils *(2,33)*. Results of molecular modeling studies suggest that stretching first occurs in the flexible domains of the collagen molecule. Studies on self-assembled type I collagen fibers show that in the absence of crosslinks, the elastic slope is reduced (2), which indicates that crosslinks are important in mechanical coupling between collagen molecules. Elastic energy storage is reported to be impaired in osteoarthritic cartilage and is associated with decreased collagen fibril lengths, suggesting that fibril length is a significant structural aspect of collagen mechanical behavior *(2,72)*.

Previous studies have examined the mechanism by which mechanical energy is translated into molecular and fibrillar deformation in the tendon *(73–75)*. Several reports show that up to a strain of 2% in tendons, molecular stretching predominates; increases in the collagen D period beyond 2% are because of molecular slippage *(73–75)*. From data reported by Mosler et al. *(73)*, it is concluded that the molecular strain is about 10% of the macroscopic strain. The remainder of the macroscopic strain is from molecular and fibrillar slippage (30%; *73*). Results of other studies demonstrate that molecular stretching and sliding alone do not explain the elastic and viscous behavior of tendons; the elastic response requires end-to-end crosslinks between collagen molecules within fibrils *(2,33)*. The magnitude of the elastic constant is directly related to the collagen fibril length and therefore, the number of collagen molecules crosslinked end-to-end in a series. The end-to-end crosslink pattern may be specific to each tissue type *(76)*, showing that energy storage in skeletal and nonskeletal tissues may be different. Although the fibril diameter does have a role in the magnitude of the elastic response, fibril length appears to be the most important parameter in dictating elastic behavior.

The role of minor collagen types, such as type XII on the mechanical properties of the tendon, is still unclear; however, recent evidence suggests that production of this collagen is high in stretched collagen matrices and suppressed in relaxed matrices *(77)*. Genes for collagen type XII and tenascin-C, another matrix component, contain stretch-responsive enhancer regions that upregulate the synthesis of these two components as a result of increased mechanical loading *(77)*. These observations imply that changes in external mechanical loading conditions to the ECM cause the synthesis of matrix components that modify the structure and possibly the mechanical properties.

Mechanical Properties of Mineralizing Tendons

The viscoelastic behavior of mineralizing turkey leg tendon has been reported during the period between 12 and 17 wk *(24,33)*. These studies indicate the elastic modulus for type I collagen is between about 3 and 7.75 GPa, similar to that found for rat-tail tendon *(24,33)*. Fibril lengths obtained from the viscous component of the stress-strain behavior are between 414 and 616 μm, which is slightly smaller than those found for rat-tail tendon, but significantly greater than those for developing chick tendons *(2,49,51)*. Mineralization appears to increase the elastic modulus for type I collagen and may lead to changes in elastic energy storage *(24)*. However, it is not clear whether tendon mineralization is an adaptive process associated with locomotion of adult birds; many similarities exist between the effectors involved in mineralization and mechanochemical transduction that occur at the cellular level. This is discussed in more detail in a later section (Mechanochemical Transduction in the Tendon, Ligament, and Capsule.

Comparative Mechanical Properties of the Tendon, Ligament, and Capsule

These mechanical properties are difficult to compare owing to the large variation in measured properties of these tissues. This variation is a result of viscoelasticity and the strain-rate dependence of the material properties *(11)*. Although the recent advance of separating the elastic and viscous contributions has yielded a value of between 4 and 8 GPa for the elastic modulus *(24,33,72)*, no reports of similar measurements have been made for the ligament and capsule. The elastic modulus for tendon models at first approximation is not strain-rate–dependent *(28)*, whereas the viscosity calculated from the viscous stress decreases with increased strain rate *(78)*.

The maximum strength for tendons and ligaments ranges from about 13 to 300 MPa, and the strain at failure and modulus values range from about 6% to 50% and 0.065 to

8 GPa, respectively (*see* ref. *11* for a review). Values for hip capsule ligament are reported to be similar to those for other ligaments and range from about 76 to 286 MPa; the reported strain to failure is between 8 and 25% *(79)*. These values are likely to depend on age and loading history through mechanochemical transduction processes.

Mechanochemical Transduction in Ligament, Tendon, and the Capsule

All dense connective tissue is loaded in tension during development under normal physiologic conditions *(3,19,26,78)*. This tension is, in part, passive tension incorporated into the collagen fibril network during development and active cellular tension that is applied by fibroblast-like cells found in the ECM. The active component of the tension exerted by fibroblasts is altered in response to changes in the external loads applied to the tissue. Thus, active cell tension balances both changes in external loading to the tissue, as well as the stresses acting at an angle to the loading direction. Therefore, the mechanism by which elastic energy is stored in dense regular connective tissue during locomotion is important not only in understanding the physiology of the tendon, ligament, and capsule but also in linking external energy storage to genetic responses that occur via fibroblast stimulation in these tissues.

ECMs found in ocular, pulmonary, musculoskeletal, cardiovascular, and dermal tissues are all under tension under normal physiologic conditions, even in the absence of external loading *(26)*. This tension fulfills cosmetic functions (i.e., smooth skin is much more appealing than wrinkled skin), and also sets up a state of dynamic mechanical loading at the collagen fibril–cell interface that stimulates mechanochemical transduction. As defined in this chapter, mechanochemical transduction refers to the effect of stresses and strains on gene expression and the regulation of cellular protein synthesis that results from changes in mechanical loading. At equilibrium, all external forces acting on tissues, organs, and collagen fibrils must sum to zero. In addition, increases in external loading cause increases in internal stresses that act on collagen fibrils and at the collagen fibril–cell interface. Beyond this effect, the observation that cells grown in collagen lattices exert a contractile force *(80)* suggests that under normal physiologic conditions, cells apply tension to the attached ECM. This tension leads to dynamic active stresses applied to the collagen network and also leads to incorporation of passive tension in the collagen fibrils during development and maturation of tissue scaffolds.

The basis of the active tension exerted by cells has been studied by growing various cell types in collagen matrices. When isolated fibroblasts are grown in a reconstituted collagen matrix, they contract the matrix because of active tension exerted by cells on the matrix *(80)*. Additionally, the cells respond differently when the matrix is stressed as opposed to unstressed *(80)*. Fibroblasts cultured in collagen matrices not only actively contract the matrix but also remodel it. These examples underscore the importance of passive and active stresses in the mechanobiology of dense connective tissue, as well as suggest the need to understand how mechanical loading is intrinsically related to genetic expression of the resident cells.

Effects of Physical Forces on Cell–ECM Interactions

The mechanical properties of dense regular connective tissue are dynamically dependent on the properties of the crosslinked collagenous network and on cell–ECM interactions. Forces are transmitted to and from cells through the ECM with changes in mechanical forces and cell shape acting as biological regulators *(81)*. Ingber hypothesized that cells use a tension-dependent form of architecture, termed tensegrity, to organize and stabilize their cytoskeleton *(81)*. Mechanical interactions between cells and their ECM appear to have a critical role in cell regulation by switching cells between different gene products *(77)*. The relationship between external loading and changes in genetic expression of cells in dense connective tissue is significant to understand joint physiology and disease.

At least two mechanisms exist by which external loads affect gene expression of resident cells in ECM: cell–ECM and cell–cell interactions *(79)*. Integrin adhesion receptors that connect ECM components and cytoskeletal elements have been implicated in mediating signal transduction through the cell membrane in both directions *(82)*. Integrin adhesion receptors are heterodimers of two different subunits termed α and β *(82)*. They contain a large ECM domain responsible for binding to substrates, a single transmembrane domain and a cytoplasmic domain that usually consists of 20–70 amino acid residues *(83)*. They mediate signal transduction through the cell membrane in both directions. Binding of ligands to integrins transmits signals into the cell and results in cytoskeletal reorganization, gene expression, and cellular differentiation (outside-in signaling). On the contrary, signals within the cell can also propagate through integrins and regulate integrin-ligand binding affinity and cell adhesion (inside-out signaling; *83,84)*.

Eukaryotic cells directly attach to ECM collagen fibers via integrin subunits, α1β1 and α1β2 *(85)*, through a six-residue (glycine-phenylalanine-hydroxyproline-glycine-glutamic acid-arginine) sequence *(86)* that is present in the b2 and d bands of the collagen-positive staining pattern (Fig. 12). Integrins are transmembrane molecules that associate via their cytoplasmic domains with a number of cytoplasmic proteins, including vinculin, paxillin, tensin, and others *(87)*. All these molecules are involved in the dynamic association with actin filaments. In cultured cells, integrin-based molecular complexes form small (0.5–1 μm) or point contacts known as focal complexes *(88)* and elongated streak-like structures (3–10 μm long). The elongated structures are associated with stress fibers containing actin and myosin, also known as focal contacts or focal adhesions *(89)*. Recent research suggests that integrin-containing focal complexes behave as mechanosensors that exhibit directional assembly in response to local force *(90)*. It has been reported that collagen binding integrins are involved in up- or downregulating collagen α1(I) and collagenase (matrix metalloproteinase 1 [MMP1]) mRNA depending on whether fibroblasts are unloaded *(91)* or loaded (*see* ref. *79* for a review).

The effects of mechanical forces have been studied on isolated fibroblasts and fibroblasts cultured in a collagen matrix. Fibroblasts were cultured on flexible-bottom surfaces coated with fibronectin, laminin, or elastin aligned perpendicular to the force vector *(92)*. Mechanically loaded cells grown on laminin, elastin, or other substrates expressed higher levels of procollagen mRNA and incorporated more labeled proline into protein than unstressed cells do *(92)*. Fibroblasts in cell culture that are not aligned with the force direction show a several-fold increase in activity of MMP1, MMP2, and MMP3, suggesting that cells unable to align with the direction of the applied load remodel their matrix more rapidly than oriented cells *(93)*.

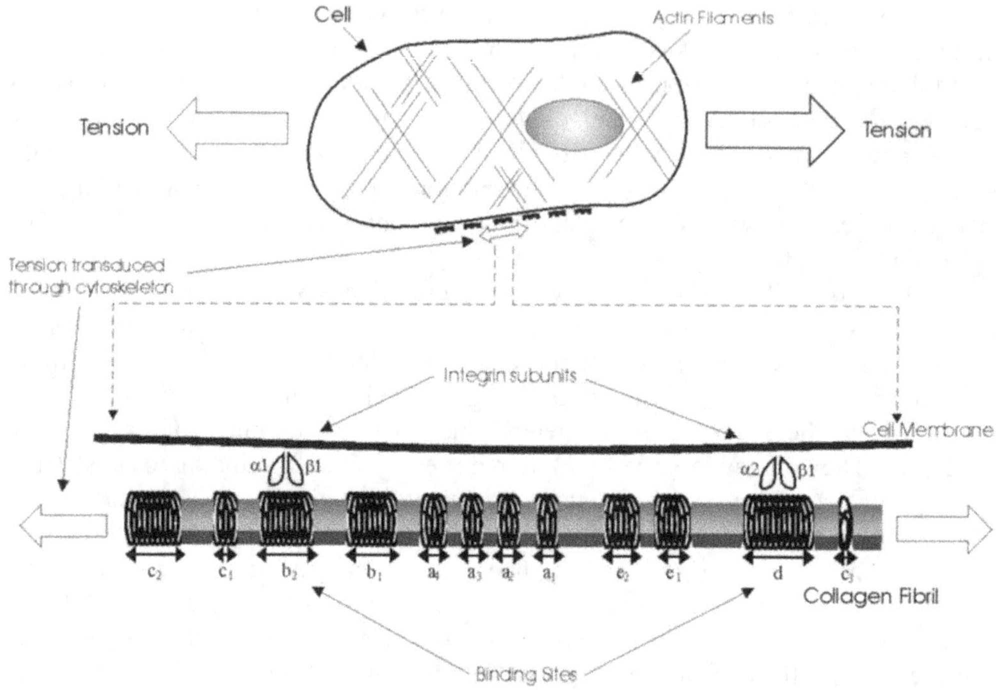

Fig. 12. Integrin-binding sites on collagen fibrils. All eukaryotic cells express integrin dimmers, α1β1 and α2β1, which bind to specific amino acid sequences found in the b_2 and d bands of the positive-staining pattern of type I collagen. This diagram illustrates the location of these integrin-binding sites relative to the flexible domains found in type I collagen fibrils. Note the integrin-binding sites are located in two of the larger flexible domains on type I collagen. Ingber *(81)* has proposed that integrins act as mechanosensors that transduce external mechanical signals into changes in gene expression and the activation of secondary messengers. External tensile and compressive forces applied to dense regular connective tissue lead to stretching of the b_2 and d bands in the type I collagen and could possibly lead to stretching and deformation of the integrin dimers in these bands. These events would lead to stimulation of mechanochemical transduction via the activation and release of secondary messengers. In this manner, external tensile forces applied to dense regular connective tissue during locomotion could cause changes in mechanochemical transduction and alteration of gene expression.

Fibroblasts grown in a three-dimensional (3D) collagen lattice have been shown to align themselves with the direction of the principal strain *(94)* and adopt a synthetic fibroblast phenotype characterized by the induction of connective tissue synthesis and inhibition of matrix degradation *(95)*. Cell contraction of 3D collagen matrices was observed in the direction opposite to the direction of applied loads *(96)*. Increased external loading was followed immediately by a reduction in cell-mediated contraction *(96)*.

Effects of External Loading on Cell–ECM and Cell–Cell Interactions

During cell adhesion to collagen in the ECM, the initial binding of integrins to their ECM ligands leads to their activation and clustering and to the assembly of focal adhesion complexes, which serve as "assembly lines" for signaling pathways. These pathways include protein kinases, adaptor proteins, guanidine-exchange factors, and small

GTPases that are recruited to these sites and may directly trigger mitogen-activated protein kinases (MAPK) pathways or growth factors, as well as activation of the nuclear factor (NF)-κB pathway *(97–99)*.

The contacts between two adjoining cell membranes are stabilized by specific cell adhesion molecules, which include the Ca^{2+}-dependent cadherins. These molecules allow cell–cell communications *(100,101)* and are involved in mechanochemical transduction via cell–cell interactions. In some cell types, cadherins are concentrated within adherens junctions that are stretch sensitive *(101,102)*, and their extracellular domains interact with cadherins on adjacent cells, whereas their cytoplasmic domains provide attachment to the actin cytoskeleton via catenins and other cytoskeletal proteins *(101,102)*. The Rho family is required for the establishment and maintenance of cadherin-based adherens junctions *(103)*. The type of cadherin expressed in a cell can affect the specificity *(102)* and physiologic properties of cell–cell interactions *(100)*.

Fibroblast–fibroblast interactions in dense connective tissue contribute to the generation of internal tension. Ragsdale et al. *(104)* showed that fibroblasts were stretched in tension after spontaneous contraction of neighboring cells. They postulated that mechanical transmission of tensile forces occurs through adherens junctions in fibroblasts. Mechanical perturbation leads to a transient increase in intracellular calcium that propagates from cell to cell *(105)*. Mechanical forces applied to fibroblast adherens junctions activate *N*-cadherin-associated, stretch-sensitive, calcium-permeable channels, which increase actin polymerization and activate MAPK pathways *(106)*.

G proteins are another family of membrane proteins believed to modulate mechanochemical transduction pathways *(107)*. Mechanical stimulation changes the conformation of G proteins, causing growth factor–like changes that initiate secondary messenger cascades that lead to cell growth *(108)*. Cyclic strain was shown to significantly decrease steady state levels of G proteins and adenylate cyclase activity in some cell types *(109)*.

In addition to the activation of signaling pathways, mechanical stress triggers the activation of stretch-activated ion channels, which have been identified in numerous cells *(110)* and were studied extensively in muscle cells *(111,112)*. Stretch-activated channels permit passage of cations, including Ca^{2+}, K^+, and Na^+, but a few anion channels are reported to be sensitive to mechanical stimulation *(110,113)*. In muscle cells, Ca^{2+} influx through voltage-gated channels induces a transient elevation in intracellular Ca^{2+} levels *(114)*. Ca^{2+} influx is activated by mechanical stimulation and catalyzes membrane depolarization and cell contraction *(112)*. The presence of extracellular Ca^{2+} appears to be a requirement for its influx owing to stretch-induced cell contraction in muscle cells *(115)*. It enhances the sensitivity of intracellular calcium on subsequent signal transduction through the activation of cascades, such as protein kinase C *(115,116)*. Strain-induced Ca^{2+} signal transmission involves the actin microfilament system because an actin polymerization inhibitor was found to abolish Ca^{2+} responses induced by mechanical strain *(117)*.

Both Ca^{2+} and K^+ channels have been implicated in mediating stretch-induced changes in cells *(107)*. Ca^{2+} ion involvement in phospholipase C (PLC) activation has been proposed, which catalyzes the generation of PLC-derived inositol phosphates and diacylglycerol necessary for phosphokinase C activation *(118,119)*. K^+ channel involvement has also been postulated (*120,121*; Fig. 13).

Many cellular processes are triggered by the application of external mechanical forces to cells found in dense connective tissue. Cell adhesion to collagen via integrin receptors, stretch activation of ion channels, changes in cell membrane structure, stretch activation of growth factor receptors, and stretch activation of cell junctions activate signaling pathways that lead to the activation of MAPK pathways and changes in gene expression. These processes are summarized in Fig. 13.

SUMMARY

The tendon, ligament, and capsule are all composed of dense regular connective tissue primarily containing types I and III collagen, proteoglycans, and cells. The physiologic function of these tissues is to store and transmit elastic energy to and from bones in the joint to aid in locomotion. Forces generated by muscle are stored as elastic strain energy during tendon deformation, then transferred to the bone to allow for joint movement. Energy is stored during joint bending as strain energy in the ligaments and capsule, which limit joint motion. Excess energy remaining after joint movement is transferred back to muscle through the attached tendon, where it is dissipated as heat.

Energy storage in dense regular connective tissue occurs by stretching flexible regions in collagen molecules and fibrils that are crosslinked into a 3D network. External forces applied to dense regular connective tissue not only cause joint bending but are also transduced into cellular changes, e.g., changes in cell division and gene expression through cell–ECM and cell–cell interactions. Cell–ECM interactions involve cell surface integrins and focal adhesion complexes that activate secondary messengers attached to the cell membrane. Once formed, focal adhesion complexes affect several pathways, including the MAPK pathway. Cell–cell interactions occur by activating cadherin-dependent cell junction stretch receptors that cause the release of intercellular calcium and activation of secondary messenger pathways. Mechanical stretching of cells also enables alterations in cell membrane ion permeability that affects cell function. All these processes affect the balance between external loading and cell-generated contractile forces, which ultimately lead to changes in composition and mechanical properties of the ECM.

ACKNOWLEDGMENTS

The authors would like to acknowledge the assistance of graduate students, Gurinder P. Seehra and Istvan Horvath, in preparing some of the figures used in this chapter.

Fig. 13. *(Opposite page)* Putative mechanisms for mechanochemical transduction in ECM. Generalized oversimplified scheme for how external mechanical stress is transduced into changes in cell genetic expression. Tensile stresses applied to the cell through direct stretching of the cell membrane, stretching of ion channels in the cell membrane, stretching of intracellular junctions, or through release of growth factors leads to the activation of secondary messengers that lead to release of factors, such as NF-κB. NF-κB binds to promoter sequences in genes (e.g., for tenascin-C and type XII collagen). *(Continued)*

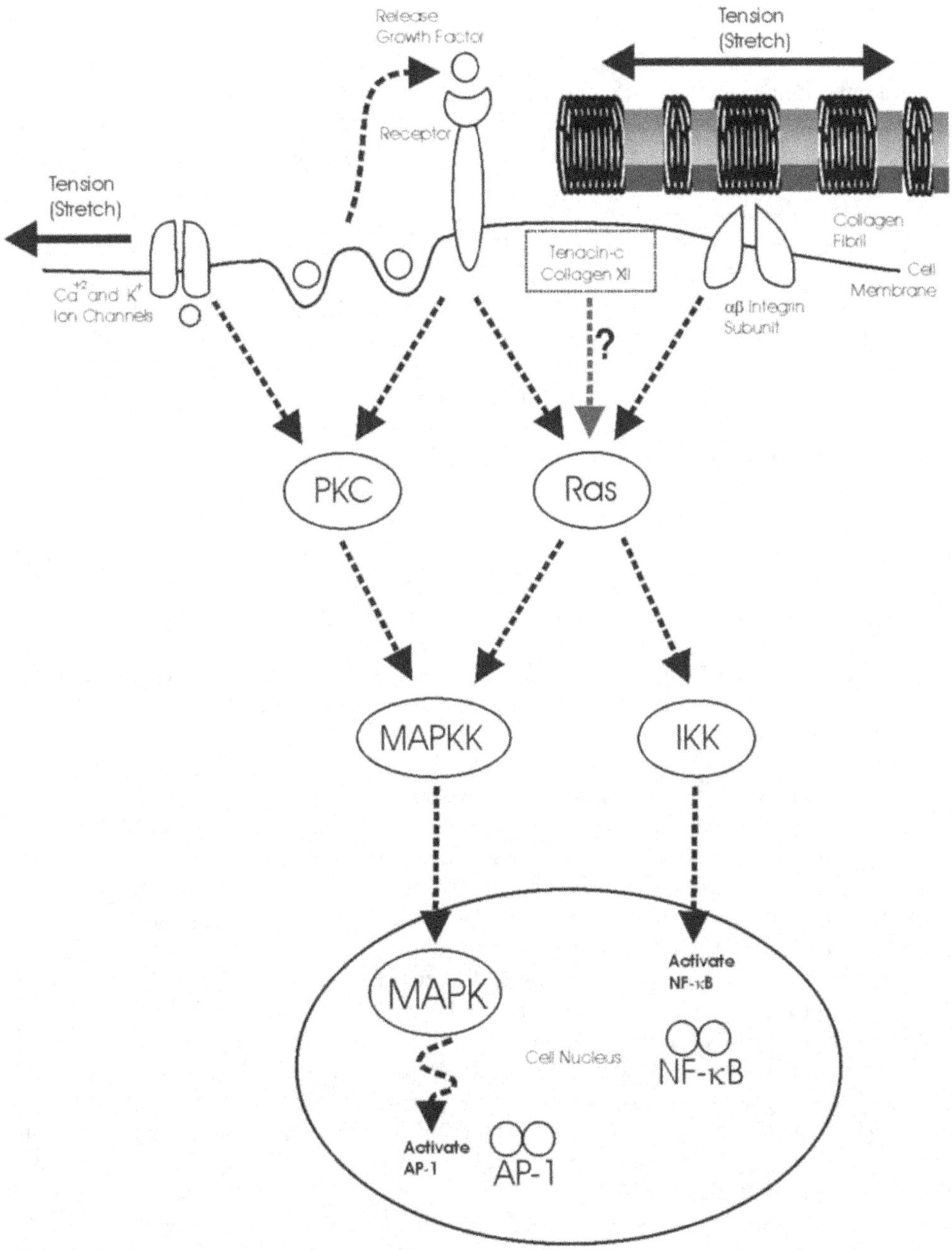

Fig. 13. *(Continued)* Stretching of ECM-integrin contacts and cell intercellular junctions are known to trigger MAPK pathways (MAPKKK, MAPKK, and MAPK) via GTPase ras. MAPKs translocate to the nucleus and activate transcription factors, such as AP-1 or SRF. Alternately, members of the MAPKKK family have been shown to activate the I-κB kinase (IKK) complex that phosphorylates I-κB and leads to the release of NF-κB, which translocates to the nucleus. In the nucleus, NF-κB binds to its target promoter sequence. Another putative route for MAPK activation is via autocrine release of growth factors and activation protein kinase C (PKC), whereas mechanical stretch also catalyzes the activation of stretch-response promoter regions in tenascin-C and type XII collagen genes in a similar manner to platelet-derived growth factor B. (Adapted from ref. *79*.)

REFERENCES

1. Roberts TJ, Marsh RL, Weyand PG, Taylor CR. Muscular force in running turkeys: The economy of minimizing work. *Science* 1997;275:113–115.
2. Silver FH, Christiansen DL, Snowhill PB, Chen Y. Role of storage on changes in the mechanical properties of tendon and self-assembled collagen fibers. *Connect Tissue Res* 2000;42:155–164.
3. Silver FH, Christiansen DL, Snowhill PB, Chen Y. Transition from viscous to elastic-dependency of mechanical properties of self-assembled collagen fibers. *J Appl Polymer Sci* 2001;7:134–142.
4. Alexander RM. *Animal Mechanics*, 2nd Ed. Blackwell Scientific, Oxford, UK, 1983.
5. Alexander RM. Elastic energy stores in running vertebrates. *A Zool* 1984;24:85–94
6. Shadwick RE. Elastic energy storage in tendons: Mechanical differences related to function and age. *J Appl Physiol* 1990;68:1033–1040.
7. Wilson AM, McGuigan MP, Su A, van den Bogert AJ. Horses damp the spring in their step. *Nature* 2001;414:895–899.
8. Silver FH, Christiansen DL. *Biomaterials Science and Biocompatibility*. Springer, New York, NY, 1999.
9. Keene DR, Lunstrum GP, Morris NP, Stoddard DW, Burgeson RE. Two type XII-like collagens localize to the surface of banded collagen fibrils. *J Cell Biol* 1991;113:971–978.
10. Kaltsas DS. Comparative study of the properties of the shoulder joint capsule with those of other joint capsules. *Clin Orthop* 1983;173:20–26.
11. Silver FH, Kato YP, Ohno M, Wasserman AJ. Analysis of mammalian connective tissue: Relationship between hierarchical structures and mechanical properties. *J LongTerm Eff Med Implants* 1992;2:165–198.
12. Niyibizi C, Visconti CS, Kavalkovich K, Woo SL-Y. Collagens in an adult bovine medial collateral ligament: Immunofluorescence localization by confocal microscopy reveals that type XIV collagen predominates at the ligament-bone junction. *Matrix Biol* 1994;14:743–751.
13. Petersen W, Tillmann B. Structure and vascularization of the cruciate ligaments of the human knee. *Anat Embryol* 1999;200:325–334.
14. Bland YS, Ashhurst DE. The hip joint: the fibrillar collagens associated with development and ageing in the rabbit. *J Anat* 2001;198:17–27.
15. Riechert K, Labs K, Lindenhayn K, Sinha P. Semiquantitative analysis of types I and III collagen form tendons and ligaments in a rabbit model. *J Orthop Sci* 2001;6:68–74.
16. Lewis AR, Ralphs JR, Kneafsey B, Benjamin M. Distribution of collagens and glycosaminoglycans in the joint capsule of the proximal interphalangeal joint of the human finger. *Anat Rec* 1999;250:281–291.
17. Moriggl B, Jax P, Milz S, Buttner A, Benjamin M. Fibrocartilage at the entheses of the suprascapular (superior transverse scapular) ligament of man—a ligament spanning two regions of a single bone. *J Anat* 2001;199:539–545.
18. Engle J. Versatile collagens in invertebrates. *Science* 1997;277:1785–1786.
19. Silver FH, Horvath I, Foran DJ. Mechanical implications of the domain structure of fibril forming collagens: Comparison of the molecular and fibrillar flexibilities of the α-chains found in types I, II and III collagen. *J Theor Biol* 2002;216:243–254.
20. Fletcher GC. Dynamic light scattering from collagen solutions. I. Translational diffusion coefficient and aggregation effects. *Biopolymers* 1976;15:2201–2217.
21. Thomas JC, Fletcher GC. Dynamic light scattering from collagen solutions. II. Photon correlation study of the depolarized light. *Biopolymers* 1979;18:1333–1352.
22. Silver FH, Langley KH, Trelstad RL. Type I collagen fibrillogenesis: Initiation via a reversible linear growth step. *Biopolymers* 1979;18:2523–2535.
23. Silver FH, Birk DE. Molecular structure of collagen in solution: Comparison of types I, II, III, and V. *Int J Biol Macromol* 1984;6:125–132.

24. Silver FH, Freeman JW, Horvath I, Landis WJ. Molecular basis for elastic energy storage in mineralized tendon. *Biomacromolecules* 2001;2:750–756.
25. Hofmann H, Voss T. Kuhn K, Engle J. Localization of flexible sites in thread-like molecules from electron micrographs: Comparison of interstitial, basement membrane and intima collagens. *J Mol Biol* 1984;172:325–343.
26. Paterlini MG. Nemethy G, Scheraga HA. The energy of formation of internal loops in triple-helical collagen polypeptides. *Biopolymers* 1995;35:607–619.
27. Silver FH. Self-assembly of connective tissue macromolecules. In: *Biological Materials: Structure, Mechanical Properties, and Modeling of Soft Tissues*, NYU Press, New York, NY, 1987, pp. 150–153.
28. Birk DE, Silver FH, Trelstad RL. Matrix assembly. In: Hay ED, ed. *Cell Biology of Extracellular Matrix*, 2nd Ed. Academic Press, New York, NY, 1991, pp. 221–254.
29. Birk DE, Fitch JM, Babiarz JP, Linsenmayer TF. Collagen type I and type V are present in the same fibril in the avian corneal stroma. *J Cell Biol* 1988;106:999–1008.
30. Andrikopoulos K, Liu X, Keene DR, Jaenisch R, Ramirez F. Targeted mutation in the col5α2 gene reveals a regulatory role for type V collagen during matrix assembly. *Nat Genet* 1995;9:31–36.
31. McBride DJ, Hahn R, Silver FH. Morphological characterization of tendon development during chick embryogenesis: Measurement of birefringence retardation. *Int J Biol Macromol* 1985;7:71–76.
32. Landis WJ. A study of calcification in the leg tendons from the domestic turkey. *J Ultrastruct Mol Struct Res* 1986;94:217–238.
33. Silver FH, Christiansen DL, Snowhill PB, Chen Y, Landis WJ. The role of mineral in the viscoelasticity of turkey tendons. *Biomacromolecules* 2000;1:180–185.
34. Hodge AJ, Petruska JA. Recent studies with the electron microscope on ordered aggregates of the tropocollagen macromolecule In: Ramachandran GN, ed. *Aspects of Protein Structure*. Academic Press, London, UK, 1963, pp 289–300.
35. Elliott DH. Structure and function of mammalian tendon. *Biol Rev* 1965;40:392–42.
36. Fessler JH, Fessler LI. Biosynthesis of procollagen. *Ann Rev Biochem* 1978;47:129–162.
37. Prockop D, Kivirikko KI, Tuderman L, Guzman NA. The biosynthesis of collagen and its disorders. *New Eng J Med* 1979;301:13–23.
38. Berg RA, Birk DE, Silver FH. Physical characterization of type I procollagen in solution: Evidence that the propeptides limit self-assembly. *Int J Biol Macromol* 1986;8: 177–182.
39. Tuderman L, Kivirikko KI, Prockop DJ. Partial purification and characterization of a neutral protease which cleaves the N-terminal propeptides from procollagen. *Biochemistry* 1977;16:3421–3429.
40. Engle J, Prockop DJ. The zipper-like folding of collagen triple-helices and the effects of mutations that disrupt the zipper. *Ann Rev Biophys Chem* 1991;20:137–152.
41. Trelstad RL, Hayashi K. Tendon collagen fibrillogenesis: intracellular subassemblies and cell surface changes associated with fibril growth. *Dev Biol* 1979;71:228–242.
42. Fleischmajer R, Olsen BR, Timpl R, Perlish JS, Lovelace O. Collagen fibril formation during embryogenesis. *Proc Natl Acad Sci USA* 1983;80:3354–3358.
43. Ruggerio F, Pfaffle M, von der Mark K, Garrone R. Retention of carboxypropeptides in type-II collagen fibrils in chick embryo chondrocyte cultures. *Cell Tissue Res* 1988;252: 619–624.
44. Fleischmajer R, Perlish JS, Olsen BR. Amino and carboxylpropeptides in bone collagen fibrils during embryogenesis. *Cell Tissue Res* 1987;247:105–109.
45. Fleischmajer R, Perlish JS, Timpl R, Olsen BR. Procollagen intermediates during tendon fibrillogenesis. *J Histochem Cytochem* 1988;36:1425–1432.
46. Holmes DF, Lowe MP, Chapman JA. Vertebrate (chick) collagen fibrils formed in vivo can exhibit a reversal in molecular polarity. *J Mol Biol* 1994;235:80–83.

47. Torp S, Baer E, Friedman B. Effects of age and of mechanical deformation on the ultrastructure of tendon. *Colston Papers* 1975;26:223–250.
48. McBride DJ. *Hind Limb Extensor Tendon Development in the Chick: A Light and Transmission Electron Microscopic Study*. MS Thesis in Physiology, Rutgers University, New Jersey, 1984.
49. Birk DE, Zycband EI, Winkelmann DA, Trelstad RL. Collagen fibrillogenesis in situ: Fibril segments are intermediates in matrix assembly. *Proc Natl Acad Sci USA* 1989;86: 4549–4553.
50. Birk DE, Southern JF, Zycband EI, Fallon JT, Trelstad RL. Collagen fibril bundles: a branching assembly unit in tendon morphogenesis. *Development* 1989;107:437–443.
51. Birk DE, Nurminskaya MV, Zycband EI. Collagen fibrillogenesis in situ: Fibril segments undergo post-depositional modifications resulting in linear and lateral growth during matrix development. *Dev Dyn* 1995;202:229–243.
52. Birk DE, Zycband EI, Woodruff S, Winkelmann DA, Trelstad RL. Collagen fibrillogenesis in situ: fibril segments become long fibrils as the developing tendon matures. *Dev Dyn* 1997;208:291–298.
53. Graham HK, Holmes DF, Watson RB, Kadler KE. Identification of collagen fibril fusion during vertebrate tendon morphogenesis. The process relies on unipolar fibrils and is regulated by collagen-proteoglycan interaction. *J Mol Biol* 2000;295:891–902.
54. Diamant J, Keller A, Baer E, Lith N, Arridge RGC. Collagen: ultrastructure and its relationship to mechanical properties as a function of ageing. *Proc R Soc Lond Bio Sci* 1972; 180:293–315.
55. Yahia L-H, Drouin G. Microscopical investigation of canine cruciate ligament and patellar tendon: Collagen fascicle morphology and architecture. *J Orthop Res* 1969;7:243–251.
56. Scott JE. The nomenclature of glycosaminoglycans and proteoglycans. *Glycoconj J* 1993;10:419–421.
57. Scott JE, Orford CR. Dermatan sulfate-rich proteoglycan associates with rat tail tendon collagen at the d band in the gap region. *Biochem J* 1981;197:213–216.
58. Cribb AM, Scott JE. Tendon response to tensile stress: An ultrastructural investigation of collagen:proteoglycan interactions in stressed tendon. *J Anat* 1995;187:423–428.
59. Scott JE, Orford CR, Hughes EW. Proteoglycan-collagen arrangements in developing rat tail tendon: An electron microscopical and biochemical investigation. *Biochem J* 1981; 195:573–581.
60. Danielson KG, Baribault H, Holmes DF, Graham H, Kadler KE, Iozzo RV. Targeted disruption of decorin leads to abnormal collagen fibril morphology and skin fragility. *J Cell Biol* 1997;136:729–743.
61. Chakravarti S, Magnuson T, Lass JH, Jepsen KJ, LaMantia C, Carroll H. Lumican regulates collagen fibril assembly: Skin fragility and corneal opacity in the absence of lumican. *J Cell Biol* 1998;141:1277–1286.
62. Nakamura N, Hart DA, Boorman RS, Kaneda Y, Shrive NG, Marchuk LL, et al. Decorin antisense gene therapy improves functional healing of early rabbit ligament scar with enhanced collagen fibrillogenesis in vivo. *J Orthop Res* 2000;18:517–523.
63. Kyriakides TR, Zhu,Y-H, Smith LT, Bain SD, Yang Z, Lin MT, et al. Mice that lack thrombospondin 2 display connective tissue abnormalities that are associated with disordered collagen fibrillogenesis, an increased vascular density, and a bleeding diathesis. *J Cell Biol* 1998;140:419–430.
64. Scott JE. Proteodermatan and proteokeratan sulfate (decorin, lumincan/fibromodulin) proteins are horsehoe shaped. Implications for their interactions with collagen. *Biochemistry* 1996;35:8795–8787.
65. Pins GD, Christiansen DL, Patel R, Silver FH. Self-assembly of collagen fibers. Influence of fibrillar alignment and decorin on mechanical properties. *Biophysical J* 1997;73:2164–2172.

66. Hart RA, Woo SL-Y, Newton PO. Ultrastructural morphology of anterior cruciate ligament and medial collateral ligaments: an experimental study in rabbits. *J Orthop Res* 1992; 10:96–103.
67. Neurath MF, Stofft E. Characterization of collagenous and elastic fiber systems and microvasculature of human cruciate ligaments. An electronmicroscopic and stereologic study. *Clin Anat* 1993;6:146–153.
68. Landis WJ, LiBrizzi JJ, Dunn MG, Silver FH. A study of the relationship between mineral content and mechanical properties of turkey gastrocnemius tendon. *J Bone Miner Res* 1995;10:859–867.
69. Nylen MU, Scott DB, Mosley VM. Mineralization of turkey leg tendon. II. Collagen-mineral relations revealed by electron and x-ray microscopy. In: Sognnaes RF, ed. *Calcification of Biological Systems*. American Academy Advanced Sciences, Washington, DC, 1960, pp. 129–142.
70. Silver FH, Horvath I, Foran D. Viscoelasticity of the vessel wall: Role of collagen and elastic fibers. *Crit Rev Biomed Eng* 2001;29:279–302.
71. Silver FH, Freeman J, Seehra GP. Collagen self-assembly and development of matrix mechanical properties. *J. Biomech* 2003;36:1529–1553.
72. Silver FH, Bradica G, Tria A. Viscoelastic behavior of osteoarthritic cartilage. *Connect Tissue Res* 2001;42:223–233.
73. Mosler E, Folkhard W, Knorzer E, Nemetschek-Gansler H, Nemetschek TH, Koch MH. Stress-induced molecular arrangement in tendon collagen. *J Mol Biol* 1985;182:589–596.
74. Sasakai N, Odajima S. Elongation mechanism of collagen fibrils and force-strain relationships of tendon at each level of structural hierarchy. *J Biomech* 1996;9:1131–1136.
75. Sasaki N, Odajima S. Stress-strain curve and Young's modulus of a collagen molecule as determined by the x-ray diffraction technique. *J Biomech* 1996;29:655–658.
76. Mechanic GL, Katz EP, Henmi M, Noyes C, Yamauchi M. Locus of a histidine-based, stable trifunctional, helix to helix collagen crosslink: Stereospecific collagen structure of type I skin fibrils. *Biochemistry* 1987;26:3500–3509.
77. Chiquet M. Regulation of extracellular matrix gene expression by mechanical stress. *Matrix Biol* 1999;18:417–425.
78. Silver FH, Ebrahimi A, Snowhill PB. Viscoelastic properties of self-assembled type I collagen fibers: Molecular basis of elastic and viscous behaviors. *Connect Tissue Res* 2002;43:569–580.
79. Silver FH, Siperko LM, Seehra GP. Mechanobiology of force transduction in skin. *Skin Res Technol* 2002;8:1–21.
80. Grinnell F. Fibroblast-collagen-matrix contraction: growth-factor signaling and mechanical loading. *Trends Cell Biol* 2000;10:362–365.
81. Ingber D. Integrins as mechanochemical transducers. *Curr Opin Cell Biol* 1991;3:841–848.
82. Liu S, Calderwood DA, Ginsberg MH. Integrin cytoplasmic domain-binding proteins. *J Cell Sci* 2000;113:3563–3571.
83. Hynes RO. Integrins: versatility, modulation, and signaling in cell adhesion. *Cell* 1992;69: 11–25.
84. Schwartz MA, Schaller MD, Ginsberg MH. Integrins: emerging paradigms of signal transduction. *Annu Rev Cell Dev Biol* 1995;11:549–599.
85. Xu Y, Gurusiddappa S, Rich RL, Owens RT, Keene DR, Mayne R, et al. Multiple binding sites in collagen type I for the integrins α1β1and α2β1. *J Biol Chem* 2000;275:38,981–38,989.
86. Knight CG, Morton LF, Peachey AR, Tuckwell DS, Farndale RW, Barnes MJ. The collagen-binding A-domains of integrins α1β1 and α2 β1 recognize the same specific amino acid sequence, GFOGER, in native (triple-helical) collagens. *J Biol Chem* 2000;275:35–40.
87. Yamada KM, Geiger B. Molecular interactions in cell adhesion complexes. *Curr Opin Cell Biol* 1997;9:76–85.

88. Nobes CD, Hall A. Rho, rac, and cdc42 GTPases regulate the assembly of multimolecular focal complexes associated with actin stress fibers, lamellipodia, and filopodia. *Cell* 1995; 81:53–62.
89. Heath JP, Dunn GA. Cell to substratum contacts of chick fibroblasts and their relation to the microfilament system. A correlated interference-reflection and high-voltage electron-microscope study. *J Cell Sci* 1978;29:197–212.
90. Riveline D, Zamir E, Balaban NO, Schwarz US, Ishizaki T, Narumiya S, et al. Focal contacts as mechanosensors: Externally applied local mechanical force induces growth of focal contacts by an mDia1-dependent and ROCK-independent mechanism. *J Cell Biol* 2001;153:1175–1186.
91. Langholz O, Rockel D, Mauch C, Kozlowska E, Bank I, Krieg T. Collagen and collagenase gene expression in three-dimensional collagen lattices are differentially regulated by α1 β1 and α2 β1 integrins. *J Cell Biol* 1995;131:1903–1915.
92. Breen EC. Mechanical strain increases type I collagen expression in pulmonary fibroblasts in vitro. *J Appl Physiol* 2000;88:203–209.
93. Mudera VC, Pleass R, Eastwood M, Tarnuzzer R, Schultz G, Khaw P, et al. Molecular responses of human dermal fibroblasts to dual cues: contact guidance and mechanical load. *Cell Motil Cytoskeleton* 2000;45:1–9.
94. Eastwood M, McGrouther DA, Brown RA. Fibroblast responses to mechnical forces. *Proc Inst Mecj Eng [H]* 1998;21:85–92.
95. Kessler D, Dethlefsen S, Haase I, Plomann M, Hirche F, Krieg T, Eckes B. Fibroblasts in mechanically stressed collagen lattices assume a "synthetic" phenotype. *J Biol Chem* 2001; 237:159–172.
96. Brown RA, Prajapati R, McGrouther DA, Yanans IV, Eastwood M. Tensional homeostasis in dermal fibroblasts: mechanical responses to mechanical loading in three-dimensional substrates. *J Cell Physiol* 1998;175:323–332.
97. Du W, Mills I, Sumpio BE. Cyclic strain causes heterogeneous induction of transcription factors. AP-1, CRE binding protein and NF-κB, in endothelial cells: species and vascular bed diversity. *J Biomech* 1995;28:1485–1491.
98. Wary KK, Mainiero F, Isakoff SJ, Marcantonio EE, Giancotti FG. The adapter protein Shc couples a class of integrins to control of cell cycle progression. *Cell* 1996;87:733–743.
99. Giancotti FG. Integrin signaling. Specificity and control of cell survival and cell cycle progression. *Curr Opin Cell Biol* 1997;9:601–700.
100. Takeichi M. Cadherin cell adhesion receptors as a morphogenetic regulator. *Science* 1991;251:1451–1455.
101. Takeichi M. Morphogenetic roles of classic cadherins. *Curr Opin Cell Biol* 1995;7:619–627.
102. Gumbiner BM. Cell adhesion: the molecular basis of tissue architecture and morphogenesis. *Cell* 1996;84:345–357.
103. Braga VM, Machesky LM, Hall A, Hotchin NA. The small GTPases Rho and Rac are required for establishment of cadherin dependent cell–cell conracts. *J Cell Biol* 1977;137: 1421–1431.
104. Ragsdale GK, Phelps J, Luby-Phelps K. Viscoelastic response of fibroblasts to tension transmitted through adherens junctions. *Biophys J* 1997;73:2798–2808.
105. Xia S-L, Ferrier J. Propagation of a calcium pulse between osteoblastic cells. *Biochem Biophys Res Commun* 1992;186:1212–1219.
106. Ko KS, Arora PD, McCulloch CA. Cadherins mediate intercellular mechanical signaling in fibroblasts by activation of stretch-sensitive calcium permeable channels. *J Biol Chem* 2001;276:35,967–35,977.
107. Takei T, Mills I, Arai K, Sumpio BE. Molecular basis for tissue expansion: clinical implications for the surgeon. *Plast Reconstr Surg* 1998;102:247–258.

108. Vandenburgh HH. Mechanical forces and their second messengers in stimulating cell growth in vitro. *Am J Physiol* 1992;262:R350–R355.
109. Wiersbitzky M, Mills I, Sumpio BE, Gewirtz H. Chronic cyclic strain reduces adenylate cyclase activity and stimulatory G protein subunit levels in coronary smooth muscle cells. *Exp Cell Res* 1994;210:52–55.
110. Yang XC, Sachs F. Mechanically sensitive, non-selective cation channels. *EXS* 1993;66: 79–92.
111. Sachs F. Mechanical transduction by membrane ion channels: A mini review. *Mol Cell Biochem* 1991;104:57–60.
112. Kirber MT, Walsh JV Jr, Singer JJ. Stretch-activated ion channels in smooth muscle: a mechanism for the initiation of stretch-induced contraction. *Pflugers Arch* 1988;412: 339–345.
113. Hu H, Sachs F. Mechanically activated currents in chick heart cells. *J Membr Biol* 1996; 154:205–216.
114. Davis MJ, Donovitz JA, Hood JD. Stretch-activated single-channel whole cell currents in vascular smooth muscle cells. *Am J Physiol* 1992;262:C1083–C1088.
115. Laher I, van Breeman C, Bevan JA. Stretch-dependent calcium uptake associated with myogenic tone in rabbit facial vein. *Circ Res* 1988;63:669–672.
116. Narayanan J, Imig M, Roman RJ, Harder DR. Pressurization of isolated renal arteries increases inositol triphosphate and diacylglycerol. *Am J Physiol* 1994;266:H1840–H1845.
117. Diamond SL, Sachs F, Sigurdson WJ. Mechanically induced calcium mobilization in cultured endothelial cells is dependent on actin and phospholipase. *Arterioscler Thromb* 1994; 14:2000–2006.
118. Dennis EA, Rhee SG, Billah MM, Hannum YA. Role of phosphoplipase in generating lipid secondary messengers in signal transduction. *FASEB J* 1991;5:2068–2077.
119. Rhee SG, Choi KD. Regulation of inositol phospholipid-specific phospholipase C isozymes. *J Biol Chem* 1992;267:12,393–12,396.
120. Brayden JE, Nelson MT. Regulation of arterial tone by activation of calcium-dependent potassium channels. *Science* 1992;256:532–535.
121. Berczi V, Stekeil WJ, Contney SJ, Rusch NJ. Pressure-induced activation of membrane K^+ current in rat saphenous artery. *Hypertension* 1992;19:725–729.

3

Tendons of the Hand

Anatomy, Repair, Healing, and Rehabilitation

Paul C. Stephens, Eddy Dona, Beata Niechoda, Tracey Clarke, and Mark P. Gianoutsos

INTRODUCTION

This chapter provides a review of the current knowledge in tendon repair, healing, and rehabilitation, which would clearly be incomplete without first reviewing tendon anatomy in the hand.

Many excellent books offer comprehensive coverage of the anatomy of the hand *(1–5)*, but this is not within the context of this chapter; only anatomy of the tendons and recent developments that have been reported are discussed.

TENDON ANATOMY

Retinacular System

The skin on the palm is the thickest in the body as a result of a thickened stratum corneum in the epidermis layer (the dermis is as thick as on the dorsum of the hand). The skin has a rich supply of sweat glands but contains no hair or sebaceous glands. Examination of the palmar hand shows a multitude of flexor creases ("lines" of the hand) and papillary ridges (fingerprints). The function of the latter is controversial, but they may function to improve grip, like the tread on a car tire. Skin of the hand is held firmly in place by its attachment to the underlying palmar fascia, and a tight network of fibrous bands connects the two.

The palmar fascia is thickest in the center of the palm, where it forms the palmar aponeurosis, which is continuous proximally with the flexor retinaculum and laterally with the thinner fascia covering the thenar and hypothenar muscles. The palmar aponeurosis is reinforced by a superficial layer of longitudinal fibers continuous with the tendon of palmaris longus; these longitudinal fibers are usually present even when palmaris longus is absent (approx 15% of patients; *6*).

The palmar aponeurosis is firmly attached to the underlying metacarpals. A fibrous medial septum extends from the medial border of the palmar aponeurosis to the fifth metacarpal, medial to which is the hypothenar compartment. A fibrous sheath also extends from the lateral border to the first metacarpal, lateral to which is the thenar compartment. A strong central fibrous band also reaches to the third metacarpal, caus-

From: *Orthopedic Biology and Medicine: Repair and Regeneration of Ligaments, Tendons, and Joint Capsule*
Edited by: W. R. Walsh © Humana Press Inc., Totowa, NJ

ing two potential spaces—the midpalmar space and the thenar space—important in predicting the spread of infection in the hand. The palmar aponeurosis widens distally in a fan-like shape before dividing into four bands, one for each finger.

A digital sheath to the thumb is usually absent, but some longitudinal fibers of the palmar fascia curve over and blend with the fascia of the thenar eminence. A transverse thickening of the palmar fascia at the metacarpal heads results in the superficial transverse metacarpal or natatory ligament. Longitudinal fibers of the palmar fascia also extend into the fingers. The pretendinous band is the longitudinal extension of the palmar aponeurosis in the fingers, inserting into the base of the proximal phalanx. At the level of the metacarpal head, it divides to blend with the spiral band and lateral digital sheet *(7,8)*. Grayson's and Cleland's ligaments are also in the digit and are essential for normal cutaneous stability during digital movements *(9)*.

Flexor Musculature and Tendons

The flexor muscles in the forearm are divided into two groups: superficial and deep. The superficial group consists of pronator teres, flexor carpi radialis, palmaris longus, flexor carpi ulnaris, and flexor digitorum superficialis (FDS). They have a common origin on the anterior surface of the medial epicondyle of the humerus. The deep group consists of flexor digitorum profundis (FDP), flexor pollicis longus (FPL), and pronator teres.

Only the FDS, FDP, and FPL cross the wrist to act on the digits; therefore, only these are further considered.

Flexor Digitorum Superficialis

The FDS has an oblique origin that arises from multiple sources on the volar surface of the humerus, ulna, and radius; its origin also defines the upper limit of the Parona space. It overlies the median nerve and ulnar vascular bundle in the forearm *(10)*. In the midpart of the forearm, the superficialis muscle belly divides into four bundles, which separate into a superficial and deep belly. The superficial layer sends tendons to the middle and ring fingers, and the deep layer sends tendons to the index and small fingers *(10)*. The FDS tendon to the little finger is not present in all individuals *(11–13)*. Cadaveric studies in Japan estimate that it is totally absent in 2% of individuals *(14)*, and a similar result of 2% was also reported in a clinical trial by Thompson et al. in 2002 *(6)*.

Flexor Digitorum Profundus

The common muscle belly of FDP arises from the medial surface of the olecranon and the upper three fourths of the ulna and interosseous membrane. The FDP to the index finger often separates in the forearm, whereas the other three tendons are usually partly together as they pass under the flexor retinaculum in the wrist. Once in the palm, the three tendons separate, such that four tendons of FDP are present in the palm, one passing to each digit. The lumbricals take their origin from the palmar section of FDP.

Flexor Pollicis Longus

The FPL arises from the anterior surface of the radius and adjacent interosseous membrane. It is a unipennate muscle whose tendon forms on the ulnar side. The tendon continues to receive muscle fibers until just above the wrist, which facilitates its identification during surgery. It is the only extrinsic flexor of the thumb.

Carpal Tunnel

The transverse carpal ligament (TCL) is a strong fibrous band that measures 2–3 cm in both its transverse and longitudinal planes. It spans the volar aspect of the wrist and proximal palm, forming the roof of the carpal tunnel. Its proximal limit is the dominant distal wrist crease. Its attachments are the hook of the hamate and pisiform medially and the tubercle of the scaphoid and ridge of the trapezium laterally. The base of the carpal tunnel is formed by the concave surfaces of the carpal bones, and the roof is formed by the TCL. Thus, the TCL and carpal bones combine to create a fibro-osseous tunnel.

The carpal tunnel is traversed by 10 structures: nine flexor tendons and the median nerve. As mentioned previously, the tendons of FDS are separate and lie in two rows, with the FDS tendons to the middle and ring fingers superficial to the tendons of the index and little finger. The tendons of FDP lie deep to the tendons of FDS in one plane, and only the FDP tendon to the index finger is separate from the others. The FDS and FDP tendons share a common flexor sheath. The median nerve traverses the carpal tunnel on the radial side of the FDS tendon to the middle finger. The FPL tendon has a separate synovial sheath and traverses the carpal tunnel lateral to the tendons of FDS and FDP, deep to the median nerve. For an illustration, *see* refs. *1–5*.

The common flexor sheath that invests the tendons of FDS and FDP in the carpal tunnel is incomplete on the radial side. This common sheath extends into the palm. In the little finger, it continues along the whole length of the flexor tendon to its insertion at the distal phalanx. In the three remaining tendons, the common flexor sheath ends just distal to the TCL. The synovial sheath of FPL (like that of the little finger) continues until its insertion on the distal phalanx *(2)*.

Palm

Upon emerging from the carpal tunnel, the four tendons of FDS and FDP fan out to enter their respective digital synovial sheaths. The FDS tendons are superficial to those of FDP in the palm. As the tendons of FDP emerge from the carpal tunnel, they give origin to the lumbrical muscles. The lumbrical muscles travel distally in the palm, inserting into the lateral bands of the digits.

Digits

The flexor tendons are covered by a thin layer of adventitia or paratenon. The tendons of FDS and FDP enter the flexor sheaths of the digits together, with the tendon of FDS palmar to the tendon of FDP. As the tendon of FDS enters the flexor sheath, it flattens out and bifurcates, allowing the tendon of FDP to continue through to its insertion at the base of the distal phalanx. The two limbs of the FDS tendon rotate away from the midline and wrap around the FDP tendon, with half the fibers crossing on the palmar surface of the phalanx to insert dorsal to the FDP tendon on the palmar surface of the proximal half of the middle phalanx (chiasma). The remaining fibers insert as radial and ulnar slips on the diaphysis of the middle phalanx *(15)*. Thus, FDS forms a tendinous bed in which the FDP tendon lies.

In the flexor sheath, both tendons are invested by a common synovial sheath that commences at the A1 pulley and terminates at their insertion. Aside from the synovial sheath of the little finger, this is continuous with the common flexor sheath of the wrist.

Flexor tendons receive their nutrition from intrinsic and extrinsic sources. The intrinsic blood supply originates from multiple sources: the musculotendinous junction, osseotendinous junction, longitudinal vessels within the paratenon and vincular vessels *(16,17)*. Extrinsic nutrition from the synovial fluid is also recognized an important source of nutrients *(18,19)* and is covered in greater detail in the Tendon Healing section.

Each tendon possesses a short and long vincula. The short vinculum of both FDS and FDP are close to their insertions. The long vinculum of FDP reaches the tendon from the palmar surface of the proximal phalanx and passes between the two halves of the FDS tendon. The long vinculum of FDS is doubled, as each half of the FDS tendon distal to the chiasma possesses a separate vinculum. They also reach the FDS tendon from the palmar surface of the proximal phalanx *(16)*.

Flexor Sheath

The digital flexor sheaths are retinacular structures that commence at the level of the metacarpal heads and terminate at the base of the distal phalanx. They function with the retinacular structures at the wrist (TCL) and in the palm (palmar aponeurosis pulley) to promote efficient flexor excursion of the tendons. These three components represent a unique and complex biomechanical system that enables complete digital flexion without limiting extension *(20)*.

The flexor tendon pulleys start to differentiate with the flexor tendons around wk 9 of intrauterine development *(21)*. Five annular and three cruciform pulleys have been identified in each of the digits. The first annular pulley (A1) is at the level of the metacarpal phalangeal joint (MCPJ). The majority of the fibers (2/3) arise from the palmar plate; the remainder (1/3) arise from the proximal portion of the proximal phalanx. The second annular pulley (A2) is located over the proximal portion of the proximal phalanx, and the third (A3) is at the level of the proximal interphalangeal joint (PIPJ) and attaches to its palmar plate. The first cruciform pulley (C1) is located between A2 and A3 over the distal portion of the proximal phalanx. The fourth annular pulley (A4) is at the midportion of the middle phalanx. The second cruciform pulley (C2) is between A3 and A4, overlying the proximal portion of the middle phalanx. The fifth annular pulley (A5) is located over the distal interphalangeal joint (DIPJ) and is attached to its palmar plate. The third cruciform pulley (C3) is located between A4 and A5 at the distal end of the middle phalanx *(20,22,23)*.

Zones of Flexor Tendon Injury

Zones of flexor tendon injury were first defined by Kleinert and Verdan in 1983 *(24)*. They divided the flexor tendon into five anatomic zones. This is the most widely used system to classify flexor tendon injuries.

Zone I: distal to the insertion of the FDS tendon.
Zone II: proximal origin of the A1 pulley to the insertion of the FDS tendon.
Zone III: from the distal edge of the TCL to the proximal edge of the A1 pulley.
Zone IV: within the carpal tunnel, deep to the TCL.
Zone V: from the musculotendinous junction to the proximal edge of the carpal tunnel.

Extensor Musculature and Tendons

Like flexion, finger extension is manifested by two muscle groups: the extrinsic and intrinsic extensors. The extrinsic extensors arise in the extensor (posterior) compartment of the forearm and are primarily responsible for extension at the MCPJs, and secondary extension at the PIPJ and DIPJ. The intrinsic muscles of the hand flex the MCPJ and extend the PIPJ and DIPJ. Thus, the intrinsic and extrinsic extensors have complimentary function at the interphalangeal joints and opposing function at the MCPJs *(25)*.

The extensor compartment of the arm contains 12 muscles arranged in two groups: a superficial and deep group.

The superficial group contains the brachioradialis, extensor carpi radialis longus (ECRL), extensor carpi radialis brevis (ECRB), extensor digitorum communis (EDC), extensor digiti minimi (EDM), extensor carpi ulnaris (ECU), anconeus, and supinator.

The deep group consists of the abductor pollicis longus (APL), extensor pollicis brevis (EPB), extensor pollicis longus (EPL), and extensor indicis propius (EIP).

The superficial muscles have a common extensor origin on the lateral epicondyle of the humerus. The deep muscles originate from the posterior surface of the radius and/or ulna and the interosseous membrane.

Functionally, they can be divided into three groups: (1) muscles that extend and abduct/adduct the wrist (ECRL, ECRB, and ECU); (2) muscles that extend the fingers (EDC, EIP, and EDM); and (3) muscles that extend and abduct the thumb (APL, EPB, and EPL).

The muscles of the posterior compartment are innervated by the posterior interosseous nerve, a branch of the radial nerve, and the radial nerve proper.

Extensor Retinaculum

At the wrist, the tendons of the extensor muscles are restrained by the extensor retinaculum—a band-like thickening of the deep fascia of the forearm. It is approx 2 cm wide and lies obliquely across the dorsum of the wrist. It functions like the flexor retinaculum to prevent bow-stringing of the tendons. It is divided into six fibro-osseous tunnels, which transmit the extrinsic extensor tendons from the extensor compartment of the forearm to the dorsum of the hand *(2)*. These are classically labeled I–VI, in a radial to ulnar fashion.

I. APL and EPB: on the lateral aspect of the radius and transmits APL and EPB, which both have a separate synovial sheath.
II. ECRB and ECRL: extends as far as the dorsal tubercle on the radius and transmits the wrist extensors, ECRB and ECRL, which also have a separate synovial sheath.
III. EPL: ulnar to the dorsal tubercle, transmits the EPL with its separate synovial sheath.
IV. EDC and EIP: a shallow groove on the dorsum of the distal radius that transmits the four tendons of EDC and the EIP tendon, all of which have a common synovial sheath.
V. EDM: over the distal radioulnar joint, transmits the EDM and its synovial sheath.
VI. ECU: at the base of the ulnar styloid, transmits the ECU and its flexor sheath.

The synovial sheaths of the tendons end distal to the extensor retinaculum; they are not continued into the hand or digits.

Extensor Digitorum Communis

The EDC has a common muscle belly that splits, giving rise to three or four tendons that pass under the extensor retinaculum in the fourth fibro-osseous tunnel, superficial to the tendon of EIP. The tendons continue across the dorsum of the hand, inserting into the extensor hood on the dorsum of the fingers. The EDC tendons to the index and long finger are usually a single tendon with a single insertion. The EDC tendon to the ring finger is usually a double tendon with a single insertion, and the EDC tendon to the little finger is variable in its presence, being absent in approx 50% of patients *(26,27)*.

Extensor Indicis Propius

The tendon of EIP is initially deep to the EDC tendons in the fourth fibro-osseous tunnel. In the dorsum of the hand, it runs distally on the ulnar side of the EDC tendon to the index finger and inserts ulnar to the EDC tendon on the dorsal aponeurosis of the index finger.

Extensor Digiti Minimi

The tendon of EDM passes through the fifth fibro-osseous tunnel alone, typically consisting of a double tendon with a double insertion into the dorsal aponeurosis of the little finger.

Juncturae Tendinum

The function of the juncturae tendinum is to interconnect the extensor tendons on the back of the hand. Its role is debated: they may be involved in spacing of the EDC tendons, force redistribution, coordination of extension or stabilization of the MCPJs *(28)*. Its presence is variable; in 2001, von Schroeder and Botte *(28)* described three subtypes:

Type 1: thin and filamentous, found primarily between the EDC tendons to the index and ring fingers and the ring and little fingers.

Type 2: thicker and well defined, found primarily between the middle and ring fingers and the ring and little fingers.

Type 3: slips between the middle and ring fingers and the ring and little finger, including EDM. Two subtypes were defined:

- Type 3y: splits and inserts into two adjacent fingers.
- Type 3r: transverse junctional connection between two tendons.

In a recent study, Hirai et al. *(29)* concluded the dissection of 548 upper limbs that the most common patterns were type 1 in the second intermetacarpal space, type 3r in the third intermetacarpal space, and type 3y in the fourth intermetacarpal space.

Dorsal Aponeurosis

The dorsal aponeurosis or extensor expansion is a complex network of multidirectional fibers that connect the extrinsic and intrinsic extensors. It can be divided into two parts, each with three insertion points: a central part that is a continuation of the extrinsic extensor tendons and a lateral part that is a continuation of the intrinsic extensors.

The central portion of the dorsal aponeurosis consists of three insertion sites into each of the three phalanges: sagittal bands into the proximal phalanx; central slip into the middle phalanx; and terminal tendon into the distal phalanx.

The long extensors insert mainly into the sagittal bands and directly into the dorsum of the proximal phalanx. The sagittal bands wrap around the distal metacarpal, MCPJ, and proximal phalanx, which inserts into the volar plate of the MCPJ and the volar periosteum of the proximal phalanx. They function primarily as extensors of the MCPJ by lifting the proximal phalanx.

Longitudinal fibers of the long extensors continue through the sagittal bands and across the dorsum of the proximal phalanx. At the midportion of the proximal phalanx, it trifurcates, giving rise to the central and two lateral slips. The central slip continues across the PIPJ to insert into the central tubercle on the dorsum of the middle phalanx. The lateral slips continue distally and coalesce to form the conjoined lateral bands (together with the lateral bands proper). The two conjoined lateral bands then coalesce with the aid of the triangular ligament to from the terminal tendon, which inserts into the dorsum of the distal phalanx. The long extensors can function to extend the interphalangeal joints but only when the MCPJ is held in partial flexion.

The lateral portion of the dorsal aponeurosis consists of three insertion sites into each of the three phalanges: transverse retinacular ligaments into the proximal phalanx; oblique retinacular ligaments and medial bands into the middle phalanx; and distal lateral band inserts into the distal phalanx.

The intrinsic muscles that control the dorsal aponeurosis include the lumbricals, interossei, and abductor digiti minimi. At the proximal lateral angles of the triangle, the insertion of the intrinsic extensors contribute to the formation of the sagittal bands. The deep transverse metacarpal ligament separates the intrinsic extensors; the interossei tendons run dorsal to it, and the lumbricals run palmer to it. The sagittal band functions to centralize the central slip of the EDC tendon over the metacarpal heads at the MCPJ level. Distal to the deep transverse metacarpal ligament, the intrinsic tendons merge to from the lateral bands.

The lateral portions of the dorsal aponeurosis attach to the proximal phalanx via the transverse retinacular ligaments. The fibers of the transverse retinacular ligaments run approximately parallel to the fibers of the sagittal band. They form a sling around the proximal phalanx, allowing it to be pulled volarly. Thus, the intrinsic muscles are primarily responsible for flexion at the MCPJ. As the interossei are inserted into the dorsal aponeurosis more proximally than the lumbricals they can make a more significant contribution to MCPJ flexion *(25,30)*. The transverse retinacular ligaments also functions to stabilize the extensor tendon over the PIPJ *(31)*.

Distal to the transverse retinacular ligaments, the lateral bands continue as the oblique retinacular ligaments and the medial bands. The oblique retinacular ligaments insert with the central slip into the central tubercle of the middle phalanx, and the medial bands insert into the dorsolateral tubercles on either side of the central slip. They function with the central slip to extend the PIPJ *(25,31)*.

The lateral band continues distally and merges with the central slips to form the conjoined lateral tendons. As mentioned previously, these merge to from the terminal tendon that inserts into the dorsum of the distal phalanx *(25)*.

Zones of Extensor Tendon Injury

Zones of extensor tendon injury were described by Kleinert and Verdan *(24)*. They defined eight zones—four odd-numbered zones overlying the digits and four even-numbered zones overlying the intervening tendon segments—increasing in number from distal to proximal. These zones overlie the following areas: zone I, DIPJ; zone II, middle phalanx; zone III, PIPJ; zone IV, proximal phalanx; zone V, MCPJ; zone VI, metacarpals; zone VII, carpal joints; and zone VIII, distal radius and ulna.

Tendons of the Thumb

Flexor Pollicis Longus

As mentioned previously, the FPL is the only extrinsic flexor of the thumb. It traverses the carpal tunnel lateral to the tendons of FDS and FDP, deep to the median nerve. Emerging from the carpal tunnel, it extends into the thumb and inserts into the base of the distal phalanx. FPL functions primarily to flex the interphalangeal joint of the thumb; however, it also flexes the metacarpophalangeal and carpometacarpal joints of the thumb and wrist. The deep head of the flexor pollicis brevis also flexes the metacarpophalangeal joint.

Thumb Pulley System

The thumb has a unique pulley system, as defined by Doyle and Blythe in 1977 *(32)*. They demonstrated the presence of one oblique and two annular pulleys (A1 and A2). The A1 pulley is a transverse retinacular pulley; its proximal 2/3 overlies the MCPJ and its distal 1/3 overlies the proximal phalanx. The A2 pulley is also a transverse retinacular pulley; its proximal 2/3 overlies the PIPJ and its distal 1/3 overlies the distal phalanx. The oblique pulley originates from the ulnar side of the proximal half of the proximal phalanx and inserts into the radial side of the base of the distal phalanx. A fourth variable annular pulley with three subtypes is recognized by some authors *(33)*.

Thumb Extension

Thumb extension is facilitated by three extrinsic muscles: APL, EPB, and EPL. However, unlike the digits, there is no dorsal aponeurosis. These are well described in *Last's Anatomy (2)*.

Abductor Pollicis Longus

APL arises from the back of the radius and ulna and the intervening interosseous membrane and passes through the first fibro-osseous tunnel at the wrist. It usually divides into two slips: one inserting into the base of the first metacarpal and the other into the trapezium. Its mechanism of action is to extend the thumb at the carpometacarpal joint, but it also assists in wrist abduction and flexion.

Extensor Pollicis Brevis

EPB arises below APL from the radius and adjacent interosseous membrane. It also passes through the first fibro-osseous tunnel with APL and it inserts into the base of the proximal phalanx. It extends the metacarpophalangeal and carpometacarpal joints of the thumb.

Extensor Pollicis Longus

EPL arises from the ulna distal to APL, crossing the wrist in the third interosseous tunnel and hooking around the dorsal tubercle (Lister's tubercle) of the radius. It inserts into the base of the distal phalanx. Its functions is to extend the interphalangeal joint of the thumb and also assists extension and abduction at the wrist.

Although there is no dorsal aponeurosis, EPL receives a fibrous expansion from both the abductor pollicis brevis and adductor pollicis, which hold the long extensor tendon in place. As such, both intrinsics are weak extensors of the thumb.

TENDON REPAIRS

Flexor Tendon Repair

One of the greatest challenges hand surgeons face is to restore normal function to the hands of patients who have sustained flexor tendon injuries.

Bunnell first coined the term "no man's land" to refer to zone II flexor tendon injuries in 1944, as results were so poor after tendon repair in this zone *(34)*. He advocated removing the injured tendon and replacing it with a tendon graft as a secondary procedure.

However, during the 1960s, several surgeons challenged this practice by performing primary tendon repairs and, by the 1970s, this had become the preferred treatment option *(35–39)*. Despite several decades of primary repair as the accepted treatment for flexor tendon injuries, achieving satisfactory postoperative hand function is still a major challenge.

It is now widely recognized that much of the outcome after flexor tendon injury is dependent on postoperative management and hand therapy. However, a sound surgical technique is the foundation upon which this is built. Unfortunately, the best method for repairing a flexor tendon is still highly debated, as each individual surgeon has their own preferred techniques and protocols. The countless number of reported surgical techniques to repair the injured flexor tendon surgery in the literature attests to this. However, despite the controversy, all surgeons would agree on several basic principles in relation to tendon repair.

- The technique should be relatively simple.
- It should involve minimal tendon handling.
- It should contain both a core and peripheral suture.
- Early postoperative mobilization by a hand therapist.

Early Mobilization

The best primary tendon repair will not restore satisfactory function if it is not accompanied with the appropriate early postoperative mobilization. Initially, protected passive finger mobilization had been the standard postoperative protocol after repair *(24,40,41)*. The motion generated by passive mobilization had been shown to improve tendon healing and reduce peritendinous adhesion formation, a significant problem associated with postoperative immobilization *(42–47)*.

With this initial insight into the benefits of passive mobilization, many authors observed the use of controlled active mobilization protocols *(48–54)*. Active mobilization generates both increased tension and motion and has been shown to offer several advantages over passive mobilization *(49,53,54)*. The main advantage is improved ultimate range of motion, thought to be caused by a decrease in adhesion between the repaired tendon and peritendinous tissues. Other advantages include minimal initial strength depression, greater tensile strength, improved tendon nutrition, and a higher rate of healing. Thus, early active motion improves the strength and gliding characteristic of healing tendons, leading to an improved hand function. However, a repair technique must be used that can withstand the tensile forces generated by active mobilization, as the risk of tendon rupture becomes a significant concern with any such protocol *(55)*.

Surgical Preparation

Tendon repair should be performed under tourniquet control and an appropriate anesthetic. The existing skin lacerations should be extended in a manner that balances access, flap vascularity, and limitation of wound length. Avoidance of longitudinal incisions passing volar to the joint axis is important in minimizing subsequent flexion contracture. Most often, a zigzag volar pattern incision is employed, as described by Bruner *(56)*. The utmost care should be taken to identify and preserve the neurovascular bundles. The tendon sheath should be opened enough to allow delivery of both proximal and distal tendon stumps. Flexing the wrist and fingers and even "milking" the palm from a proximal to distal direction to deliver a retracted proximal tendon stump is a way to facilitate this. Fine artery forceps passed down the flexor sheath can also be used; however, avoid blindly grasping down the sheath. A thrombus visible within the sheath indicates that the tendon stump is not too far away as these are often found on the end of the stump. If such measures fail to produce the tendon stump, an incision should be made within the palm or even at the wrist level (if necessary) to find it. Once found, it can then be passed distally down the sheath with the help of a fine catheter, such as an infant-feeding tube.

Once both tendon stumps are within the surgical field, they can be secured in position by passing a fine needle through each and adjacent soft tissues, taking care to avoid the neurovascular bundles. If the tendon ends are jagged, these can be "cleaned" by excising a minimal amount, ensuring that the tendons are not shortened too much as this will result in a permanent finger flexion contracture. In the uncommon situation where the tendon is lacerated at a very oblique angle (greater than 10 mm of the length of the tendon) the repair could be performed using the Becker method *(57)*. This method was proposed as a means of repairing all tendon injuries via beveling the ends, and although it provided a strong repair, it created a problematic shortening of the tendon and is therefore no longer routinely used. An alternate method of such oblique lacerations is to excise a minimal amount from each end to reduce the angle of the point of division. Then proceed to repair the tendon with both a "core" and a "peripheral" suture, as this is the preferred technique for all flexor tendon injuries.

The aim is to have a repair site that is smooth enough to allow minimal gliding resistance within the sheath, and strong enough to withstand early mobilization so it does not rupture or allow significant gap formation. The gap retarding qualities of flexor tendon repair techniques are important; studies have shown that gap formation of as little as 1–3 mm can result in increased peritendinous adhesion formation and adverse clinical outcomes *(58–60)*.

Core Repair

The most widely recognized form of tendon repair is that described by Kessler in 1973 *(61)*. It is a two strand repair with two lateral "grasping" components on each side of the tendon division. Pennington *(62)* described the "locking" loop modification of the Kessler repair, where the transverse component of the suture passes anterior to the longitudinal strands, locking onto a bundle of tendon fibers when the tendon is subject to tensile forces. Locking repairs have been shown to afford more strength to the repair than simple "grasping" loops *(63–65)*.

Hatanaka and Manske *(66)* further demonstrated that increasing the cross-sectional area of the locking component increased the strength of the repair. Modified forms of the Kessler technique are probably the most commnonly applied surgical techniques in tendon repair.

Numerous other techniques have been described, all of which aim to provide a stronger repair *(48,50,67–74)*. One typical theme from these techniques is that the strength of the repair is proportional to the number of strands crossing it, with a four-stranded repair being twice as strong as a two-stranded repair and, consequently, a six-stranded repair being almost three times stronger. Several authors have even described eight-stranded repair techniques *(73,74)*. Unfortunately, increasing the strands per repair also increases the techniqual complexity and, more importantly, the bulk of the repair. Therefore, many of these multistrand techniques have not yet been used in common practice.

Four-stranded repair techniques are usually favored because they provide sufficiently increased strength without the bulk or tissue handling requirements of six- or eight-stranded repairs *(48,67,68,71)*. Kubota et al. *(67)* described a four-strand single-knot modified Kessler repair, which provides four "locking" segments on either side of the tendon division. However, McLarney's *(72)* four-strand cruciate repair is perhaps ideal. Although it is not as strong as Kubota's four-strand modified Kessler technique *(65)*, it does provide the strength of a four-strand repair with the simplicity and tendon handling requirements of only a two-stranded repair.

Suture material and caliber are also important aspects of tendon repair. Various materials have been employed for the core suture. Larger caliber sutures are obviously stronger than those that are smaller. But again, a balance between suture size and minimal bulk must be met. For this reason, 3/0 or 4/0 suture material is generally preferred. The ideal suture material would be a monofilament for handling ease (to allow easy sliding within the tendon), maximal stiffness (to minimize the amount of stretch), and bioresorbable. Unfortunately, no suture material yet fulfils all these criteria.

Uncertainties regarding the longevity of bioresorbable sutures, and the tissue reaction they may provoke during resorption, has generally precluded their use. Prolene and, to a lesser extent, Nylon, are typically the perferred sutures, as they are nonresorbable monofilaments and are thus easy to handle. However, they are flawed by their relatively poor stiffness qualities, resulting in a greater potential for stretch, with subsequent gap formation and repair failure. Braided sutures, e.g., Ticron and Ethibond, confer greater stiffness when compared with Prolene but can be difficult to handle, especially when using four or more strands in the repair. This difficulty relates to their inability to "slide" within the tendon once placed; therefore, adjusting individual suture strand lengths and tension is extremely difficult. This is an important issue, as Trail et al. *(75)* demonstrated that differential suture strand loading could reduce the repair strength.

Ketchum et al. *(76)* showed that Supramid, a polyfilament ensheathed caprolactan (Supramid, S. Jackson, Inc., Alexandria, VA), is a good suture material. It is nonresorbable, slides within the tendon well, and has minimal extensibility. It is also one of the few sutures available with two strands per needle, thus making multistrand repairs relatively easy.

Another area of debate is the placement of the suture knot. Aoki et al. *(77)* have shown using canine cadaver tendons that knots placed within the repair site can reduce the strength of the repair. They also demonstrated that the greater the number of knots, the worse the tensile strength. Using a canine in vivo study, Pruitt et al. *(53)* also showed that the early tendon tensile strength was worse when knots were placed within the repair site. However, at 6 wk, there was no significant difference between those that had knots placed either within or outside of the repair site.

Despite the early biomechanical advantages of knot placement outside of the repair site, this does result in greater gliding resistance *(78)*, with knots possibly catching on the tendon pulleys. McLarney's *(72)* original description of the cruciate four-strand repair used an intratendinous placement of the suture knot, consequently avoiding these issues. However, in our experience, most surgeons prefer to place the knot between the two tendon ends. Ideally, utilizing a single continuous suture; thus, only one knot is required.

Peripheral Suture

Much to the disappointment of the surgeon new to flexor tendon repair, the diagrammatic perfection of coaptation is not usually met in practice. To this end, a circumferential suture was used, originally as a tidy-up suture *(35)*. However, it has been shown to confer significant biomechanical advantages to the overall integrity of the repair, improving the resistance to gap formation and providing as much as 50% of the ultimate load to failure and stiffness *(3,67,68,79–81)*. This makes it an important consideration, particularly in those patients likely to commence on an early finger mobilization program.

Although originally described as an epitenon repair *(35)*, as it only involved the epitenon, Mashadi and Amis *(82)* showed the importance of the suture passing through the tendon fibers. Therefore, it is preferably referred to as a circumferential component of repairs, because all currently advocated methods pass through the tendon fibers. The suture material of choice is generally a 6/0 or even a 5/0 monofilament, such as Prolene.

The simple running technique is likely the most commonly employed circumferential suture. The suture strands of this repair run along the line of the tendon fibers. Attempts to improve this technique have been described with Diao et al. *(79)*, who found an 80% increase in repair strength when the bite depth was increased. Several other modifications of the simple running repair have been described but are not routinely used by most surgeons *(83)*.

Another method that has widespread use is the cross-stitch repair, described by Silfverskiold and Anderson in 1993 *(84)*. The transverse component of this method provides a stronger hold on the tendon as it runs perpendicular to the orientation of the tendon fibers. A further development is the interlocking horizontal mattress technique, recently described by some authors *(85)*. This relatively easy method "locks" around the periphery of the tendon when subject to tensile forces and has been shown to be biomechanically superior to the simple running and cross-stitch repairs in vitro. Various other horizontal mattress methods have been reviewed that provide greater biomechanical properties in comparison to the simple running suture *(35,82,86,87)*; however, many are flawed by their complexity in design and are therefore not routinely used by many surgeons.

Like the core suture, studies have demonstrated that increasing the number of strands crossing the repair site increases the repair strength *(53)*.

Sheath and Pulley

Every effort should be made to repair all aspects of the sheath, but this can be technically challenging. Theoretically, this would be expected to reduce peritendinous adhesion formation, yet, no strong evidence exists to support this. If a decision to repair has been made, then this should be with a nonresorbable suture, such as 6/0 Prolene.

Evidence exists to encourage preserving and repairing the pulleys; as discussed earlier, they are essential for normal finger functioning *(10,78,88–90)*. An absent or incompetent pulley results in an increased moment arm, owing to tendon bowstringing, requiring increased tendon excursion to produce the same arc of motion. Clinically, this is associated with the loss of power, reduced range of motion, the risk of additional pulley rupture, and the development of fixed flexion contractures *(91)*.

Biomechanically the most important pulleys are the A2 and A4 pulleys *(88,89,92)*. It may be necessary to open (otherwise known as "vent") one of the pulleys to permit greater access for tendon repair. If this is necessary, then this should be performed dorso-laterally, allowing sufficient dorsal cuff to aid in its closure after the tendon itself has been repaired. A repaired tendon that cannot move passively through its full excursion with minimal resistance is another reason a pulley may need to be vented or even partially excised. Kwai and Elliot *(93)* showed that in a series of 126 complete zone II tendon transections, venting was required in 64% of A2 (56%) and A4 (8%) pulleys. The mean size of their venting was 52% of the pulley length. Other biomechanical studies have shown that up to 75% of both the A2 and A4 pulleys can be sacrificed with minimal decrease in the total finger flexion and without significant risk of rupture *(94–96)*.

In contrast to the A2 and A4 pulleys, the A3 pulley is considered to be of little biomechanical importance. However, Tang and Xie *(97)* demonstrated that A3 and the adjacent sheath spanning A2 to A4 does have an important part in restraining tendon bowstringing at the PIPJ.

Zone Injuries

If sufficient distal stump exists, then tendon repair should be performed in the same manner as described for zone II injuries. However, if the laceration is very distal, or if the FDP has avulsed from the distal phalanx, then a different approach should be taken. The traditional repair method was the pull-out suture tied over a button on the nail plate, originally described by Bunnell *(98)*. As it is a pullout method, the preferred suture is therefore limited to a monofilament, such as Prolene. The duration of removal is usually 6 wk, at which stage, sufficient healing at the tendon bone interface should have occurred. Unfortunately, this technique has many disadvantages; it is unsightly, requires a second, albeit minor, procedure to remove the suture and button, can act as a source of suture tract infection, and it can cause discomfort to the nail region. Additionally, the results of this repair method are poorly reported. Moiemen and Elliot *(99)* in a series of 14 such repairs, noted that six regained less than 50% of their normal DIPJ flexion.

Much like zone II injuries, methods have been proposed to increase the strength of the pull-out repair through various suture techniques or by increasing the suture strands involved *(17,100)*. However, this does not eliminate the problems encountered with pull-out techniques.

Small bone anchors have been developed to secure soft tissues to bone, and several have been advocated for use in FDP tendon fixation *(101–103)*. Bone anchors potentially make it a simple one-stage repair and allow the use of more than two strands per repair *(103)*. As suture pull-out is not required, braided, less extensible sutures can be used with the potential for less gap formation at the tendon bone interface. But, like the pull-out button technique, there is still a paucity of clinical trials in the literature.

Zones III–V injuries should be repaired in the same manner as zone II injuries already described. They tend to be less challenging in the absence of the digital sheath.

Partial Lacerations

The treatment of partially lacerated flexor tendons has been controversial. The possible complications associated with an unrepaired partial laceration include triggering, entrapment, or rupture *(104–110)*. Triggering creates discomfort during finger motion, as the laceration site gets caught on the pulley edge. Entrapment is caused by the inability of the laceration site to enter the pulley, resulting in limited range of motion.

Several authors have demonstrated that suturing of a partially divided tendon causes a reduction of the tensile strength of the tendon in vivo *(111,112)*. Other authors have shown that the threshold load levels to rupture human flexor tendons with major divisions of their cross-sectional area (CSA) of up to 75% are higher than the physiologic load levels measured during active motion, suggesting that these partial lacerations can withstand in vivo forces associated with active mobilization *(113)*.

In a clinical study of 34 patients by Wray and Weeks *(114)*, functional results with partial lacerations of up to 95% were excellent in 92% of cases. A similar study of 15 patients by Al-Qattan *(115)* with a mean partial laceration of 71% (range 55–90%) showed an excellent outcome in 93% at 6 mo.

The logical approach to partial flexor tendon lacerations would be to intraoperatively assess for any triggering. If such triggering exists, and the laceration is less than 75% of the tendon CSA, then the edges should be trimmed or beveled. If the laceration is greater than 75% of the tendon CSA, then a standard core and circumferential suture should be employed to coapt the edges. Although the remaining intact portion of the tendon is almost certainly biomechanically superior than any repair technique, it does facilitate tendon healing and maintains a normal caliber.

Extensor Tendon Repair

Extensor tendon injuries are more frequently encountered than flexor tendon injuries, because they are less protected than flexor tendons. As highlighted previously, their different anatomy entails that the treatment of such injuries differs to that of flexor tendons. The type of injury, surgical approach, and potential deformity vary according to the injury zone. Injuries and their respective treatments are categorized into the eight zones described by Verdan *(116)*.

Zone I Injury (Mallet Finger)

Disruption of the extensor tendon over the DIPJ produces the characteristic flexion deformity known as a mallet finger. A mallet finger may be open, but it is more commonly closed. They are classified into four types:

Type I: closed, with or without an avulsion fracture.
Type II: laceration at or proximal to the DIPJ with loss of tendon continuity.
Type III: deep abrasion with loss of skin, subcutaneous cover and tendon substance.

Type IV: which is designated into three categories:
- A: transepiphyseal plate fracture of the distal phalanx in children.
- B: hyperflexion injury with fracture of the articular surface of 20–50%.
- C: hyperextension injury with fracture of the articular surface usually greater than 50% and with early or late palmar subluxation of the distal phalanx.

Each type of injury warrants a different treatment, but in the majority of cases, splinting alone will suffice.

Type I: continuous splinting of the DIPJ in full extension for 6 wk, followed by 2 wk of night splinting.

Type II: a simple figure-of-eight suture to repair the tendon. The DIPJ is then splinted in extension for 6 wk, followed by 2 wk of night splinting.

Type III: immediate soft tissue coverage and primary grafting or late reconstruction using a free tendon graft.

Type IV: with the following treatments:
- A: closed reduction. The extensor mechanism is attached to the basal epiphysis; thus, closed reduction followed by splinting for 3–4 wk results in correction of the deformity.
- B: splinting for 6 wk with 2 wk of night splinting.
- C: owing to the palmar subluxation, this injury is best managed operatively with open reduction and internal fixation with a Kirschner wire. This should also be protected with a splint for 6 wk, followed by wire removal and DIPJ mobilization.

Zone II Injury (Middle Phalanx)

A zone II injury is usually secondary to a laceration or crush mechanism. If less than 50% of the tendon width is divided, then treatment involves routine wound care and splintage for 7–10 d, followed by active mobilization. Injuries greater than 50% of the tendon should be repaired with either a continuous running suture or several figure-of-eight sutures using a nonresorbable 4-0 or 5-0 suture, which is followed by 6 wk of splinting.

Zone III Injury (Boutonniere Deformity)

Disruption of the central slip overlying the PIPJ results in a Boutonniere deformity with loss of extension of the PIPJ and hyperextension of the DIPJ. This may be a closed or open injury. As a general rule, all open injuries over the PIPJ should be explored in the operating theater. An early injury may not necessarily be associated with a Boutonniere deformity, as this usually develops 10–14 d after the initial injury, especially in closed trauma *(117)*. As the tendon ends do not retract in this area, treatment is relatively simple and requires several figure-of-eight sutures using a nonresorbable 4-0 or 5-0 suture, followed by up to 6 wk of splinting.

In closed injuries, localized swelling without the classic deformity are characteristically seen early. Diagnosis is best made by splinting the finger in extension for a few days and reexamining the finger after the swelling settles down. Weak or absent extension of the PIPJ suggests central slip disruption *(118)*. Initial treatment of closed injury should be splinting the PIPJ in extension for 4–6 wk and reapplication of a splint if the deformity recurs.

Surgical indications for a closed Boutonniere deformity are: displaced avulsion fracture at the base of the middle phalanx; axial and lateral instability of the PIPJ associated with loss of active or passive extension of the joint *(119)*; and failed nonoperative treatment.

Surgical treatment consists of securing the central slip to the middle phalanx with or without the bony fragment. This may be helped by the use of a bony anchor in a nonfracture avulsion injury. Splinting the PIPJ in extension is then required. If a bony fracture is involved, mobilization is usually commenced after radiographic evidence of union exists. If primary repair of the central slip is not possible, both lateral bands can be longitudinally split and sutured together along the dorsal midline, thus recreating the central slip. Another option is to create a turnover flap from the proximal portion of the central slip, which is sutured to the distal end of the central slip. The proximal defect is then closed primarily. These methods help prevent the development of a Boutonniere deformity and will allow active flexion of the PIPJ.

Zone IV Injury (Proximal Phalanx)

These injuries are more often partial and tend to only involve the broad extensor retinaculum, not the lateral bands. For such partial injuries, if no loss of extension is present, then repair is often not required, and early motion should be considered. Alternatively, a simple running or figure-of-eight suture using a nonresorbable 5-0 suture to coapt the edges may be used. For complete lacerations, primary repair should be performed followed by 6 wk of splinting in extension.

Zone V Injury (MCPJ)

An important aspect of injuries in this zone is that they are often owing to human bites, and the potential complications can be significant. When associated with a human bite, the incidence of complications is directly related to the time from injury to treatment. Surgical exploration, thorough irrigation, and primary repair are indicated. Arthrotomy should be considered if there are any concerns regarding MCPJ involvement. All involved structures, including partial injuries, should be repaired. Lateral bands should be repaired to prevent lateral migration of the extensor digitorum communis tendon and subsequent loss of metacarpophalangeal extension *(120,121)*. Repairs are satisfactorily carried out using figure-of-eight sutures with a nonresorbable 4-0 or 5-0 suture.

For definite bite-related injuries, broad-spectrum antibiotics are always required, and the wound is usually left open to heal by secondary intention or closed several days if no clinical infection has developed.

Zone VI Injury (Dorsal Hand)

As the tendons are thicker and more oval shaped, repair should be performed using a four-strand core suture with a nonresorbable 4-0 suture similar to that used in flexor tendons. A peripheral suture is not required. Importantly, single or partial tendon lacerations in this zone may not result in a loss of extension at the MCPJ, because extensor forces are transmitted from adjacent extensor tendons through the juncturae tendinum. Hence, clinical examination cannot be relied on to assess tendon integrity, and all wounds must be formally inspected with appropriate anesthetic support.

Zone VII Injury (Wrist)

Exposure in this region is limited because of the coverage by the extensor retinaculum. Therefore, partial division or venting of the retinaculum is required to enable a formal tendon repair, which should consist of a four-strand core suture as per zone VI injuries. Efforts should be made to preserve some segment of the retinaculum to prevent tendon bowstringing.

Zone VIII Injury (Dorsal Forearm)

Repair of this zone can be difficult with complications in identifying individual tendons with multiple tendon injuries and fibrous septa retracting into the muscle bellies when the division occurs at the musculotendinous junction. Significant consideration should be given to restoring wrist and thumb extension. For muscle bellies, multiple figure-of-eight sutures are required. Splinting of the wrist in 45° extension, the metacarpophalangeal joint in 15–20° flexion, and, occasionally, the elbow at 90° of flexion is required.

TENDON HEALING IN THE HAND

Microanatomy and Nutrition of the Tendon in the Hand

Tendons are remarkably organized structures adapted to transmit force generated by muscle. Ancient surgeons commented on the tendon injuries and proposed various treatments, including tendon repair. Due to Galen's work and his profound influence on the practice of surgery, tendon injuries were allowed to heal without intervention—this method of treatment continued until the 19th century. Although early observations on tendon morphology date back to the 18th and 19th centuries, it was not until the 20th century that knowledge was truly advanced *(122)*.

The complexity of tendon structure can be appreciated on histological sectioning. The major constituent of tendons is type I collagen (>80% of dry weight). Three chains of collagen are coiled in a right-handed triple helix that are held together by covalent bonds, forming a collagen molecule. The molecule is approx 1.5 nm in diameter and 300 nm long. By arranging collagen molecules in a quarter-stagger, oppositely charged amino acids are aligned. Collagen molecules combine to form very strong structures: microfibrils. Microfibrils combine to form subfibrils, which then form fibrils. Fibrils are immersed in a matrix that is rich in proteoglycans, glycoproteins, and water. Tightly packed fibrils become fascicles (Fig. 1).

The living components of the tendon—collagen-producing fibroblasts—reside between fibrils. The longitudinal histological section demonstrates cell bodies, which appear characteristically spindle-shaped and are orientated in rows between collagen bundles (Fig. 2). Fibroblasts stain darkly when using basic histological stains, such as hematoxylin and eosin. Fascicles within the tendon are bound by loose connective tissue: the endotenon. The endotenon contains fibroblasts, microvessels, lymphatics, and nerve endings. The cross-section of the intrasynovial flexor tendon also reveals the existence of a loose connective tissue layer surrounding the tendon, which constitutes the visceral synovial membrane or epitenon. Tendons that are not supported by the synovial sheath have a layer of loose connective tissue surrounding them: the paratenon.

Early observations regarding the vascular pattern of tendons were linked to those of tendon healing and the formation of adhesions. However, the German and French anatomists presented more systematic investigative work in the mid-19th century. Following his cadaveric studies, Berkenbush in 1887 *(122)* first described the vascular pattern of the human flexor tendon. He concluded that the blood supply to the sheathed tendon comes from the perimysium, periosteum, and the surrounding tissue via vessels in the

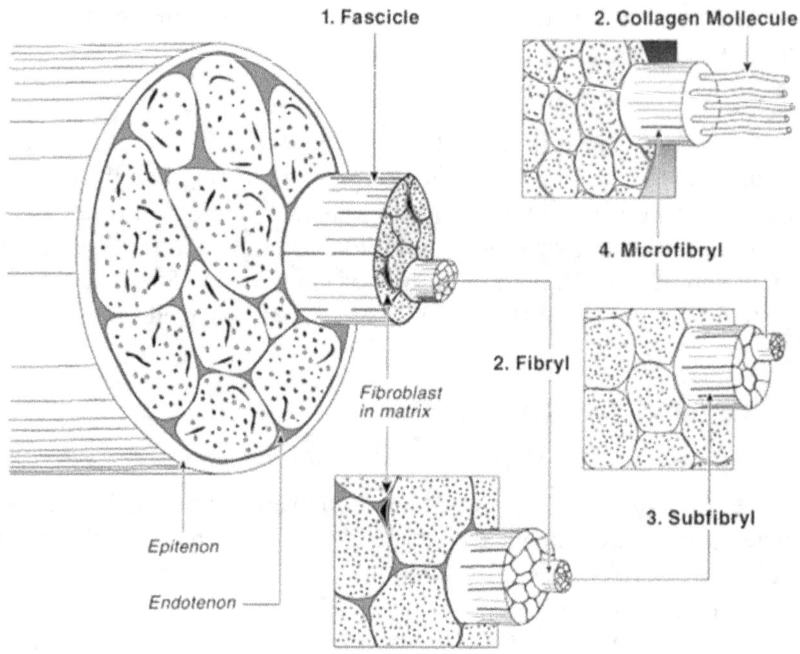

Fig. 1. Tendon structure.

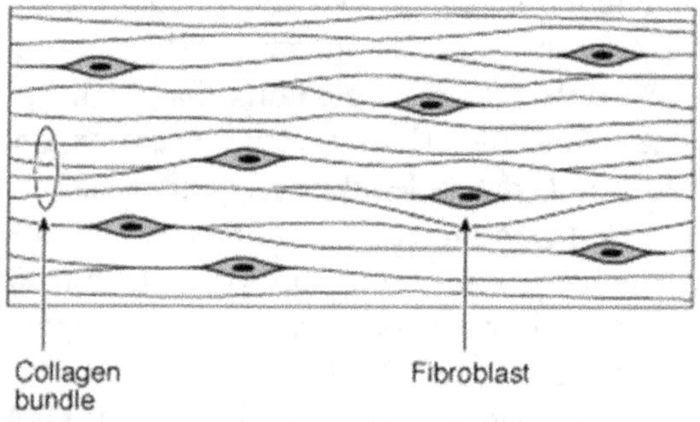

Fig. 2. Longitudinal section of a tendon.

sheath. Berkenbush was probably the first investigator to establish that both superficialis and profundus tendons had consistent areas of avascularity. He also postulated that the tendon was poorly nourished owing to this pattern of vascular supply.

Research by Arai in the early 20th century confirmed Berkenbush's findings and suggested the importance of diffusion in the process of tendon nutrition. In the 1960s and 1970s several investigators revisited and further examined the theory of nutrition by diffusion. In 1963 Potenza *(123)* and later Lundborg et al. *(124)* confirmed that the avascular segments in the tendons are predominantly nourished by diffusion, whereas the vascular parts derive their nutrition from vascular perfusion *(122)*.

Manske and coauthors *(90,125)* further defined and compared the effectiveness of both processes in several animal species. Their work published in the 1980s concluded that although both diffusion and perfusion were important nutrient pathways to the flexor and extensor tendons, diffusion was more effective than perfusion and could, in the absence of perfusion, support most of the tendon *(19,90,126)*. Others, including Lundborg et al. and Hooper et al. *(124,127–129)*, further quantified the relative efficiency of both processes using radioactive tracers.

Tendon Healing

The healing process of the injured tendon has been well documented *(130)*. After the tendon has been incised and sutured, the healing process is initiated. It consists of three stages: the inflammatory stage, collagen production, and scar maturation and remodelling.

Following surgical repair, the incision site fills with a blood clot containing the inflammatory cells, their mediators, and fibrin. Within the next few days, fibroblasts arrive into the area. Collagen production can be detected on the third postoperative day. Initially, the collagen products can be detected in the cytoplasm, but within days, the collagen fibrils are visible under the microscope. The angiogenic activity in the tendon stumps is markedly increased by d 7 *(131)*. After 2 wk, the tendon stumps appear fused by the fibrous bridge that is formed by the migrating collagen type I fibers. At this stage collagen fibers are positioned perpendicularly to tendon fibrils. Within the next 2 wk, the remodeling process ensures a progressive parallel organization of collagen fibers. Interestingly, only the collagen fibers within and around the tendon organize in this parallel manner.

The fibroblasts in the repair zone appear to be of both intrinsic and extrinsic origin. Further remodeling coincides with increased strength and reduced mass of scar tissue and continues only in the presence of longitudinal stressing. The remodeling process continues for approx 4 mo.

In the 1960s and 1970s, many researchers made significant contributions to the current understanding of the healing cascade. Peacock *(132–137)* focused predominantly on the cellular aspects of the healing and recognized the three phases of the healing cascade as previously described. Potenza *(123,138,139)* examined the importance of proliferation and migration of the fibroblasts into the repair site. Both Peacock and Potenza believed that the formation of fibrous attachments or adhesions was significant in the delivery of cells and nutritional support to the repair zone. Later, cells external to the tendon were identified as also having a role in the repair process, the extrinsic repair *(140–145)*.

Lindsay identified the inflammatory nature of adhesions and disputed their importance for the healing process. For the first time, his work demonstrated the existence of the intrinsic and extrinsic processes of the cellular repair in chickens *(146–148)*.

Lundborg and associates *(124,149–151)* then examined the intrinsic contribution to the healing cascade. They investigated the cellular behavior of cut rabbit tendons by placing the excised segment in remote in vivo locations like the synovial cavity or subcutaneously in the dialysing pouch. The results of these studies, which confirmed the intrinsic capacity of the tendons to heal in the absence of adhesions, were later disputed, as the environment in which tendons were placed was found to influence the healing. However, it was not long before the in vitro studies of Becker and Graham *(152,153)* once again demonstrated that the injured chicken tendons were capable of migrating intrinsic fibroblasts into the defect. These fibroblasts were responsible for the production of new collagen fibrils.

Manske et al. and Gelberman et al. *(18,19,46,122,125,154–156)* validated the previous findings and confirmed the existence of the intrinsic reparative process in many other species, including rabbit, dog, chicken, and monkey Harwood et al. and Boyer et al. *(130,131,157,158)* further defined the molecular aspects of fibroblast behavior and the angiogenesis process in the injury zone.

The healing process can be affected by several factors; one is the presence of a longitudinal mechanical force at the time of tendon healing and regeneration. If the force applied exceeds the strength of the early repair, this can cause separation of the injured tendon at the weakest point. However, moderate physiological forces applied longitudinally to regenerating intrasynovial tendon can be beneficial. Several researchers confirmed that early mobilization of repaired intrasynovial tendons reduces the occurrence of adhesions and improves results of the repair *(47,60,159–161)*.

Experimental studies comparing low and high levels of in vivo force during rehabilitation of dogs by Boyer et al. *(162,163)* showed that tensile properties of repaired tendons did not differ between the low- and high-force rehabilitation groups. In fact, it was the suture technique that was primarily important in providing the strength of the repair in the early postoperative period of 1– 6 wk.

Adhesions

Tendons surrounded by sheaths are always at risk of forming adhesions. Adhesions to the surrounding sheath are the most common complication of flexor tendon healing. Adhesions limit the smooth gliding motion of the tendon within the sheath and are believed to be responsible for impaired hand function following flexor tendon repair. Many aspects of adhesion formation have been studied to develop algorithms of treatment that would avoid or minimize their formation *(60,144,145,160,164–166)*.

Several investigators have concluded the importance of the sheath continuity as an inevitable element in the process of tendon healing *(167–169)*. Peterson et al. *(166)* concluded in his experimental studies in 1986 that continuity of the sheath had no effect on flexor tendon healing; results of clinical studies *(35,170)* have also supported this point of view.

Various anti-inflammatory pharmaceuticals, e.g., antihistamines, steroids, and hyaluronic acid, have been attempted to improve the clinical outcome *(154,171)*. These have proved to be of little clinical use. Several different synthetic mechanical barriers have also been used with mixed results *(172,173)*.

Particular attention was devoted to various regimes of postoperative tendon mobilization. Cooney et al. *(174)* and Brunelli et al. *(175)* reported success using passive motion protocols. However, over the last two decades, the protocols of early active motion have been accepted as the standard of care because of their superior results.

Until the biochemical model of the healing cascade of the intrasynovial tendon is fully described, only marginal improvement in the surgical outcome of tendon injuries will likely be observed.

Yet, some mediators clearly demonstrate key influence over the healing process. Lactate has been shown to have a stimulatory effect on collagen production. Tissue hypoxia stimulates lactate production by macrophages, whose presence in the area is known to

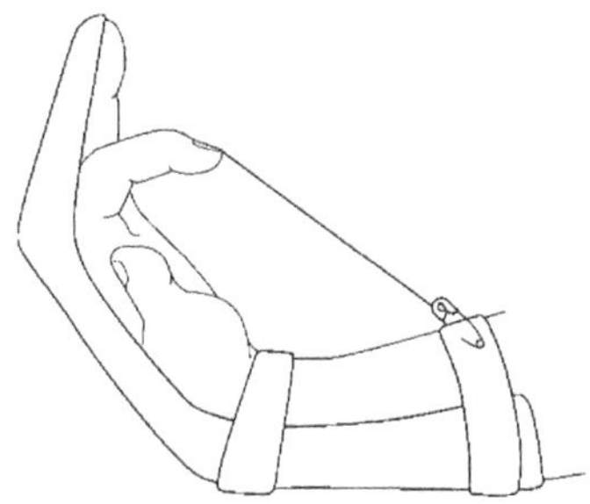

Fig. 3. Splint position described by Kleinert. The wrist is flexed to 20° short of full flexion. MP joints are flexed to 40°. Rubber band traction is applied only to the injured digit.

stimulate collagen production. Lactate is capable of further stimulating other growth factors with positive influence on collagen production, such as transforming growth factor-β (TGF-β). Klein et al. *(158)* used flexor tendon fibroblasts harvested from the rabbit tendon, which were placed in tissue culture with an increased level of lactate. The epitenon and tendon sheath fibroblasts have all proven to significantly increase their collagen production in vitro in response to high lactate levels. Collagen I production by epitenon cells increased 15% and production by endotenon tenocytes by 12%.

TENDON REHABILITATION

Flexor Tendon Rehabilitation

The ultimate goal of flexor tendon repair is to restore normal digital function. Historically, repaired flexor tendons were treated with immobilization *(161)*. This produced a strong repair but also led to uncontrolled tendon adhesion, loss of tendon gliding, secondary joint contracture, and unsatisfactory digital function.

Scientific and clinical research since this time has demonstrated the beneficial effects of applying early controlled stress to the healing tendon *(43,45,49,160,176)*. Mobilized tendons gain greater tensile strength, form fewer adhesions, and have better excursion, resulting in improved digital function.

Rehabilitation programs that employ early motion principles have almost invariably replaced immobilization and can be broadly categorized into three groups: passive flexion/active extension, passive flexion/passive extension, and active flexion/active extension.

Passive Flexion/Active Extension

The first results of early passive motion were reported by Kleinert and associates *(38)*. Good to excellent results were achieved in 87% of cases using a postoperative technique of passive flexion and active extension of the repaired digit *(39)*.

After carefully controlled surgical repair, patients were placed in a dorsal forearm based splint with the wrist flexed to 20° short of full flexion, the metaphalangeal (MP) joints in 40° flexion, and the interphalangeal joints fully extended. Rubber band traction was applied to the tip of the injured digit and pulled toward a fixed point on the forearm (Fig. 3). During exercise, the patient actively extended against the rubber band, which passively returned the digit to a posture of flexion. The splint was discontinued after 6 wk, at which time gentle active flexion exercises were commenced.

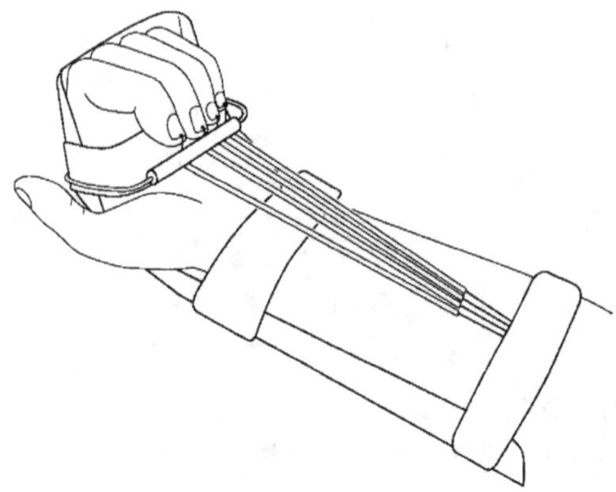

Fig. 4. Modifications to the original Kleinert splint. Wrist is flexed to 20°. MP joints are flexed to 90°. Rubber band traction is applied to all four fingers, and a palmar pulley is used to increase distal joint flexion.

The Kleinert concept of passive controlled motion using rubber band traction has remained among the most popular methods of rehabilitation, but many modifications to the original regimen have been introduced (Fig. 4). Wrist flexion has been reduced to neutral, lowering the tensile load at the repair site *(177)*. MP flexion has been increased to 90°, facilitating the action of the intrinsic musculature in extending the interphalangeal (IP) joints *(161)*. A palmar pulley has been added to redirect the line of pull of the traction toward the palm, increasing DIPJ flexion and improving FDP excursion at this joint *(178,179)*. All four digits are placed in rubber band traction, reducing restriction on tendon glide caused by adjacent digits not brought into full flexion *(180)*.

The complication of PIPJ flexion contracture, seen as a result of the sustained flexion digit posture in the splint, has been addressed in several ways. First, patients are encouraged to manually reduce rubber band tension to allow full active IP joint extension during exercise sessions. Second, traction is reduced or disconnected during sleep.

Exercise parameters have remained largely unchanged despite the numerous splint modifications. Patients are instructed to perform 10 active extension exercises each waking hour, and the splint is worn for 6 wk. After this, active movement is commenced. Return to full activity is not advised until 10–12 wk postoperatively, but reducing the postoperative period to 8 wk has not been found to be detrimental *(181)*.

Passive Flexion/Passive Extension

An alternative method of rehabilitation that incorporated the concept of early motion was described by Duran and Houser *(159)*. Immediately following repair, the patient was placed in a dorsal forearm–based splint that extended to the proximal phalanges but did not include the PIPJs. The wrist was held in 20° flexion. Rubber band traction was applied to the injured digit and fixed to the distal forearm (Fig. 5).

Unlike the previously described programs, the rubber band traction was removed for exercises performed twice daily and consisted of six to eight repetitions of passive digital motion, designed to maximize differential tendon glide (Fig. 6). The dorsal splint was removed at 4.5 wk, and the rubber band was attached to a wrist cuff. Passive

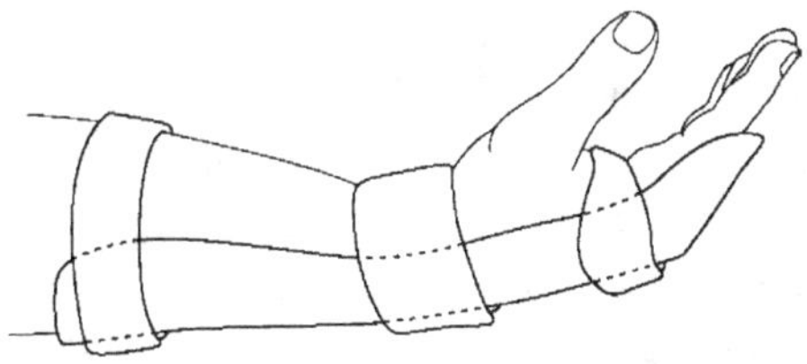

Fig. 5. Dorsal-blocking splint used for the passive flexion/passive extension protocol. The splint extends to the proximal phalanx and holds the wrist in 20° flexion.

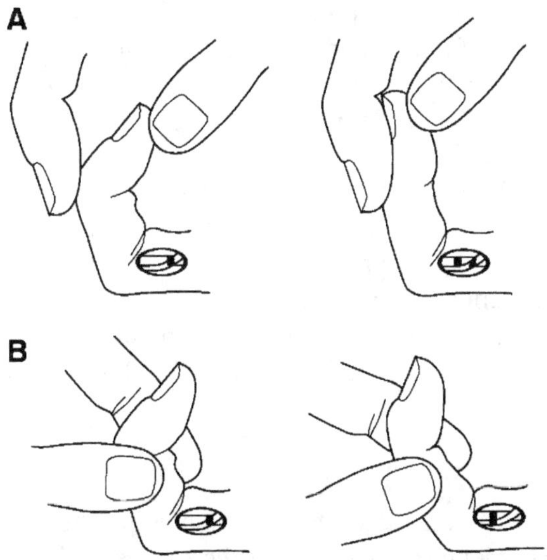

Fig. 6. Passive flexor tendon-gliding exercises. **(A)** Passive extension of the DIPJ glides the FDP repair distal to the FDS repair. **(B)** Passive extension of the PIPJ glides both repairs distal to the laceration site.

motion was continued and active extension commenced. The rubber band traction was discontinued at 5.5 wk when active motion was permitted.

Although Duran and Houser's *(159)* original passive motion protocol is now rarely followed in its entirety, passive digital motion is frequently incorporated into current dynamic traction programs, and the more recently devised active motion programs.

Active Flexion/Active Extension

Excellent results using passive motion protocols have not been universally achieved *(182,183)*. This has raised doubts about the ability of passive digital motion to produce adequate excursion at the repair site, particularly in the presence of postoperative hematoma and edema *(122,165)*. The addition of an active component to postoperative mobilization has increased the excursion of tendon repair *(184,185)*.

These findings have led to the development of early active mobilization programs. However, the force generated by active muscle contraction is not easy to control, and the challenge of such programs has been in maximizing tendon excursion without exceeding the tensile limit of the repair.

Early reports of active motion protocols demonstrate favorable motion outcomes but unacceptably high rates of rupture *(51,52,54,55,186)*. Ruptures may be attributable to the use of repair techniques inadequate to withstand the tensile demands of active motion, which is discussed previously in the section on tendon repairs.

In a typical program *(187)*, the patient is placed in a dorsal protective splint with the wrist in neutral, MP joints in approx 40° flexion, and the IP joints extended. Therapy is commenced 48 h postoperatively to allow time for the resolution of edema, which may otherwise increase the resistance to tendon glide during active motion and contribute to repair site deformation.

Under therapist supervision, the splint is removed, the wrist is placed in 20° extension to reduce the work of flexion, and the patient is asked to gently actively flex the fingers through a limited range of motion over approx 10 repetitions. Flexion efforts are alternated with passive digital flexion; active digital extensions are with the wrist in modest flexion.

The patient is seen two to three times a week and supplements therapy sessions with a home exercise program of passive digital motion within the splint. Active motion may be added to the home exercise program after the first session *(188)*, or delayed for up to 3 wk *(187)*. Treatment is progressed by the addition of place and hold exercises in wk 2, active fist making in wk 4, and light pick-up activities in wk 5. The splint is discontinued after the fifth postoperative week and light-resisted activities are introduced at wk 6.

Extensor Tendon Rehabilitation

The extensor tendons' contribution to the balance, power, dexterity, and range of hand activities is fundamental, but injury to the extensors is often regarded as less serious than injury to the flexors *(189)*. This attitude is reflected in the convention of managing extensor injuries with postoperative immobilization. The extensor tendons proximal to the extensor retinaculum are broad and flat, with a relatively high tendon-to-bone interface, making them prone to peritendinous adhesion when immobilized after injury. Long-term complications, such as extensor lag and loss of digital flexion, have been observed as a result of static immobilization of repaired extensor tendons *(190)*. Efforts to prevent adhesion and restore the normal gliding function of repaired extensor tendons have seen the development of postoperative programs incorporating the concepts of early motion, thus effective in the management of repaired flexor tendons *(38,39,43,45,49,160,161,176)*.

The anatomical and biomechanical characteristics of the extensor tendons vary from their origin in the distal forearm to their insertion into the terminal phalanx. Therefore, a single postoperative program would be unsuitable to adequately treat all levels of injury.

Rehabilitation programs will be described for each zone, following on from the discussion previosly in section "Extensor Tendon Repairs."

Zone I

A disruption of the conjoined lateral bands in zone I results in an extensor lag at the DIPJ. The deformity is commonly referred to as a mallet finger. Injuries may be closed or open.

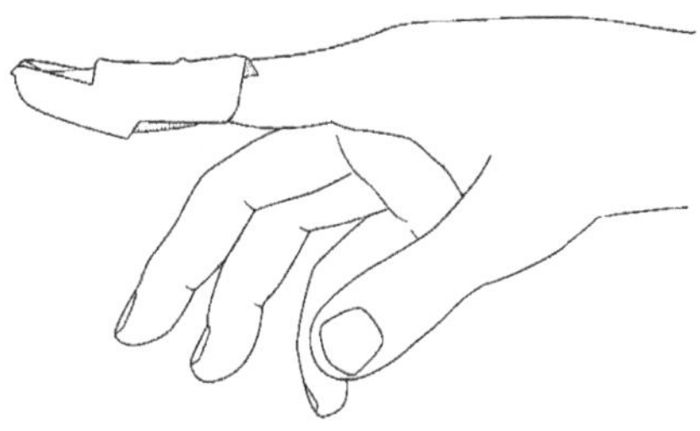

Fig. 7. The prefabricated Stack splint immobilizes the DIPJ in slight hyperextension.

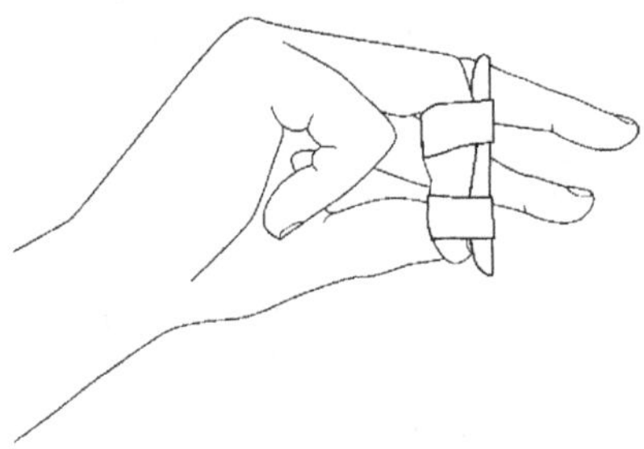

Fig. 8. A dorsal mallet finger splint maintains distal joint extension while allowing full flexion of the PIPJ.

Treatment of the closed injury involves immobilization of the DIPJ in extension or slight hyperextension. This may be achieved by the application of a suitable splint. Prefabricated plastic splints are available for this purpose and have been found to be highly effective (Fig. 7; *191,192*).

More commonly, a custom-molded thermoplastic splint is applied to the digit to ensure an exact fit. The splint extends from the tip of the finger to the PIPJ and may be placed dorsally, volarly, or in the design of the prefabricated styles circumferentially. The dorsal splint (Fig. 8) has the advantage of allowing unrestricted PIPJ flexion *(191,192)* and interferes the least with sensory feedback from the finger tip during hand function. It is customary to splint the DIPJ in some hyperextension, but care must be taken to avoid pressure necrosis of the dorsal skin from a position of extreme hyperextension *(193)*.

The splint is worn continuously for a period of 6–8 wk, then for a further 2 wk at night *(191,194,195)*. During the final 2 wk, additional splint-weaning measures may be employed. The patient may be instructed to apply the splint during the day if a lag is observed and leave the splint in place until the next day. Alternatively, a sling of strapping tape may be applied to gently support the DIPJ in extension.

Splint treatment is effective in restoring or improving extension in 50–75% of cases *(194,196,197)*. The remainder have persistent extensor lag and/or loss of terminal joint flexion *(198)*. Gradual reduction of extensor lag has been observed in the months following treatment as the scar tissue bridging the extensor defect contracts *(195)*. While it is recommended that splinting of the mallet finger be initiated as soon as possible after injury, splinting has been shown to be beneficial even after delay in commencing treatment *(199,200)*.

Open injuries may be satisfactorily treated in the same manner as the closed injury. Alternatively, a longitudinal K-wire can be placed through the extended DIPJ at the time of repair *(201)*. The wire is removed at 6 wk, and a night splint is worn for a further 2 wk. No difference has been found in the outcome between Stack splintage and K-wire fixation *(202)*.

Zone II

Injuries from disruption of the lateral bands in zone II are splinted in the same manner as for zone I. In the case of a single lateral-band injury, the digital extension splint is usually removed at 10–14 d, and active movement is resumed *(192)*.

Zone III

Disruption of the central slip in zone III results in a loss of active extension at the PIPJ, and associated hyperextension of the DIPJ. The consequent posture is referred to as a "boutonniere deformity," thus named because of the apparent "button-holing" of the PIPJ between the volarly displaced lateral bands in the space created by the injured central slip. The injury can be closed or open.

Empirically, the boutonniere deformity (either open or closed) has been treated by 4–6 wk of immobilization in a static PIPJ extension splint *(203,204)*. The DIPJ is kept free to allow active and/or passive movement to prevent adhesions of the lateral bands and contracture of the oblique retinacular ligaments.

Results of treatment by immobilization are frequently disappointing, particularly after complex and open injuries. Characteristic extensor lag and loss of flexion of the IP joints are attributable to extensor tendon adhesion at the proximal phalanx *(190,196,205)*.

To reduce tendon adhesion and improve outcome, early controlled motion programs for open zone III injuries have been developed. Both passive *(206–209)* and active *(210)* controlled motion programs have been described. Both are initiated within 5 d of repair.

The passive motion program reported by Crosby and Wehbe *(204)* requires the application of a dorsal, hand-based dynamic splint that holds the MP joints in neutral. Rubber band traction provides passive PIPJ extension (Fig. 9). The patient is instructed to flex the finger through a limited range of 30°, 10 times every waking hour in the dynamic splint. The splint is discontinued after 4–6 wk when active motion is commenced.

The active motion program, termed "short-arc motion" *(210)*, uses a series of static digital splints for rest and exercise (Fig. 10). When not exercising, the involved digit is immobilized in extension in a static volar digital splint. The immobilization splint is removed every waking hour to allow 20 repetitions of PIPJ flexion through a range of 30°, guided by the first exercise splint. A second exercise splint is used to support the PIPJ in extension, whereas the DIPJ is flexed 20 times through an unrestricted range of motion.

If no lag develops during the first 2 wk of treatment, the first exercise splint is altered to allow 40° of PIPJ motion in the third postoperative week and 50° during the fourth. Splinting is discontinued 4–6 wk postoperatively. During exercise, the wrist is positioned in 30° of flexion, and the MP joint is supported in 0° of flexion to reduce the workload on the EDC throughout the activity.

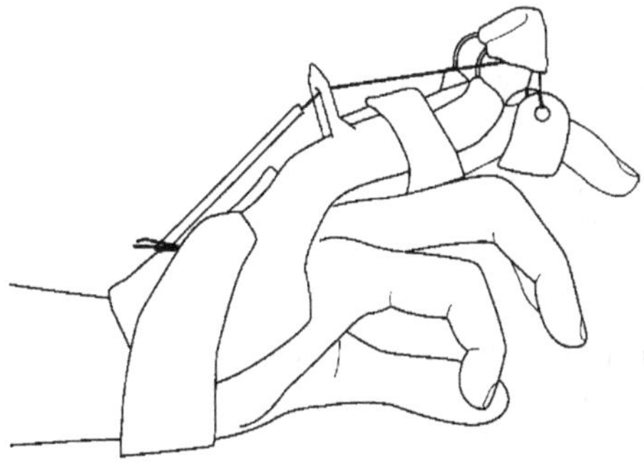

Fig. 9. A hand-based dynamic splint for zone III extensor tendon injury. The splint allows active PIPJ flexion, and the rubber band traction provides passive PIPJ extension.

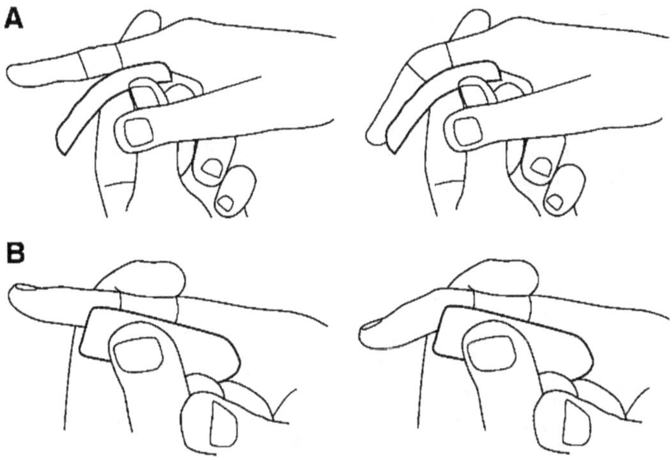

Fig. 10. Exercise splints for "short-arc motion". **(A)** The first splint allows 30° of PIPJ flexion. **(B)** The second splint supports the PIPJ in extension and allows unrestricted DIPJ flexion.

Zones IV–VII

Disruptions to the extensor tendons in the region extending from the proximal phalanges to the wrist have been empirically managed by postoperative immobilization *(211)*. Techniques of early passive mobilization and, more recently, controlled active mobilization *(212–214)* have yielded improved outcomes.

Immobilization

Following exploration and repair, the forearm is immobilized in a volar splint (Fig. 11) with the wrist in approx 40° extension, the MP joints in 0–20° of flexion, and the IP joints extended. The splint is discontinued after 3 wk, and standard rehabilitation techniques follow to restore maximum active range of motion.

Early Passive Mobilization

Within the first five postoperative days, a dorsal forearm–based dynamic extension splint (Fig. 12) is applied with the wrist in 20–40° extension. Rubber band traction

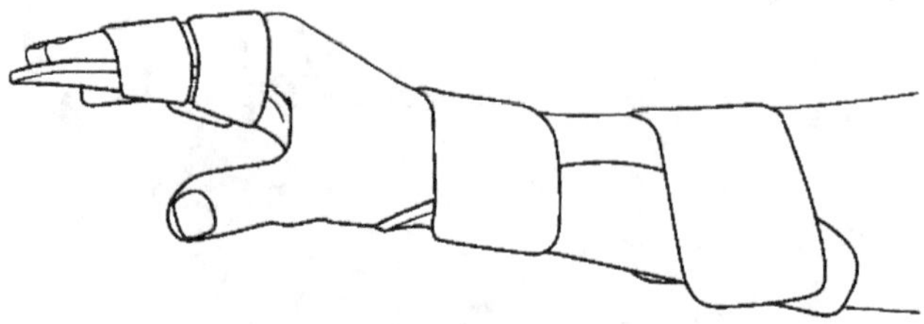

Fig. 11. Volar immobilization splint for zones V–VII extensor tendon injury. The wrist is held in 40° extension and the MP joints in 20° flexion.

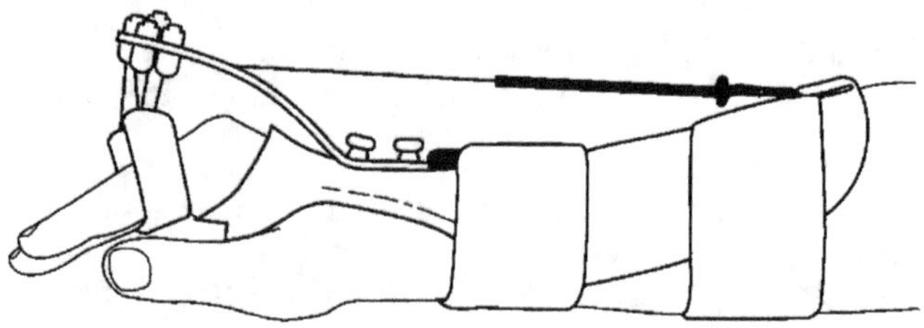

Fig. 12. Forearm-based dynamic extension splint. The splint allows active MP joint flexion, and the rubber band traction passively extends the MP joints.

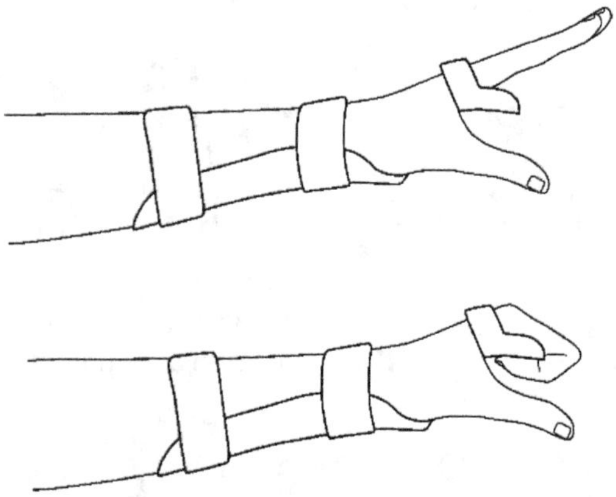

Fig. 13. Static volar splint for controlled active motion. The splint allows active MP joint flexion to 45°. IP joint flexion is unrestricted.

holds the MP joint in extension. The patient is instructed to actively flex the MP joints 10 times every hour, with the traction device passively extending the joint to neutral. The range of flexion is initially limited to 30° by a blocking device, which is progressively adjusted each week to allow an increased range of flexion until the splint is removed at 6 wk.

Controlled Active Mobilization

During the first three to four postoperative days, a palmar blocking splint (Fig. 13) is applied, in which the hand rests in 30° and the MP joints in 45° flexion. The IP joints are unsupported and able to move freely.

The patient is instructed to actively flex and extend the MP and IP joints simultaneously within the confines of the splint 10 times every hour. MP extension is limited to neutral during the first 2 wk. In the third week, the MP flexion block is increased to 70° and hyperextension exercises of the MP joints are added. The splint is discontinued after 4 wk.

No difference exists in the outcome between dynamic extension splinting and controlled active mobilization in patients with simple extensor tendon injuries in zones V and VII. Therefore, controlled active mobilization is recommended in this patient group, as it is simpler, cheaper, and requires less therapy time.

In practice, dynamic splinting remains the preferred treatment for multiple tendon lacerations, complex injuries involving damage to underlying bone or joint, or injuries associated with a loss of dorsal skin.

CONCLUSION

Advances in the understanding of the beneficial effects of early controlled stress on the healing tissue revolutionized the management of tendon injuries. Repaired tendons were once uniformly immobilized, and expectations of the restoration of digital function were poor. Now tendon repairs are subject to early motion rehabilitation protocols, and recovery of good to excellent function of 80% or more is expected *(215)*. Developments in suture techniques and materials have improved the tensile strength of tendon repairs and have allowed the transition from passive mobilization to active mobilization rehabilitation protocols after repair.

Despite these advancements, tendon rehabilitation remains a relatively complex undertaking, requiring the application of a splint, treatment by a skilled hand therapist, and a compliant and motivated patient. The future of tendon repair lies in the ability to produce a repair that is immediately robust enough to withstand the demands of unprotected hand function.

REFERENCES

1. Moore KL, Agur AMR. *Essential Clinical Anatomy*. Williams & Wilkins, Baltimore, MD, 1995.
2. Sinnatamby CS. *Last's Anatomy: Regional and Applied*, 10th Ed.: Churchill Livingstone, New York, NY, 1999, p. 539.
3. Williams PL. *Gray's Anatomy*, 38th Ed. Churchill Livingstone, New York, NY, 1995, p. 2092.
4. Green DP, Hotchkiss RN, Pederson WC. *Green's Operative Hand Surgery*. 4th Ed. Churchill Livingstone, New York, NY, 1998.
5. Smith P. *Lister's The Hand*, 4th Ed. Churchill Livingstone, New York, NY, 2001, p. 624.
6. Thompson NW, et al. Functional absence of flexor digitorum superficialis to the little finger and absence of palmaris longus—is there a link? *J Hand Surg [Br]* 2002;27:433–434.
7. Rayan GM. Palmar fascial complex anatomy and pathology in Dupuytren's disease. *Hand Clin* 1999;15:73–86,vi–vii.
8. Saar JD, Grothaus PC. Dupuytren's disease: an overview. *Plast Reconstr Surg* 2000;106: 125–136.
9. Chrysopoulo MT, et al. Cleland's ligaments: an anatomic study. *Plast Reconstr Surg* 2002; 109:566–575.
10. Idler RS. Anatomy and biomechanics of the digital flexor tendons. *Hand Clin* 1985;1:3–11.

11. Austin GJ, Leslie BM, Ruby LK. Variations of the flexor digitorum superficialis of the small finger. *J Hand Surg [Am]* 1989;14:262–267.
12. Baker DS, et al. The little finger superficialis—clinical investigation of its anatomic and functional shortcomings. *J Hand Surg [Am]* 1981;6:374–378.
13. Stein A, Lemos M, Stein S. Clinical evaluation of flexor tendon function in the small finger. *Ann Emerg Med* 1990;19:991–993.
14. Ohtani O. Structure of the flexor digitorum superficialis. *Okajimas Folia Anat Jpn* 1979; 56:277–288.
15. Boyer MI, et al. Flexor tendon repair and rehabilitation. State of the art in 2002. *Instr Course Lect* 2003;52:591–605.
16. Brockis JG. The blood supply of the flexor tendon and extensor tendons of the fingers in man. *J Bone Joint Surg Br* 1953;35:131–138.
17. Boyer MI, et al. Repair of flexor digitorum profundus tendon avulsions from bone: an ex vivo biomechanical analysis. *J Hand Surg [Am]* 2002;27:594–598.
18. Gelberman RH, Manske PR. Factors influencing flexor tendon adhesions. *Hand Clin* 1985; 1:35–42.
19. Manske PR, Lesker PA. Flexor tendon nutrition. *Hand Clin* 1985;1:13–24.
20. Doyle JR. Palmar and digital flexor tendon pulleys. *Clin Orthop* 2001;383:84–96.
21. Sbernardori MC, et al. Histogenesis and morphology of the flexor tendon pulley system in the human embryonic hand. *J Hand Surg [Br]* 2000;25:175–179.
22. Doyle JR. Anatomy of the finger flexor tendon sheath and pulley system. *J Hand Surg [Am]* 1988;13:473–484.
23. Doyle JR. Anatomy of the flexor tendon sheath and pulley system: a current review. *J Hand Surg [Am]* 1989;14:349–351.
24. Kleinert HE, Verdan C. Report of the Committee on Tendon Injuries (International Federation of Societies for Surgery of the Hand). *J Hand Surg [Am]* 1983;8:794–798.
25. von Schroeder HP, Botte MJ. Anatomy and functional significance of the long extensors to the fingers and thumb. *Clin Orthop* 2001;383:74–83.
26. Schenck R. Variations of the extensor tendons of the fingers: Surgical significance. *J Bone Joint Surg Am* 1964;46:103–110.
27. von Schroeder HP, Botte MJ. Anatomy of the extensor tendons of the fingers: variations and multiplicity. *J Hand Surg [Am]* 1995;20:27–34.
28. von Schroeder HP, Botte MJ. The functional significance of the long extensors and juncturae tendinum in finger extension. *J Hand Surg [Am]* 1993;18:641–647.
29. Hirai Y, et al. An anatomic study of the extensor tendons of the human hand. *J Hand Surg [Am]* 2001;26:1009–1015.
30. von Schroeder HP, Botte MJ. Functional anatomy of the extensor tendons of the digits. *Hand Clin* 1997;13:51–62.
31. Rockwell WB, Butler PN, Byrne BA. Extensor tendon: anatomy, injury, and reconstruction. *Plast Reconstr Surg* 2000;106:1592–1603.
32. Doyle JR, Blythe WF. Anatomy of the flexor tendon sheath and pulleys of the thumb. *J Hand Surg* 1977;2:149–151.
33. Bayat A, et al. The pulley system of the thumb: anatomic and biomechanical study. *J Hand Surg [Am]* 2002;27:628–635.
34. Bunnell S. Injuries of the hand. In *Surgery of the Hand*. JB Lippincott, Philadelphia, PA, 1944, pp. 449–502.
35. Lister GD, et al. Primary flexor tendon repair followed by immediate controlled mobilization. *J Hand Surg [Am]* 1977;2:441–451.
36. Kessler I, Nissim F. Primary repair without immobilization of flexor tendon division within the digital sheath. An experimental and clinical study. *Acta Orthop Scand* 1969; 40:587–601.
37. Verdan CE. Primary repair of flexor tendons. *J Bone Joint Surg Am* 1960;42:647–657.

38. Kleinert HE, Kutz JE, Ashbell TS. Primary repair of lacerated flexor tendons in no man's land (abstract). *J Bone Joint Surg Am* 1967;49:577.
39. Kleinert HE, et al. Primary repair of flexor tendons. *Orthop Clin North Am* 1973;4: 865–876.
40. Ejeskar A. Flexor tendon repair in no-man's-land: results of primary repair with controlled mobilization. *J Hand Surg [Am]* 1984;9:171–177.
41. Strickland JW, Glogovac SV. Digital function following flexor tendon repair in Zone II: A comparison of immobilization and controlled passive motion techniques. *J Hand Surg [Am]* 1980;5:537–543.
42. Woo SL, et al. The importance of controlled passive mobilization on flexor tendon healing. A biomechanical study. *Acta Orthop Scand* 1981;52:615–622.
43. Feehan LM, Beauchene JG. Early tensile properties of healing chicken flexor tendons: early controlled passive motion versus postoperative immobilization. *J Hand Surg [Am]* 1990;15:63–68.
44. Takai S, et al. The effects of frequency and duration of controlled passive mobilization on tendon healing. *J Orthop Res* 1991;9:705–713.
45. Gelberman RH, et al. Effects of early intermittent passive mobilization on healing canine flexor tendons. *J Hand Surg [Am]* 1982;7:170–175.
46. Gelberman RH, et al. The early stages of flexor tendon healing: a morphologic study of the first fourteen days. *J Hand Surg [Am]* 1985;10:776–784.
47. Gelberman RH, et al. The effects of mobilization on the vascularization of healing flexor tendons in dogs. *Clin Orthop* 1980;153:283–289.
48. Lee H. Double loop locking suture: a technique of tendon repair for early active mobilization. Part I: Evolution of technique and experimental study. *J Hand Surg [Am]* 1990;15: 945–952.
49. Aoki M, et al. Biomechanical and histologic characteristics of canine flexor tendon repair using early postoperative mobilization. *J Hand Surg [Am]* 1997;22:107–114.
50. Savage R, Risitano G. Flexor tendon repair using a "six strand" method of repair and early active mobilization. *J Hand Surg [Br]* 1989;14:396–399.
51. Small JO, Brennen MD, Colville J. Early active mobilization following flexor tendon repair in zone II. *J Hand Surg [Br]* 1989;14:383–391.
52. Cullen KW, et al. Flexor tendon repair in zone II followed by controlled active mobilization. *J Hand Surg [Br]* 1989;14:392–395.
53. Kubota H, et al. Mechanical properties of various circumferential tendon suture techniques. *J Hand Surg [Br]* 1996;21:474–480.
54. Bainbridge LC, et al. A comparison of post-operative mobilization of flexor tendon repairs with "passive flexion-active extension" and "controlled active motion" techniques. *J Hand Surg [Br]* 1994;19:517–521.
55. Elliot D, et al. The rupture rate of acute flexor tendon repairs mobilized by the controlled active motion regimen. *J Hand Surg [Br]* 1994;19:607–612.
56. Bruner JM. The zig-zag volar-digital incision for flexor-tendon surgery. *Plast Reconstr Surg* 1967;40:571–574.
57. Becker H, Davidoff M. Eliminating the gap in flexor tendon surgery. A new method of suture. *Hand* 1977;9:306–311.
58. Seradge H. Elongation of the repair configuration following flexor tendon repair. *J Hand Surg [Am]* 1983;8:182–185.
59. Ejeskar A, Irstam L. Elongation in profundus tendon repair. A clinical and radiological study. *Scand J Plast Reconstr Surg* 1981;15:61–68.
60. Gelberman RH, et al. The effect of gap formation at the repair site on the strength and excursion of intrasynovial flexor tendons. An experimental study on the early stages of tendon-healing in dogs. *J Bone Joint Surg Am* 1999;81:975–982.
61. Kessler I. The "grasping" technique for tendon repair. *Hand* 1973;5:253–255.

62. Pennington DG. The locking loop tendon suture. *Plast Reconstr Surg* 1979;63:648–652.
63. Mashadi ZB, Amis AA. The effect of locking loops on the strength of tendon repair. *J Hand Surg [Br]* 1991;16:35–39.
64. Hotokezaka S, Manske PR. Differences between locking loops and grasping loops: effects on 2-strand core suture. *J Hand Surg [Am]* 1997;22:995–1003.
65. Wada A, et al. The mechanical properties of locking and grasping suture loop configurations in four-strand core suture techniques. *J Hand Surg [Br]* 2000;25:548–551.
66. Hatanaka H, Manske PR. Effect of the cross-sectional area of locking loops in flexor tendon repair. *J Hand Surg [Am]* 1999;24:751–760.
67. Kubota H, et al. Effect of a new repair technique on biomechanical properties of canine flexor tendons: in vitro study. *Hand Surg* 1998;3:247–255.
68. Greenwald DP, Hong HZ, May Jr. JW. Mechanical analysis of tendon suture techniques. *J Hand Surg [Am]* 1994;19:641–647.
69. Taras JS. Primary flexor tendon repair. *Oper Tech Orthop* 1993;3:270–277.
70. Ketchum LD. Suture materials and suture techniques used in tendon repair. *Hand Clin* 1985;1:43–53.
71. Shaieb MD, Singer DI. Tensile strengths of various suture techniques. *J Hand Surg [Br]* 1997;22:764–767.
72. McLarney E, Hoffman H, Wolfe SW. Biomechanical analysis of the cruciate four-strand flexor tendon repair. *J Hand Surg [Am]* 1999;24:295–301.
73. Dinopoulos HT, et al. The resistance of a four- and eight-strand suture technique to gap formation during tensile testing: an experimental study of repaired canine flexor tendons after 10 days of in vivo healing. *J Hand Surg [Am]* 2000;25:489–498.
74. Winters SC, et al. The effects of multiple-strand suture methods on the strength and excursion of repaired intrasynovial flexor tendons: a biomechanical study in dogs. *J Hand Surg [Am]* 1998;23:97–104.
75. Trail IA, Powell ES, Noble J. The mechanical strength of various suture techniques. *J Hand Surg [Br]* 1992;17:89–91.
76. Ketchum LD, Martin NL, Kappel DA. Experimental evaluation of factors affecting the strength of tendon repairs. *Plast Reconstr Surg* 1977;59:708–719.
77. Aoki M, et al. Effect of suture knots on tensile strength of repaired canine flexor tendons. *J Hand Surg [Br]* 1995;20:72–75.
78. Momose T, et al. The effect of knot location, suture material, and suture size on the gliding resistance of flexor tendons. *J Biomed Mater Res* 2000;53:806–811.
79. Diao E, et al. Effect of peripheral suture depth on strength of tendon repairs. *J Hand Surg [Am]* 1996;21:234–239.
80. Wade PJ, Muir IF, Hutcheon LL. Primary flexor tendon repair: the mechanical limitations of the modified Kessler technique. *J Hand Surg [Br]* 1986;11:71–76.
81. Kim PT, et al. Tensile strength of cross-stitch epitenon suture. *J Hand Surg [Br]* 1996; 21:821–823.
82. Mashadi ZB, Amis AA. Strength of the suture in the epitenon and within the tendon fibres: development of stronger peripheral suture technique. *J Hand Surg [Br]* 1992;17: 172–175.
83. Leddy JP. Flexor tendon-acute injuries. In Green DP, ed. *Operative Hand Surgery*, Churchill Livingstone, New York, NY, 1993, pp. 1823–1851.
84. Silfverskiold KL, Andersson CH. Two new methods of tendon repair: an in vitro evaluation of tensile strength and gap formation. *J Hand Surg [Am]* 1993;18:58–65.
85. Dona E, et al. *The Biomechanical Properties of Two New Flexor Tendon Circumferential Suture Techniques*. British Society for Surgery of the Hand Autumn Meeting, Edinburgh, Scotland, 2002.
86. Wade PJ, Wetherell RG, Amis AA. Flexor tendon repair: significant gain in strength from the Halsted peripheral suture technique. *J Hand Surg [Br]* 1989;14:232–235.

87. Lin GT, et al. Biomechanical studies of running suture for flexor tendon repair in dogs. *J Hand Surg [Am]* 1988;13:553–558.
88. Peterson WW, et al. Effect of pulley excision on flexor tendon biomechanics. *J Orthop Res* 1986;4:96–101.
89. Lin GT, et al. Functional anatomy of the human digital flexor pulley system. *J Hand Surg [Am]* 1989;14:949–956.
90. Manske PR, Lesker PA. Comparative nutrient pathways to the flexor profundus tendons in Zone II of various experimental animals. *J Surg Res* 1983;34:83–93.
91. Bowers WH, Kuzma GR, Bynum DK. Closed traumatic rupture of finger flexor pulleys. *J Hand Surg [Am]* 1994;19:782–787.
92. Doyle JR, Blythe W. Macroscopic and functional anatomy of the flexor sheath. Proceedings of the 29th Annual American Society for Surgery of the Hand. *J Bone Joint Surg Am* 1974;56:1094.
93. Kwai Ben I, Elliot D. "Venting" or partial lateral release of the A2 and A4 pulleys after repair of zone II flexor tendon injuries. *J Hand Surg [Br]* 1998;23:649–654.
94. Mitsionis G, et al. Feasibility of partial A2 and A4 pulley excision: residual pulley strength. *J Hand Surg [Br]* 2000;25:90–94.
95. Mitsionis G, et al. Feasibility of partial A2 and A4 pulley excision: effect on finger flexor tendon biomechanics. *J Hand Surg [Am]* 1999;24:310–314.
96. Tomaino M, et al. The effect of partial excision of the A2 and A4 pulleys on the biomechanics of finger flexion. *J Hand Surg [Br]* 1998;23:50–52.
97. Tang JB, Xie RG. Effect of A3 pulley and adjacent sheath integrity on tendon excursion and bowstringing. *J Hand Surg [Am]* 2001;26:855–861.
98. Bunnell S. *Surgery of the Hand*, 2nd Ed. JB Lippincott, Philadelphia, PA, 1948, pp. 381–466.
99. Moiemen NS, Elliot D. Primary flexor tendon repair in zone 1. *J Hand Surg [Br]* 2000;25: 78–84.
100. Silva MJ, et al. Flexor digitorum profundus tendon-to-bone repair: an ex vivo biomechanical analysis of 3 pullout suture techniques. *J Hand Surg [Am]* 1998;23:120–126.
101. Skoff HD, et al. Bone suture anchors in hand surgery. *J Hand Surg [Br]* 1995;20:245–248.
102. Buch BD, et al. The Mitek Mini G2 suture anchor: biomechanical analysis of use in the hand. *J Hand Surg [Am]* 1995;20:877–881.
103. Brustein M, et al. Bone suture anchors versus the pullout button for repair of distal profundus tendon injuries: a comparison of strength in human cadaveric hands. *J Hand Surg [Am]* 2001;26:489–496.
104. Hueston JT, Wilson WF. Flexor fibre protrusion through the digital fibrous flexor sheath. *Hand* 1973;5:39–42.
105. Janecki Jr CJ. Triggering of the finger caused by flexor-tendon laceration. *J Bone Joint Surg Am* 1976;58:1174–1175.
106. Bilos ZJ, Hui PW, Stamelos S. Trigger finger following partial flexor tendon laceration. *Hand* 1977;9:232–233.
107. Schlenker JD, Lister GD, Kleinert HE. Three complications of untreated partial laceration of flexor tendon—entrapment, rupture, and triggering. *J Hand Surg [Am]* 1981;6:392–398.
108. Minami A, Ogino T. Trigger wrist caused by a partial laceration of the flexor superficialis tendon of the ring finger. *J Hand Surg [Br]* 1986;11:457–459.
109. Frewin PR, Scheker LR. Triggering secondary to an untreated partially-cut flexor tendon. *J Hand Surg [Br]* 1989;14:419–421.
110. al-Qattan MM, Posnick JC, Lin KY. Triggering after partial tendon laceration. *J Hand Surg [Br]* 1993;18:241–246.
111. Ollinger H, Wray Jr RC, Weeks PM. Effects of suture on tensile strength gain of partially and completely severed tendons. *Surg Forum* 1975;26:63–64.
112. Reynolds B, Wray Jr RC, Weeks PM. Should an incompletely severed tendon be sutured? *Plast Reconstr Surg* 1976;57:36–38.

113. Hariharan JS, et al. Partial lacerations of human digital flexor tendons: a biomechanical analysis. *J Hand Surg [Am]* 1997;22:1011–1015.
114. Wray Jr RC, Weeks PM. Treatment of partial tendon lacerations. *Hand* 1980;12:163–166.
115. al-Qattan MM. Conservative management of zone II partial flexor tendon lacerations greater than half the width of the tendon. *J Hand Surg [Am]* 2000;25:1118–1121.
116. Verdan CE. Primary and secondary repair of flexor and extensor tendon injuries. In Flynn JE, ed. *Hand Surgery*. Williams & Wilkins, Baltimore, MD, 1975.
117. Minamikawa Y, et al. Wrist position and extensor tendon amplitude following repair. *J Hand Surg [Am]* 1992;17:268–271.
118. Elson RA. Rupture of the central slip of the extensor hood of the finger. A test for early diagnosis. *J Bone Joint Surg Br* 1986;68:229–231.
119. Tubiana R. Surgical repair of the extensor apparatus of the fingers. *Surg Clin North Am* 1968;48:1015–1031.
120. Hart RG, Uehara DT, Kutz JE. Extensor tendon injuries of the hand. *Emerg Med Clin North Am* 1993;11:637–649.
121. Blair WF, Steyers CM. Extensor tendon injuries. *Orthop Clin North Am* 1992;23:141–148.
122. Manske PR. Flexor tendon healing. *J Hand Surg [Brit]* 1988;13:237–245.
123. Potenza AD. Critical evaluation of flexor tendon healing adhesion formation within artificial digital sheaths. *J Bone Joint Surg Am* 1963;45:1217–1233.
124. Lundborg G, Eiken O, Rank F. Synovium as a nutritional medium in tendon grafting. *Handchirurgie* 1977;9:107–111.
125. Manske PR, Lesker PA. Histologic evidence of intrinsic flexor tendon repair in various experimental animals. An in vitro study. *Clin Orthop* 1984;182:297–304.
126. Kain CC, et al. The effect of vascularization on avian flexor tendon repair. A biochemical study. *Clin Orthop* 1988;233:295–303.
127. Lundborg G. The vascularization of the human flexor pollicis longus tendon. *Hand* 1979; 11:28–33.
128. Lundborg G, Myrhage R, Rydevik B. The vascularization of human flexor tendons within the digital synovial sheath region—structureal and functional aspects. *J Hand Surg [Am]* 1977;2:417–427.
129. Hooper G, Davies R, Tothill P. Blood flow and clearance in tendons. Studies with dogs. *J Bone Joint Surg Br* 1984;66:441–443.
130. Buckwalter JA, Einhorn TA, Sheldon SR. *Orthopaedic Basic Science. Biology and Biomechanics of the Musculoskeletal System*, 2nd Ed. American Academy of Orthopedic Surgeons, Rosemont, IL, 2003.
131. Boyer MI, et al. Quantitative variation in vascular endothelial growth factor mRNA expression during early flexor tendon healing: an investigation in a canine model. *J Orthop Res* 2001;19:869–872.
132. Peacock Jr EE. Inter- and intramolecular bonding in collagen of healing wounds by insertion of methylene and amide cross-links into scar tissue: tensile strength and thermal shrinkage in rats. *Ann Surg* 1966;163:1–9.
133. Peacock Jr EE. Biology of tendon repair. *N Engl J Med* 1967;276:680–683.
134. Peacock Jr EE. Dynamic aspects of collagen biology. I. Synthesis and assembly. *J Surg Res* 1967;7:433–445.
135. Peacock Jr EE. Dynamic aspects of collagen biology. II. Degradation and metabolism. *J Surg Res* 1967;7:481–497.
136. Peacock Jr EE, Madden JW. Human composite flexor tendon allografts. *Ann Surg* 1967;166:624–629.
137. Peacock Jr EE, Madden JW. Some studies on the effects of beta-aminopropionitrile in patients with injured flexor tendons. *Surgery* 1969;66:215–223.
138. Potenza AD. Flexor tendon injuries. *Orthop Clin North Am* 1970;1:355–373.

139. Potenza AD, Melone C. Evaluation of freeze-dried flexor tendon grafts in the dog. *J Hand Surg [Am]* 1978;3:157–162.
140. Whitson TC, Peacock Jr EE. Effect of alpha alpha dipyridyl on collagen synthesis in healing wounds. *Surg Gynecol Obstet* 1969;128:1061–1064.
141. Craver JM, Madden JW, Peacock Jr EE. Biological control of physical properties of tendon adhesions: effect of beta-aminopropionitrile in chickens. *Ann Surg* 1968;167:697–704.
142. Potenza AD, Herte MC. The synovial cavity as a "tissue culture in situ"—science or nonsense? *J Hand Surg [Am]* 1982;7:196–199.
143. Potenza AD. Philosophy of flexor tendon surgery. *Orthop Clin North Am* 1986;17:349–352.
144. Potenza AD. Digital sheath excision. *J Hand Surg [Am]* 1991;16:765–766.
145. Potenza AD. Flexor sheath continuity. *J Hand Surg [Am]* 1992;17:581–583.
146. Lindsay WK, Thomson HG. Digital flexor tendons: an experimental study, Part I. The significance of each component of the flexor mechanism in tendon healing. *Br J Plast Surg* 1960;12:289–319.
147. Lindsay WK, Thomson HG, Walker FG. Digital flexor tendons: an experimental study, Part II. The significance of a gap occuring at the line of suture. *Br J Plast Surg* 1960;13: 1–9.
148. Lindsay WK, McDougall EP. Digital flexor tendons: an experimental study, Part III. The fate of autogenous digital flexor tendon grafts. *Br J Plast Surg* 1961;13:293–304.
149. Lundborg G, Rank F. Experimental intrinsic healing of flexor tendons based upon synovial fluid nutrition. *J Hand Surg [Am]* 1978;3:21–31.
150. Lundborg G, et al. Superficial repair of severed flexor tendons in synovial environment. An experimental, ultrastructural study on cellular mechanisms. *J Hand Surg [Am]* 1980;5: 451–461.
151. Rank F, et al. Flexor tendon specimens in organ cultures. *Scand J Plast Reconstr Surg* 1980;14:179–183.
152. Becker H, et al. Intrinsic tendon cell proliferation in tissue culture. *J Hand Surg [Am]* 1981;6:616–619.
153. Graham MF, et al. Intrinsic tendon fibroplasia: documentation by in vitro studies. *J Orthop Res* 1984;1:251–256.
154. Manske PR, et al. Intrinsic flexor-tendon repair. A morphological study in vitro. *J Bone Joint Surg Am* 1984;66:385–396.
155. Manske PR, Lesker PA. Biochemical evidence of flexor tendon participation in the repair process—an in vitro study. *J Hand Surg [Brit]* 1984;9:117–120.
156. Gelberman RH, et al. Flexor tendon repair in vitro: a comparative histologic study of the rabbit, chicken, dog, and monkey. *J Orthop Res* 1984;2:39–48.
157. Harwood FL, Goomer RS, Gelberman RH, Silva MJ, Ameil D, et al. Regulation of alpha(v)beta3 and alpha5beta1 integrin receptors by basic fibroblast growth factor and platelet-derived growth factor-BB in intrasynovial flexor tendon cells. *Wound Repair Regen* 1999;7:381–388.
158. Klein MB, et al. Flexor tendon wound healing in vitro: the effect of lactate on tendon cell proliferation and collagen production. *J Hand Surg [Am]* 2001;26:847–854.
159. Duran RH, Houser RG. Controlled passive motion following flexor tendon repair in zones II and III. In *AAOS Symposium on Flexor Tendon Surgery in the Hand.* CV Mosby, St. Louis, 1975.
160. Gelberman RH, et al. The excursion and deformation of repaired flexor tendons treated with protected early motion. *J Hand Surg [Am]* 1986;11:106–110.
161. Wang AW, Gupta A. Early motion after flexor tendon surgery. *Hand Clin* 1996;12:43–55.
162. Goldfarb CA, et al. The effect of variations in applied rehabilitation force on collagen concentration and maturation at the intrasynovial flexor tendon repair site. *J Hand Surg [Am]* 2001;26:841–846.

163. Boyer MI, et al. Intrasynovial flexor tendon repair. An experimental study comparing low and high levels of in vivo force during rehabilitation in canines. *J Bone Joint Surg Am* 2001;83A:891–899.
164. Farkas LG, Lindsay WK. Digital flexor tendon graft healing: pseudosheath and functional return. *Surg Forum* 1979;30:539–541.
165. Lane JM, Black J, Bora Jr FW. Gliding function following flexor-tendon injury. A biomechanical study of rat tendon function. *J Bone Joint Surg Am* 1976;58:985–990.
166. Peterson WW, et al. Effect of flexor sheath integrity on tendon gliding: a biomechanical and histologic study. *J Orthop Res* 1986;4:458–465.
167. Matthews P. The pathology of flexor tendon repair. *Hand* 1979;11:233–242.
168. Matthews P, Richards H. Factors in the adherence of flexor tendon after repair: an experimental study in the rabbit. *J Bone Joint Surg Br* 1976;58:230–236.
169. Strickland JW. Flexor tendon injuries. Part 1. Anatomy, physiology, biomechanics, healing, and adhesion formation around a repaired tendon. *Orthop Rev* 1986;15:632–645.
170. Tonkin MA. Primary flexor tendon repair: surgical techniques based on the anatomy and biology of the flexor tendon system. *World J Surg* 1991;15:452–457.
171. Szabo RM, Younger E. Effects of indomethacin on adhesion formation after repair of zone II tendon lacerations in the rabbit. *J Hand Surg [Am]* 1990;15:480–483.
172. Kapetanos G. The effect of the local corticosteroids on the healing and biomechanical properties of the partially injured tendon. *Clin Orthop* 1982;163:170–179.
173. Peterson WW, et al. Effect of various methods of restoring flexor sheath integrity on the formation of adhesions after tendon injury. *J Hand Surg [Am]* 1990;15:48–56.
174. Cooney WP, et al. Management of acute flexor tendon injury in the hand. *Instr Course Lect* 1985;34:373–381.
175. Brunelli G, Vigasio A, Brunelli F. Slip-knot flexor tendon suture in Zone II allowing immediate mobilization. *Hand* 1983;15:352–358.
176. Wada A, et al. Comparison of postoperative early active mobilization and immobilization in vivo utilising a four-strand flexor tendon repair. *J Hand Surg [Br]* 2001;26:301–306.
177. Savage R. The influence of wrist position on the minimum force required for active movement of the interphalangeal joints. *J Hand Surg [Br]* 1988;13:262–268.
178. McGrouther DA, Ahmed MR. Flexor tendon excursions in "no-man's land." *Hand* 1981;13:129–141.
179. Chow JA, et al. A combined regimen of controlled motion following flexor tendon repair in "no man's land". *Plast Reconstr Surg* 1987;79:447–455.
180. May EJ, Silfverskiold KL, Sollerman CJ. Controlled mobilization after flexor tendon repair in zone II: a prospective comparison of three methods. *J Hand Surg [Am]* 1992;17:942–952.
181. Adolfsson L, et al. The effects of a shortened postoperative mobilization programme after flexor tendon repair in zone II. *J Hand Surg [Br]* 1996;21:67–71.
182. Edinburg M, Widgerow AD, Biddulph SL. Early postoperative mobilization of flexor tendon injuries using a modification of the Kleinert technique. *J Hand Surg [Am]* 1987;12:34–38.
183. Gault DT. A review of repaired flexor tendons. *J Hand Surg [Br]* 1987;12:321–325.
184. Hagberg L, Selvik G. Tendon excursion and dehiscence during early controlled mobilization after flexor tendon repair in zone II: an x-ray stereophotogrammetric analysis. *J Hand Surg [Am]* 1991;16:669–680.
185. Silfverskiold KL, May EJ. Gap formation after flexor tendon repair in zone II. Results with a new controlled motion programme. *Scand J Plast Reconstr Surg Hand Surg* 1993;27:263–268.
186. Allen BN, et al. Ruptured flexor tendon tenorrhaphies in zone II: repair and rehabilitation. *J Hand Surg [Am]* 1987;12:18–21.

187. Steelman P. Treatment of flexor tendon injuries: therapist's commentary. *J Hand Ther* 1999;12:149–151.
188. Hatanaka H, et al. Aggressive active mobilization following zone II flexor tendon repair using a two-strand heavy-gauge locking loop technique. *J Orthop Sci* 2002;7:457–461.
189. Rosenthal EA. The extensor tendons: anatomy and management. In Hunter JM, Mackin EJ, Callahan AD, eds., *Rehabilitation of the Hand: Surgery and Therapy*. CV Mosby, St. Louis, MO, 1984, pp. 519–564.
190. Newport ML, Blair WF, Steyers Jr CM. Long-term results of extensor tendon repair. *J Hand Surg [Am]* 1990;15:961–966.
191. Stack G. Mallet finger. *Lancet* 1968;2:1303.
192. Evans RB. An update on extensor tendon management. In Hunter JM, Mackin EJ, Callahan AD, eds., *Rehabilitation of the Hand: Surgery and Therapy*. CV Mosby, St. Louis, MO, 1984, pp. 565–608.
193. Rayan GM, Mullins PT. Skin necrosis complicating mallet finger splinting and vascularity of the distal interphalangeal joint overlying skin. *J Hand Surg [Am]* 1987;12:548–552.
194. Abouna JM, Brown H. The treatment of mallet finger. The results in a series of 148 consecutive cases and a review of the literature. *Br J Surg* 1968;55:653–667.
195. Stack HG. A modified splint for mallet finger. *J Hand Surg [Br]* 1986;11:263.
196. Stern PJ, Kastrup JJ. Complications and prognosis of treatment of mallet finger. *J Hand Surg [Am]* 1988;13:329–334.
197. Warren RA, Kay NR, Norris SH. The microvascular anatomy of the distal digital extensor tendon. *J Hand Surg [Br]* 1988;13:161–163.
198. Evans D, Weightman B. The Pipflex splint for treatment of mallet finger. *J Hand Surg [Br]* 1988;13:156–158.
199. Patel MR, Desai SS, Bassini-Lipson L. Conservative management of chronic mallet finger. *J Hand Surg [Am]* 1986;11:570–573.
200. Garberman SF, Diao E, Peimer CA. Mallet finger: results of early versus delayed closed treatment. *J Hand Surg [Am]* 1994;19:850–852.
201. Brzezienski MA, Schneider LH. Extensor tendon injuries at the distal interphalangeal joint. *Hand Clin* 1995;11:373–386.
202. Auchincloss JM. Mallet-finger injuries: a prospective, controlled trial of internal and external splintage. *Hand* 1982;14:168–173.
203. Coons MS, Green SM. Boutonniere deformity. *Hand Clin* 1995;11:387–402.
204. Crosby CA, Wehbe MA. Early motion after extensor tendon surgery. *Hand Clin* 1996;12:57–64.
205. Okafor B, et al. Mallet deformity of the finger. Five-year follow-up of conservative treatment. *J Bone Joint Surg Br* 1997;79:544–547.
206. Hung LK, et al. Early controlled active mobilization with dynamic splintage for treatment of extensor tendon injuries. *J Hand Surg [Am]* 1990;15:251–257.
207. O'Dwyer FG, Quinton DN. Early mobilization of acute middle slip injuries. *J Hand Surg [Br]* 1990;15:404–406.
208. Saldana MJ, et al. Results of acute zone III extensor tendon injuries treated with dynamic extension splinting. *J Hand Surg [Am]* 1991;16:1145–1150.
209. Walsh MT, et al. Early controlled motion with dynamic splinting versus static splinting for zones III and IV extensor tendon lacerations: a preliminary report. *J Hand Ther* 1994;7: 232–236.
210. Evans RB. Immediate active short arc motion following extensor tendon repair. *Hand Clin* 1995;11:483–512.
211. Lovett WL, McCalla MA. Management and rehabilitation of extensor tendon injuries. *Orthop Clin North Am* 1983;14:811–826.
212. Browne Jr EZ, Ribik CA. Early dynamic splinting for extensor tendon injuries. *J Hand Surg [Am]* 1989;14:72–76.

213. Chow JA, et al. A comparison of results of extensor tendon repair followed by early controlled mobilization versus static immobilization. *J Hand Surg [Br]* 1989;14:18–20.
214. Ip WY, Chow SP. Results of dynamic splintage following extensor tendon repair. *J Hand Surg [Br]* 1997;22:283–287.
215. Strickland JW. Development of flexor tendon surgery: twenty-five years of progress. *J Hand Surg [Am]* 2000;25:214–235.

4

Evolution of Concepts in Flexor Tendon Surgery of the Hand

Randip R. Bindra

INTRODUCTION

Recovering function after a tendon injury to the hand continues to remain a challenge in clinical practice. Although suturing the two ends of a severed tendon may seem to be the most intuitive method today, tendon lacerations have been controversial for two centuries. Various researchers in both clinical and experimental fields have held contrasting views on all aspects of tendon injuries, from physiology of the normal tendon and its response to injury to the timing and technique of repair and subsequent mobilization. This chapter aims to present a historical timeline of evolving concepts of tendon surgery to provide insight into the parallel development of experimental research and surgical techniques that are behind the current fundamental principles of tendon surgery.

The turning point in modern flexor tendon surgery came with the controversial report by Kleinert and coworkers presented at the annual meeting of the American Society of Surgeons of the Hand in 1967 *(1)*. The authors reported better results with primary tendon repair than was then thought possible. The initial report was met with disbelief, as it challenged scientific concepts of tendon healing of that time period *(2)*. Further improvements in surgical techniques led to more clinical reports of success with primary tendon repair, resulting in a new wave of experimental investigations into the healing process that brought on the modern concepts of tendon healing and repair.

Tendons Should Not Be Repaired

The physician philosopher Galen (129–ca210 AD) began his work, the "Ars parva," in the ancient civilization of Pergamum in Greece and later found fame in Rome. Likely the result of an inadvertent suture of a lacerated median nerve, he warned that attempts to suture a tendon would result in severe pain, twitching, and, in extreme instances, convulsions and death *(3)*. At the time, there was no clear distinction between nerves and tendons—a white tubular structure (the nerve) entered the muscle and a similar looking structure (the tendon) exited at the opposite end. Galen called the latter a "neuron". Galean concepts (and misconceptions) dominated medicine for over a thousand years in Europe, to such an extent that little heed was paid to Avicenna, an Arab physi-

From: *Orthopedic Biology and Medicine: Repair and Regeneration of Ligaments, Tendons, and Joint Capsule*
Edited by: W. R. Walsh © Humana Press Inc., Totowa, NJ

cian from Hamadan, Persia, around the 10th century who was the first to recommended tendon repair after laceration or rupture.

Tendons Can Heal if Repaired

Avicenna's prescription of tendon repair found a following 600 yr later when Italian Arabist Surgeons of the 17th century, such as Roger of Parma and Roland of Milan, began to practice and advocate the operation of tendon repair. William of Salicet noted that the two ends of a cut tendon could be brought into approximation and stitched as was then done for skin and flesh to allow a better union and cicatrix. He also dispelled the belief that the pain caused by the nerve and needle would lead to convulsions. This belief spread to the French school, which developed during the Renaissance with Guy de Chulise who recommended the repair of nerves and tendons in defense of the doctrine of William. Ambroise Paré, the famed French surgeon of the time, wrote about the success of primary tendon repair that healed by first intention. Near the same period, the Italian surgeon Andre Della Croce also advocated tenorrhaphy more decidedly, devoting several pages to the operation in his work on surgery and reporting several cases with success. In 1682, Meekren demonstrated the absence of pain in tendons when he experimentally crushed tendon fibers and partially divided them in experimental animals *(3)*. However, other surgeons continued to follow Galean concepts and wrote about the pain, swelling, inflammation, and convulsions that could be caused by the needle penetrating nerves and tendons as it was directly transmitted to the brain. The concern of a sharp needle prick in the tendon was such that Bienase developed a technique to bring severed tendon ends together by placing silk sutures around them.

Tendons Are Insensitive

A clear distinction between nerves and tendons was first proposed in 1752 by Von Haller. His publication on the sensibility and irritability of various tissues conclusively demonstrated that tendons were insensitive *(4)*. This work received approval from the French Academy of Science, paving the way for acceptance of tenorrhaphy in mainland Europe. In the late 17th and early 18th Centuries, tenorrhaphy was given a further boost by several animal experimentations that showed successful healing of Achilles and wrist tendons in dogs. This success then spread to England with Hunter's experiments on canine Achilles tendon, which illustrated healing with an encircling callus similar to healing bone. His compilation of observations during the Seven Years' War (1756–1763) when he served as surgeon with the British army was entitled, *A Treatise on the Blood, Inflammation, and Gun-Shot Wounds*. Published posthumously in 1794, his book outlined fundamental principles of inflammation and tissue healing.

Antiseptic Surgery

In 1865, Louis Pasteur suggested that decay was caused by living organisms in the air, which upon entering matter, caused it to ferment. Joseph Lister in Scotland made the connection with wound sepsis and began to apply it in his practice with the use of carbolic acid to disinfect wounds and to prepare the operative site for surgery. In 1867, he established principles for "antiseptic" surgery, including tenets, e.g., instruments must be disinfected, surgeons must wash their hands and wear clean clothes. German surgeons led by Robert Koch followed Lister's antiseptic practices in surgery with success in the Franco-Prussian War from 1870–1872. The turning point in antiseptic surgery was the successful surgical wiring of a closed fracture of the patella by Lister (1877) without infection. It became clear that it was possible to operate on extremities without complication of infection and ensuing gangrene.

Tendons Can Be Reconstructed With Grafted Tissue

Experimental studies in the end of the 19th century demonstrated that it was possible to directly transplant tendons between different species of animals. Peyrot (1886) and Monod (1887) successfully used animal tendons to reconstruct tendon defects in their patients. Following Mainzer's report in 1902 of tendon lengthening using portions of paralyzed tendons for poliomyelitis, several reports of tendon transfers began to appear in the literature *(4)*. Experimental studies of transplantation of tendon and fascia became common in the early 1900s with reports by Kirschner and Rehn in Germany and Lewis and Davis in the United States. The rapid progress in tendon surgery then came upon an unexpected and apparently insurmountable complication—adhesion and scarring of the grafted tissue. Biesalski (Berlin, 1910) offered some hope when he found that adhesions could be avoided by using the autogenous sheaths of tendons.

Tendon Injuries are Best Repaired With Tendon Grafts

Surgery on flexor tendons in the hand for repair or reconstruction became standard practice by the first quarter of the 20th century. The use of palmaris longus and toe extensors as tendon grafts in the hand were first reported by Lexer in Germany, in 1912 *(4)*. Lexer effectively reconstructed flexor tendons lost after sepsis, ischemic contractures, and untreated lacerations. He established principles, such as placing the tendon anastomosis distant from the skin incision, use of local skin flaps to prevent skin-tendon adherence, and commencement of motion as early as 6 d after repair.

In 1916, Leo Mayer published classic articles on tendon transplantation that describe the science of tendon healing and the principles of surgical technique *(5–7)*. Most of Mayer's work was done on the foot and ankle, and he demonstrated the anatomy of the tendon sheath, blood supply of the tendon, and the concept of tendon and tendon–sheath motion. In 1918, Sterling Bunnell wrote his first of several articles reviewing the anatomy and physiology of tendons and the importance of the paratenon in providing an adequate gliding mechanism. He stressed that the basis for successful surgery in the hand was the atraumatic surgical technique using a bloodless field with perfect asepsis and careful assistance to avoid tissue damage. He also stressed the importance of postoperative immobilization with planned mobilization delayed until 3 wk postsurgery *(8)*. Bunnell refined his surgical technique over the next 3 yr and described an atraumatic suture technique to repair tendons.

In 1928, Bunnell presented further refinements in surgical techniques in hand surgery *(9)*. He demonstrated that not only tendons could be repaired but also damaged digital nerves. He found that flexor tendons severed opposite the proximal phalanx—the region he later called the "no man's land" did not do well after suture, as the junction became adherent in the narrow fixed channel, and the healed tendon did not glide. He recommended that it was better to excise the entire tendon and replace it with a smooth graft with paratenon. The graft was sutured in place in the palm and at the tip of the finger with more satisfactory gliding and function after healing. His technique involved the use of braided silk placed in the tendon for a distance of three or four zigzag stitches, starting a centimeter from the cut end of the tendon, and burying the knots within the tendon leaving minimum silk on the tendon surface. For rehabilitation, he suggested keeping the wrist in the flexion for 1 mo by means of an adhesive band or a flat metal dorsal splint while allowing active motion with the concept that the flexion of the wrist steals the muscle's strength but allows full amplitude of motion.

Timely Mobilization Benefits Healing

By now it had become clear that prolonged immobilization would lead to the formation of significant adhesions and scarring with loss of motion. When Mason and Allen studied the timeline of tendon healing in 1941, the prevailing belief was that tendons healed simply by scar tissue formation that under physiological stresses converted to tendon-like tissue *(10)*. A wrist tendon in a canine model was divided and immediately repaired with a silk suture using a technique that incorporated two transversely running sutures placed 1 cm from the cut end in each part of the tendon. Sutures from either end were tied securely to bring the tendon ends together to allow placement of a few fine approximating sutures. In contradiction to Bunnell's philosophy of burying the suture within the repair, their suture lay outside the tendon with one knot on either side. The cut ends were closely approximated with a few fine silk sutures. It was felt that this method of suture would leave tendon ends free to participate in the healing process. They examined the healing tendons at intervals varying from 2 to 68 d by histological examination and tensile strength testing using a spring scale.

Mason and Allen found two histological stages of tendon healing with cellular contribution from both the tendon and surrounding tissues. The first stage involved proliferation to form a fibroblastic cuff between and around the ends of the tendon. They referred to this as the "stage of hyperplasia" which lasted about 14–16 d. The second stage of repair resulted in the formation of tendon callus that ultimately converted into the tendon and was referred to as the stage of "organization and differentiation." They concluded that connective tissues both around and within the tendon were important in the healing process. However, variations in tensile strength over the period of tendon healing demonstrated three distinct phases. During the first 4 or 5 d after suture, the tensile strength of the sutured tendon dropped considerably. At this time, the tendon ends were soft and held together by a gelatinous exudate, and the repair failed by suture pull-out of the tendon. This first healing phase was the "exudative stage". The tensile strength rose rapidly after 5 d until d 14–16 to reach a plateau by the d 19–21. This corresponded to the histological phase of fibroplasia. They found that tendons allowed unrestricted use after 3 wk showed a sharp rise in tension and were becoming 50% stronger than immobilized tendons after as little as 1 wk of motion. Mason and Allen concluded that the application of motion very early after repair would be harmful, but at the 3-wk phase, motion was beneficial to the repair process. They made the following recommendations regarding movement after repair: motion too early is liable to cause marked reaction and thickening, and motion

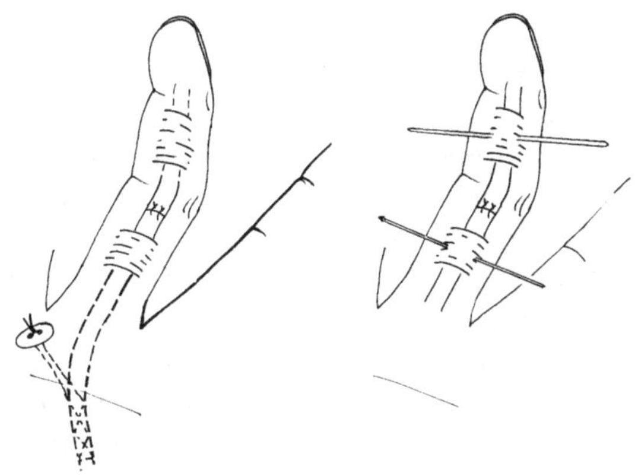

Fig. 1: The "suture at a distance" technique that was first employed for primary tendon repair. Bunnell used a pullout suture placed in the proximal tendon to take tension off the tendon repaired with fine sutures. The suture was tied over a button in the palm. Verdan placed a transfixing needle in each part of the tendon for the same purpose. The needles were removed after 3 wk.

must be built up gradually with active guarded motion followed by unrestricted use later. This publication firmly established the concept of delayed active mobilization after tendon repair and that motion begun in the first 2–3 wk postrepair was harmful.

Injured Flexor Tendons Can Be Repaired Primarily in Selected Cases

Near the same time period, Bunnell published his technique for primary repair of severed tendons in the hand *(11)*. He excised the sublimis tendon to allow better gliding of the repaired profundus. The laceration itself was repaired with very fine coapting silk sutures. Tension was taken off the repair by placing a stainless steel pull-out suture proximally in the tendon at the palm level (Fig. 1). The wire ends were delivered at the interdigital web and tied over a button to allow removal after healing. In the first edition of his book, *Surgery of the Hand*, published 4 yr later, Bunnell presented the prerequisites for primary repair of severed tendons: repair must be done within 6 h (infection was a prime concern in the preantibiotic era) by a surgeon skilled in this type of surgery and with thorough debridement and covering of all vulnerable tissues *(12)*.

Sumner Koch used the Mason-Allen technique to perform primary repair of divided flexor tendons under ideal circumstances *(13)*. Only five of 46 patients in this series met his strict criteria for primary tendon repair and included fingers free from excessive scar formation; uninjured synovial sheath to allow smooth gliding of the repair; and intact pulley mechanism and mobile joints. If primary end-end repair could not be achieved, he used the excised sublimis or a toe extensor as a bridge graft run through the digit and connecting the profundus tendon in the distal finger and in the palm. The injured hand was immobilized in a plaster with the wrist and elbow flexed for 6 or 7 d with dressing changes at 3- or 4-d intervals. Active motion was allowed at the end of the wk 3. A key principle in the postoperative period was that relaxation at the suture line was achieved by flexion of the wrist and moderate flexion of the metacarpophalangeal joints, never at the interphalangeal joints, to avoid permanent flexion contractures in them. Physical therapy began at the end of wk 4 with the purpose to stimulate circulation by hydrotherapy and massage of the flexor muscle and to maintain passive mobility of the finger joints.

Infection was the most common cause of failure in Boyes' series of primary digital flexor tendon repair published in 1947 *(14)*, followed by adhesion of the repaired digital flexor tendons in what he called the "critical zone." The third cause of failure was complications from poorly placed surgical incisions. Using Bunnell's techniques, he recommended exposure by midlateral incisions in the digits with additional transverse incisions in the palm. He suggested primary tendon repair only in those cases in which the wound was sharp, of short duration, and without any accompanying fractures or soft tissue damage. In these ideal conditions, Boyes recommended removal of the sublimis down to its insertion and repair of the profundus tendon alone. He advocated removal of the sheath overlying the repair and a lateral release of the pulleys to relieve tension and prevent ischemic necrosis of the tendon ends. If conditions were less than ideal, the wound was closed primarily after the excision of devitalized tissue. Joint motion was maintained passively with a plan to return for a delayed repair of the tendons 3 or 4 wk later using the Bunnell method of "suture at a distance" with fine interrupted sutures at the repair site and stainless steel wire pullout placed proximally in the palm.

In 1947, Littler reported successful management of flexor tendon injuries by reconstruction with a free graft *(15)*. His principles for successful tendon grafting were (1) excision of the entire fibrous flexor sheath except for the pulleys at the base of the proximal and middle phalanges; (2) use of a Bunnell stainless steel pullout suture for the distal juncture and a silk or nylon Bunnell suture at the proximal juncture in the palm; and (3) suturing the graft at the lumbrical level in the palm and covering the juncture with this muscle. He recommended complete immobilization for the first 3 wk, followed by removal of the skin sutures and pullout wire. Passive joint exercises were started at 3 wk, progressing to active flexion exercises by wk 4. He believed primary repair of the profundus tendon could be attempted if the tendon was divided at the middle phalanx level. However, he thought that it was better to place the repair junction as close to the profundus insertion as possible, even if it meant sacrificing a portion of the distal tendon.

Guy Pulvertaft reiterated these principles in the Hunterian lecture delivered to the Royal College of Surgeons in London in 1948. He recommended primary tendon repair only when ideal circumstances existed; in these cases, he advised excision of the sublimis tendon and repair of the profundus alone. If immediate repair could not be preformed, Pulvertaft felt that treatment with a tendon graft was appropiate once the wounds had healed, the acute inflammation had resolved, and when full digital mobility was restored *(16)*.

In his editorial (*Journal of Bone and Joint Surgery*, 1959), Mason pointed out the strict criteria for primary repair of flexor tendons in the fibrous flexor sheath. In most cases, it was best to simply cleanse and close the wound to promote healing to occur and carry out repair by a tendon graft as a secondary procedure *(17)*. In the same issue, Boyes reiterated that secondary reconstruction with a tendon graft done properly would result in a higher output of satisfactory function than direct repair *(18)*. In the largest series of the time, Kelly and coworkers retrospectively reviewed the outcome of 789 tendon injuries. They recommended that injuries of the flexor tendons should be repaired primarily in the carpal tunnel and at the palmar level when the character of the wound permitted. However, they felt that flexor tendons cut within the area of the annular ligament had to adhere to survive, and the results of primary repair were significantly poorer than those after secondary repair by tendon grafting *(19)*.

Other reports in the 1950s further consolidated the principles established by Sterling Bunnell over three decades earlier *(20–22)*:

1. Successful repair of both sublimis and profundus tendons in the finger was impossible, and the flexor sublimis should be excised.
2. Primary suture of the flexor profundus within zone II or "no man's land" rarely succeeded, and the preferred treatment was a tendon graft extending from the palm to the tip of the finger.
3. It was unsafe to commence motion before 3 wk.

Use of Prophylactic Antibiotics in Flexor Tendon Surgery

Although Fleming discovered penicillin as early as 1928, it was only in the 1940s that it began to be produced on a large scale for widespread use. However, the scarcity of drugs during World War II and a lack of universal agreement on the prophylactic use of antibiotics saw little use of the drug after surgery, such as tendon repair, until the 1950s. Thereafter, it became routine practice to administer prophylactic penicillin intramuscularly for 6 d after tendon repair surgery *(21)*.

Primary Repair and Early Motion for All Flexor Tendon Injuries

Verdan from Switzerland felt that the policy of free tendon graft in preference of tendon repair after injury was too rigorous *(23)*. He felt that delayed tendon grafting was only justified when general or local conditions did not allow immediate repair. He proposed a technique of tendon repair that involved a 1-cm excision of the fibrous flexor sheath, placement of two percutaneous transfixing needles in each segment of the tendon, and accurate approximation of the tendon ends with four small epitenon stitches using 6/0 arterial silk (Fig. 1). He removed the pins and splint 3 wk postoperatively to start motion and reported results comparable to tendon grafting. The premise for this technique was relaxation of the repair by sutures placed some distance from the division site, fine sutures at the repair site, and in-growth of healing elements from surrounding tissues through the window in the tendon sheath.

Thus, the concept of primary tendon repair first began with the basic tenets of (1) relaxation of the repair by sutures placed some distance from the site of division; (2) accurate tendon reapproximation with a few fine sutures; and (3) excision of the fibrous sheath to leave a window over the healing area to allow the in-growth of elements of healing and blood supply.

In Israel, Kessler believed that tendon repair with a secure suture allowing early motion would lead to primary healing without adhesions *(24)*. He described a new type of grasping suture and attempted controlled motion from the third day. His suture technique was not very different from that described by Mason and Allen two decades earlier; in Kessler's stitch, the longitudinal components of the suture were contained within the tendon (Fig. 2). Experimenting on chicken tendons, he found that mild adhesions did occur around the repaired tendon, but they were fine bundles aligned with the direction of movement and did not significantly affect tendon excursion. He reported

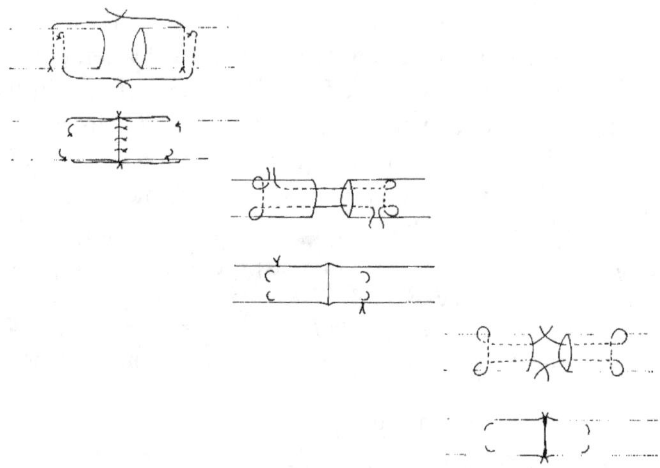

Fig. 2. The Mason-Allen core suture grasped the tendon with a transverse pass, and longitudinal limbs of the suture were tied to approximate the tendon. The Kessler stitch was based on the same concept, but the longitudinal limbs were placed within the tendon. Tajima further refined the Kessler suture by burying the knots within the repair.

similar success in a small series using the same "grasping" stitch followed by early motion.

Around the same time as Kessler's report, Kleinert and Associates presented their 10-yr experience with primary repair of both flexor tendons in No Man's Land. The paper presented at the 1967 meeting of the American Society for Surgery of the Hand became one of the most controversial presentations of the time *(25)*. All lacerations were sharp with minimal soft tissue damage, no contamination, and no associated bone injuries. After tendon repair, their patients started immediate mobilization in an indigenous splint with rubber band traction that provided passive-finger flexion and allowed active extension by the patient. They reported that 87% of results were good to excellent on private service patients compared with 76% poor results on teaching service patients, demonstrating that patient compliance was an important factor in the final outcome of these injuries. In his discussion of the paper, Boyes found these estimates to be the most outstanding results to date *(26)*. Such astonishment and controversy arose after the presentation that a committee of the society went to Louisville to examine patients and review the results for themselves *(2)*! The original presentation was never published, and the first written article from Louisville appeared in 1973, where the authors stressed the importance of early tendon mobilization—abolishing the concept of postoperative immobilization for 3 wk as proposed by Mason 30 yr earlier *(27)*. Since the late 1960s, the practice of primary tendon repair followed by early motion became popular and has been reported by several authors *(28–31)*.

Duran proposed a controlled passive motion regime starting 2–5 d after surgery with intermittent passive flexion and active extension of the digits *(32)*. The advantage of this regime was the reduced likelihood of joint contracture from continual flexion maintained by rubber bands in the Kleinert program. Duran's regime resulted in improved results over delayed mobilization in a comparative clinical study *(33)*.

First reports of early *active* mobilization after repair were proposed in separate reports by Becker and Savage, who developed stronger repairs that could withstand more aggressive rehabilitation *(28,34)*. Small and colleagues in Belfast, Northern Ireland were the first to propose a simple protocol for *controlled early active* mobilization of flexor tendons 48 h after routine repair using a Kessler core suture *(29)*. This regime required both active flexion and extension while protected in a splint and is now referred to as the "controlled active motion" or "Belfast regime." Subsequent studies have confirmed its simplicity, safety, and effectiveness with even more active repetitions every hour than originally proposed *(30,35)*.

To provide more synergistic active digital motion, Strickland proposed a modification of splinting as part of the controlled active motion protocol *(36)*. A splint is fashioned to hold the metacarpophalangeal joints in 60° of flexion. A hinge at the wrist level allows full flexion and 30° extension of the wrist. The patient then passively bends the digits into a composite fist and extends the wrist, actively maintaining the fingers in a flexed position. The digits are then extended as the wrist is actively flexed. This method provides more excursion and a physiological motion of the repaired tendon but requires fabrication of a special splint and sufficient understanding of this synergistic movement by the patient.

The improved techniques of tendon repair supported by clinical reports of the safety of active motion after repair has led to the adoption of controlled active mobilization protocols that are started 1 or 2 d after routine flexor tendon repair.

The Flexor Tendon has Intrinsic Healing Capabilities

Early research into the process of tendon healing in the middle of the 20th century suggested that tendon healing was mainly the result of reparative efforts of the surrounding tissue and that adhesions were important for tendon healing. Peacock pointed out the phases of tendon healing and felt that the tendon cells were not capable of collagen production, and the migration of peripheral cells provided the blood vessels and fibroblasts for collagen production *(37,38)*. Supporting these observations, Potenza further demonstrated that if blocking tubes were placed about the repair sites, preventing migration of granulation tissue from the sheath to the site of repair, healing was delayed or prevented *(39)*.

Successful clinical results that demonstrated tendon healing without adhesions in the 1970s and 1980s challenged conventional beliefs and stimulated new research into the science. Most prominent among investigators of the time were Gelberman, Lundborg, and Manske.

The first issue that required clarification was the vascularity of the tendon. How could an avascular structure heal without in-growth of vessels or adhesions to the synovial sheath? As far back as 1887, Berkenbusch established that flexor tendons were poorly vascularized within the sheaths *(40)*. The short vincular vessels mainly remained on the surface of the tendons, and watershed areas in between were avascular, leading to the belief that synovial fluid diffusion was responsible for all or most of tendon nutrition *(39)*. Further clarification was provided by Manske and his associates with the use of tracer uptake to study flexor tendon nutrition in experimental animals of different species *(41)*. They noted a dual source of nutrition with diffusion more effective than perfusion and responsible for nutrition to the avascular segments of the tendon. With demonstration of tendon healing in the avascular environment of the knee joint and tissue culture media, it became clear that the reparative process of tendon healing could proceed on nutrition derived from diffusion alone *(42,43)*.

Experimental studies had previously suggested that revascularization of the flexor tendons and grafts during the healing process took place from peritendinous tissues via adhesions with minor contribution from the tendons' own vessels *(44,45)*. Gelberman and coauthors were the first to document the vascular response associated with the healing of flexor tendons without extrinsic vessel in-growth *(46)*. In their canine study, they showed extension of pre-existing vessels that initially extended on the tendon surface and then penetrated the substance as intratendinous vessels through normally avascular regions to reach the site of repair by 17 d postinjury. This vascular in-growth phase coincided with an increase in the strength at the repair site and was positively influenced by motion.

Effect of Motion on the Healing Process

In 1927, Garlock recommended active motion within limits of pain on the fifth postoperative day after tendon repair *(47)*. He felt that active motion was safer, because it was limited by pain and that early motion would prevent adhesions with the sheath. He based this on his experimental studies on the repair process in dogs, where he demonstrated that scar tissue between the divided ends of the tendons progressively increased in strength and density following d 5 without any initial weakening.

Unfortunately, Garlock's work never seemed to gain clinical favor, and Bunnell's doctrine of immobilization for 3 wk prevailed. This was reinforced by Mason and Allen's experimental work in 1941 that demonstrated weakening of immobilized tendons for several days after repair, and surgeons continued the practice of delaying mobilization until 3 wk postrepair *(10)*.

Following successful clinical reports of early motion in the 1970s, Gelberman and coworkers studied the effects of mobilization with a comparative study in a canine model *(48)*. Tendons continuously immobilized did not show any significant increase in strength until 12 wk. Tendons that were mobilized passively after a delay showed increased strength in comparison to the immobilized groups at each time interval beyond 3 wk. The most encouraging finding was that tendons passively mobilized immediately after repair showed remarkably higher values to ultimate load at each time interval than the two previous groups. In addition, tendon gliding measured by angular rotation was low in immobilized tendons and notably higher in tendons in both immediate and delayed mobilization groups at 6 wk, reaching normal values by 12 wk. Gelberman proceeded with microangiographic studies to correlate motion with revascularization. Early tendon mobilization was associated with an increased number of vessels within the sheath, around the repair site and within the tendon at the site of suture *(49)*. Immobilization beyond 3 wk had a deleterious effect on the healing process with a significant reduction in tendon vascularity *(50)*. The same group then examined DNA content as an index of tissue cellularity to assess the effect of mobilization on cellular response *(51)*. The results paralleled those of strength and vascularity with significantly higher total DNA content at the repair site and in the tendon sheath in mobilized versus immobilized tendons with the difference between the groups progressively greater with time. Repair site cellularity was 140% greater;

the sheath cellularity was 60% greater than the immobilized tendons at 12 wk. Immobilized tendons showed no change in DNA content during the entire period studied.

Motion also changes the morphology of the healing tendon *(51)*. In a canine experiment, tendons in early stages of healing were studied by light and electron microscopy. Within 10 d after repair, mobilized tendons demonstrated a proliferative response of the epitenon with a smooth covering over the repair and adhesion-free healing by 42 d. The predominant origin of the repair site cell was the surface epitenon cell, rather than the endotenon, and cells aligned along the motion axis. Little healing was noted in the immobilized group by 10 d with predominance of collagen absorption between 21 and 42 d with few signs of protein synthesis. There was a lack of early epitenon response, and tendon healed mainly by a delayed proliferation of endotenon cells.

The outcome of these studies is clear. Intrinsic tendon healing is possible independent of in-growth of adhesions providing physiological loads are applied to the tendon to stimulate vascularity, cellular activity, and collagen synthesis.

Evolution of the Surgical Incision

When surgeons first considered repair of flexor tendons in the hand, they simply chose the direct approach, incising the finger down the middle, over the tendon, and away from the important neurovascular structures. In his landmark paper on reconstruction of the hand published in 1924, Bunnell was the first to condemn the anterior approach because of the flexion contracture that inevitably resulted *(52)*. He also pointed out that the incision risked damaging flexor pulleys and created increased potential for scarring over the repaired tendon. He recommended a lateral incision that was neutral in respect to flexion extension of the digit or one that was placed zigzag across flexion creases and, hence, would not contract longitudinally. He later termed the lateral approach the "midlateral incision" and recommended that the incision be placed dorsal to the neurovascular bundle to avoid injury to the digital nerve, which was elevated anteriorly with the flap.

The other approach popular at the time was the "anterolateral incision" described by Kanavel and Mason in 1939 *(53)*. The latter was centered over the digital nerve and mobilized the volar skin flap, leaving the nerve (and digital artery) in place. The anterolateral incision was notable for reduced bleeding, as the dorsal branch of the digital artery was not violated but did cause some compromise of sensation in the volar flap.

Around 1952, an anteriorly placed zigzag approach began to find favor among hand surgeons treating Dupuytren's disease. Initially used for palmar fasciectomy, it was also subsequently found to be useful for disease extending into the finger. Julian Bruner first started using the zigzag approach for flexor tendon surgery in 1965 with its advantages of direct access, extensibility, and preservation of neurovascular bundles *(54)*. The report presented at the Anglo-Scandinavian Symposium of Hand Surgery in 1967 saw the acceptance of this incision that now bears his name. Most hand surgeons currently use one of the three incisions previously described.

Evolution of the Core Stitch

The goal of hand surgeons has been to create a tendon repair strong enough to withstand immediate active motion regimes and allow an early return to normal activity. Since Kleinert's report of successful early mobilization after tendon repair, the litera-

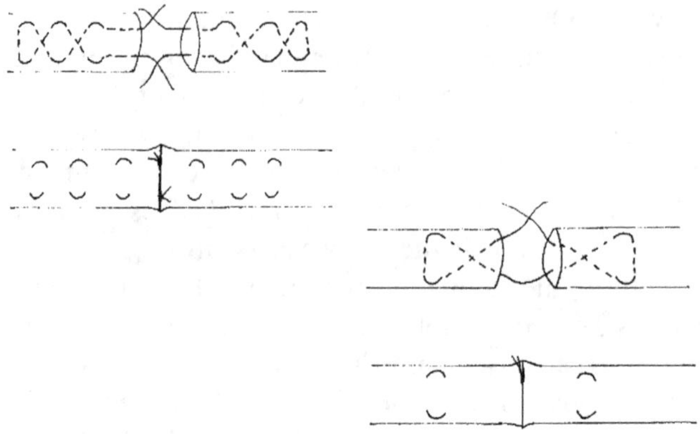

Fig. 3. The original Bunnell zigzag suture was utilized for securing the tendon-graft junction in tendon graft surgery. Kleinert modified the suture for use in primary tendon repairs.

ture on hands surgery has been inundated with reports of various modifications of core sutures with comparative biomechanical studies.

In the early 1920s, both Garlock and Bunnell described a similar technique to suture tendons using a zig-zag suture placed within the tendon substance *(9,47)*. However, Bunnell did not suture the tendon ends together with this stitch. Instead, he approximated the tendon ends with a few fine sutures and used a zig-zag pullout suture in the proximal tendon stump to take tension off the repair *(9)*.

With the 1940s came the use of the Mason stitch with two transverse passes within each tendon stump and longitudinal limbs of the suture running outside the tendon from where they were knotted (Fig. 2; *10*). This was the first description of an end-end repair that was adopted for clinical use.

Kleinert and coworkers started to use a shorter version of the Bunnell suture for primary end-end approximation of tendons in the 1950s and reported their series in 1967 (Fig. 3; *1*). In 1969, Kessler described his stitch, a modification of the Mason stitch, where the entire suture was placed within the tendon. His technique had the knots placed outside the tendon at opposite ends (Fig. 2; *24*).

Kleinert and coworkers supplemented the "core" stitch with a simple running epitenon stitch to tidy the tendon. Tajima modified the Kessler core stitch by inserting the suture through the cut end of the tendon to allow the knots to be buried within the repair site (Fig. 2; *55*). This technique of suture placement within the tendon had the additional advantage of providing a hold in each tendon end to enable manipulation through a pulley (if necessary) without direct handling of the tendon itself. Later reports from the Louisville group described the use of this modified Kessler stitch with a simple running epitenon or a bowel-type Lembert inverting epitenon stitch *(56)*.

Pennington indicated that correct placement of the transverse component of the Kessler suture was critical to obtaining a "locking" stitch. It was essential to place the transverse pass of the suture superficial to the longitudinal part of the suture. Longitudinal traction applied to the suture would result in a tightening loop around the enclosed tendon fibers, effectively locking the suture in place *(57)*.

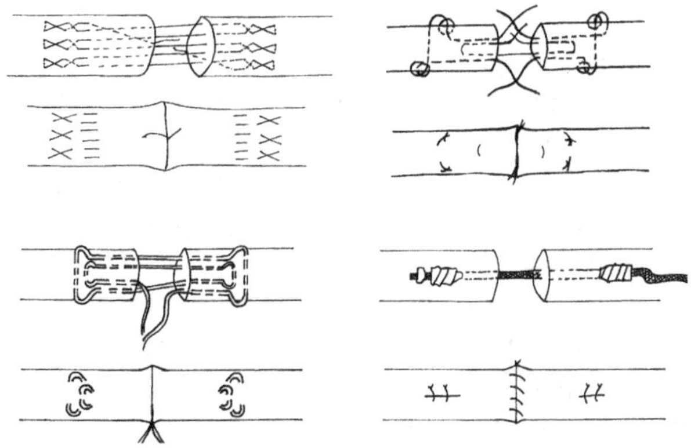

Fig. 4. The Savage was the first multistrand core stitch introduced to increase repair strength. Strickland added a second suture loop to his locking suture modification of the Kessler stitch to create a four-strand repair. Using a double-armed looped suture, Silva et al. obtained an eight-strand repair. The Tenofix uses a multistrand steel wire held between an anchor fixed in each end of the tendon.

Urbaniak was one of the first researchers to compare mechanical properties of suture materials and techniques that were in use in 1975 *(58)*. Both in vitro and vivo studies in a canine model demonstrated that Ethilon (monofilament nylon) had the lowest tensile strength and Tevdec, a braided polyester suture, was the strongest. He noted that tying a knot in a suture markedly altered its tensile strength, reducing it by 22–47% in all materials except steel, which only lost 10% of its original strength. Sutures placed parallel to the collagen bundles of the tendon failed by pullout; sutures oriented obliquely or transversely failed by breaking. The in vivo study in dogs (immobilized after repair) showed that repair strength dropped during the first 10 d, more so in the Bunnell suture, which he attributed to its strangling effect. Urbaniak measured the normal forces in intact human digital flexor tendons and found that the Kessler technique maintained adequate strength to withstand early motion against mild resistance.

Tsuge from Japan introduced a new core suture that utilized looped nylon placed within the tendon substance with its purported advantage of minimizing disturbance to circulation. He recommended a few additional epitenon sutures (if required) for better approximation *(59)*. After 2 yr, he reported success in a clinical series using a simplified version of the stitch, but the stitch has not been widely adopted *(60)*.

In 1978, Becker proposed conversion of the laceration to an oblique one, followed by accurate approximation of the tendon ends with multiple fine interrupted sutures. This suture did not find much use in clinical practice *(61)*.

The use of multiple strands in the core stitch became popular after Savage demonstrated increased strength of a suture construct when the number of strands was increased *(62)*. He devised a strong suture technique that involved multiple grasps of the tendon with six strands across the repair site and subsequently reported good results with early motion in a clinical series (Fig. 4; *28*). Using in vivo experimental studies, others have confirmed that strength of the repair ultimately depends on the amount of strands utilized and a six-strand repair, such as the Savage repair or newer eight-strand repairs that are the strongest *(63,64)*.

In 1989 Strickland reported a further modification to the Kessler core stitch, adding a locking loop to the Kessler stitch at each grasp in the tendon and burying the knots within the repair *(65)*. A few years later, he recommended an increase in the strands across the repair site by adding a horizontal mattress stitch to the modified Kessler stitch within the tendon (Fig. 4; *66*).

Hotokezaka and coworkers reemphasized Pennington's concept of the locking suture technique when they experimentally showed that the locking loop configuration tightens around bundles of tendon fibers under tension, providing greater tensile strength than the grasping configuration, which does not tighten around but pulls through bundles of fibers *(67)*. Hatanaka then showed that using a larger core suture results in a greater increase in the ultimate and gap strength values of locking loop core sutures. When a smaller suture (e.g., 4-0) is used, the strength of the suture is the weakest factor; locking loops do not provide any additional benefit over a grasping suture *(68)*.

Lubbers recently developed a novel method of tendon repair—the device termed "TenoFix," which consists of two stainless steel anchors connected with a multifilament 2-0 stainless steel suture (Fig. 4). An anchor is placed in each tendon end by a small tenotomy that is 1 cm away from the laceration, and the steel suture is threaded through the anchors. Once the tendon ends are approximated, the is suture fixed in place by crimping a stop bead threaded onto the suture. Early clinical trials have demonstrated equal efficiency when compared with a four-strand suture and lower rupture rates *(69)*.

Based on these studies, the most appropriate method to consider is a core suture with a diameter as large as possible that employs a locking technique to provide better resistance to gapping and a higher tensile strength.

Evolution of the Epitenon Stitch

In 1954, Kyle emphasized the importance of good coaptation of the tendon ends to prevent the "unsatisfied fibers" not buried within the repair from growing outward and forming adhesions with surrounding tissues *(70)*. The earliest descriptions of repair techniques always included fine "epitenon sutures" at the repair site to provide a neat suture line and invert the tendon ends. Lister and colleagues suggested the use of a simple running suture or a Lembert running suture as used in the bowel to invert the epitenon *(55)*. Mechanical studies in vitro, especially with the use of cyclic loading, have demonstrated the significance of the epitenon stitch in the prevention of gapping at the repair site *(71,72)*. Thus, it became clear that the epitenon stitch served three functions: a smooth repair that would glide easily, reinforce strength, and prevent gapping of the repair when mobilized.

In a chicken study, Lindsey illustrated that gap formation at the site of tendon repair was associated with increased "callus" formation, leading to poor clinical function from the increased adhesion formation and impaired tendon gliding *(73)*. Seradge confirmed this in a clinical series, which found the incidence of tenolysis correlated with the amount of gap present at the repair site *(74)*. Poorer clinical results were found in gaps larger than 2 mm. Canine studies have demonstrated that gap size has a strong negative effect on tensile properties, and tendons with gaps greater than 3 mm do not accrue

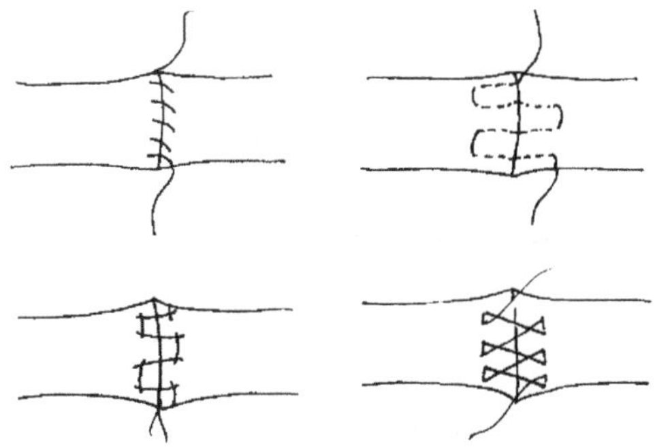

Fig. 5. The simple running or the horizontal mattress epitenon stitches can tidy tendon ends but pull out under tension. Locking looped epitenon sutures, such as the Lin or Silfverskiold, add significant strength to the repair.

stiffness or strength from 10 to 42 d. Further studies by the same group have shown that tendons with gaps larger than 3 mm have a 35% lower ultimate force and 53% lesser rigidity in comparison to tendons with no gap or gaps less than 3 mm. However, adhesions expected to develop in the presence of a gap are prevented if early motion is instituted after repair *(75)*.

Lin and coauthors suggested modification of the epitenon suture to create a locking configuration that would significantly increase the repair strength *(76)*. Subsequent reports of various types of epitenon repairs have an increased strength up to 50% (Fig. 5; *77,78*).

Most authors recommend a strong core suture using a locking configuration with four strands across the repair *(79)*. Kessler-type core sutures that run parallel with the tendon do not seem to withstand gapping even with four strands. It is essential to consider the addition of a circumferential locking loop epitenon repair *(80)*.

Evolution of Delayed Emergency

The concept of primary tendon repair within 6 h of injury as proposed by earlier authors was challenged by Iselin in 1958 when he proposed that fresh hand wounds could be closed late as a "delayed emergency" as long as they were kept clean *(81)*. Further confirmation of this concept was obtained from Madsen in 1963 when he reported that wounds could be treated as a delayed emergency with infection rates lower than 3% *(82)*. He applied similar principles to flexor tendon injuries, demonstrating that after cleansing the wound and daily dressing changes, tendon repair could be delayed by 1–3 d with good results in 79% of a series of 53 flexor tendons *(83)*.

Years later, delayed emergency was further modified. With cleansing and closure of the wound on the day of the injury, Schneider and colleagues reported repair of flexor tendons up to 3 wk later with results comparable to repair done primarily on the same day of surgery *(84)*. They did not use any antibiotics but only advocated tetanus prophylaxis on the day the injury occurred.

Thus, the concept of modern tendon surgery was set. It was possible and indeed preferable to delay the primary tendon repair for experienced surgeons and trained personnel during daytime hours.

CONCLUSION

During the past 2000 yr, several concepts have evolved in the field of tendon injury and repair. Although the most notable advances have occurred in the last 25 yr, the efforts of earlier surgeons and scientists with limited resources and techniques must not be compromised, as it is the controversy raised in previous studies that has led to the stimulation of thought and proposal of new techniques.

It is now known that tendons can heal without the development of adhesions if approximated with a good surgical technique and rehabilitated early in the postoperative period. A good repair that is strong and can resist gapping and rupture after active motion initiated soon after surgery will yield excellent results in the majority of cases.

REFERENCES

1. Kleinert H, Kutz J, Ashbell TS, Martinez E. Primary repair of lacerated flexor tendons in "No Man's Land" (abstract). *J Bone Joint Surg* 1967;49A:577.
2. Newmeyer III W, Manske P. No man's land revisited: The primary flexor tendon repair controversy. *J Hand Surg* 2004;29A:1–5.
3. Gratz C. The history of tendon suture. *Medical Journal and Record* 1928;127:156–157, 213–215.
4. Adamson J, Wilson J. The history of flexor tendon grafting. *J Bone Joint Surg* 1961;43A: 709–716.
5. Mayer L. The physiological method of tendon transplantation I. Historical, anatomy and physiology of tendons. *Surg Gynaecol Obstet* 1916;22:182–197.
6. Mayer L. The physiological method of tendon transplantation. II. Operative technique. *Surg Gynaecol Obstet* 1916;22:298–306.
7. Mayer L. The physiological method of tendon transplantation. III. Experimental and clinical experiences. *Surg Gynaecol Obstet* 1916;22:472–481.
8. Bunnell S. Repair of tendons in the fingers and description of two new instruments. *Surg Gynaecol Obstet* 1918;26:103–110.
9. Bunnell S. Repair of nerves and tendons of the hand. *J Bone Joint Surg* 1928;10:1–26.
10. Mason ML, Allen HS. The rate of healing of tendons. *Ann Surg* 1941;113:424–459.
11. Bunnell S. Primary repair of severed tendons. The use of stainless steel wire. *Am J Surg* 1940;47:502–516.
12. Bunnell S. *Surgery of the Hand*. JB Lippincott, Philadelaphia, PA, 1944.
13. Koch SL. Division of the flexor tendons within the digital sheath. *Surg Gynaecol Obstet* 1943;78:9–22.
14. Boyes JH. Immediate vs delayed repair of the digital flexor tendons. *Ann West Med Surg* 1947;1:145–152.
15. Littler JW. Free tendon grafts in secondary flexor tendon repair." *Am J Surg* 1947;74: 315–321.
16. Pulvertaft GR. Repair of tendon injuries in the hand. *Ann Royal Coll Surg* 1948;3:3–14.
17. Mason ML. Primary tendon repair. *J Bone Joint Surg* 1959;41A:575–577.
18. Boyes JH. Why tendon repair? *J Bone Joint Surg* 1959;41A:577–579.
19. Kelly AP. Primary Tendon Repairs. *J Bone Joint Surg* 1959;41A:581–598.
20. Allen HS. Management of lacerations of flexor tendons within the digits. *Surg Clin North Am* 1955;35:189–194.
21. Siler VE. Primary tenorrhaphy of flexor tendons in the hand. *J Bone Joint Surg* 1950;32A: 218–225.
22. White WL. Secondary restoration of finger flexion by digital tendon grafts. *Am J Surg* 1956;91:662–668.

23. Verdan CE. Primary repair of flexor tendons. *J Bone Joint Surg* 1960;42A:647–657.
24. Kessler I, Nissim F. Primary repair without immobilization of flexor tendon division within the flexor sheath. *Acta Orthop Scand* 1969;40:587–601.
25. Kleinert HE, Kutz JE, Ashbell TS, Martinez E . Primary repair of lacerated flexor tendons in "No Man's Land" (abstract). *J Bone Joint Surg* 1967;49A:577.
26. Boyes JH. Discussion of Kleinert/Kutz/Ashbell/Martinez paper. *J Bone Joint Surg* 1967; 49A:577.
27. Kleinert HE, Kutz JE, Atasoy E, Stormo A. Primary repair of flexor tendons. *Orthop Clin North Am* 1973;4:865–876.
28. Savage R, Risitano G. Flexor tendon repair using a "six strand" method of repair and early active mobilisation. *J Hand Surg* 1989;14B:396–399.
29. Small JO, Brennen MD, Colville J. Early active mobilisation following flexor tendon repair in zone 2. *J Hand Surg* 1989;14B:383–391.
30. Bainbridge LC, Robertson C, Gillies D, Elliot D. A comparison of postoperative mobilization of flexor tendon repairs with "passive flexion- active extension" and "controlled active motion" techniques. *J Hand Surg* 1994;19B:517–521.
31. Kitsis CK, Wade PJF, Krikler SJ, Parsons NK, Nicholls LK. Controlled active motion follwoing primary flexor tendon repair: A prospective study over 9 years. *J Hand Surg* 1998;23B:344–349.
32. Duran RJ, Houser RG. *Controlled Passive Motion Following Flexor Tendon Repair in Zones II and III*. CV Mosby, St. Louis, MO, 1975.
33. Strickland JW, Glogovac SV. Digital function following flexor tendon repair in Zone ll: A comparison of immobilization and controlled passive mobilization techniques. *J Hand Surg [Am]* 1980;5:537–543.
34. Becker H. Primary repair of flexor tendons in the hand without immobilization—preliminary report. *The Hand* 1978;10:37–47.
35. Elliot D, Moiemen NS, Flemming AFS, Harris SB, Foster AJ. The rupture rate of acute flexor tendon repairs mobilized by the controlled active motion regimen. *J Hand Surg* 1994;19B:607–612.
36. Strickland JW. Flexor tendon repair: Indiana method. *The Indiana Hand Center Newsletter* 1993;1:1–12.
37. Potenza AD. Tendon healing within the flexor digital sheath in the dog. *J Bone Joint Surg* 1962;44A:49–64.
38. Peacock EE. Biological principles in the healing of long tendons. *Surg Clin North Am* 1965;45:461–176.
39. Potenza A. Critical evaluation of flexor tendon healing and adhesion formation within artificial digital sheaths. *J Bone Joint Surg* 1963;5A:1217–1233.
40. Manske PR. Flexor tendon healing. *J Hand Surg* 1988;13B:237–245.
41. Manske PR, Bridwell K, Whiteside LA, Lesker PA. Nutrition of flexor tendons in monkeys. *Clin Orthop* 1978;136:294–298.
42. Lundborg G, Rand F. Experimental intrinsic healing of flexor tendons based upon synovial fluid nutrition. *J Hand Surg* 1978;3A:21–31.
43. Manske PR, Gelberman RH, Vande Berg JS, Lesker PA. Intrinsic flexor tendon repair. *J Bone Joint Surg* 1984;66A:385–396.
44. Lindsay W, Thomson H. Digital flexor tendons: An experimental study. Part I. The significance of each component of the flexor mechanism in tendon healing. *Br J Plast Surg* 1960;12:289–316.
45. Chaplin D. The vascular anatomy within normal tendon, divided tendons, free tendon grafts and pedicle tendon grafts in rabbits. A microangiographic study. *J Bone Joint Surg* 1973;55B:369–389.
46. Gelberman RH, Khabie V, Cahill CJ. The revascularization of healing flexor tendons in the digital sheath. *J Bone Joint Surg* 1991;73A:868–881.

47. Garlock J. The repair process in wounds of tendons and in tendon grafts. *Ann Surg* 1927;85:92–103.
48. Gelberman RH, Woo SL, Lothringer K, Akeson WH, Amiel D. Effects of early intermittent passive mobilization on healing canine flexor tendons. *J Hand Surg [Am]* 1982;7:170–175.
49. Gelberman RH, Amifl D, Gonsalves M, Woo S, Akeson WH. The influence of protected passive mobilization on the healing of flexor tendons: a biochemical and microangiographic study. *Hand* 1981;13:120–128.
50. Gelberman RH, Menon J, Gonsalves M, Akeson WH. The effects of mobilization on the vascularization of healing flexor tendons in dogs. *Clin Orthop* 1980;153:283–289.
51. Gelberman RH, Vande Berg JS, Lundborg GN, Akeson WH. Flexor tendon healing and restoration of the gliding surface. *J Bone Joint Surg* 1983;65A:70–80.
52. Bunnell S. Reconstructive surgery of the hand. *Surg Gynaecol Obstet* 1924;39:259–274.
53. Bruner J. Incisions for plastic and reconstructive (non-septic)surgery of the hand. *Br J Plast Surg* 1951;4:49–55.
54. Bruner J. The zig-zag volar-digital incision for flexor-tendon surgery. *Plast Reconst Surg* 1967;40:571–574.
55. Tajima T. History, current status and aspects of hand surgery in Japan. *Clin Orthop* 1984;184: 41–49.
56. Lister GD, Kleinert HE, Kutz JE. Primary flexor tendon repair followed by immediate controlled mobilization. *J Hand Surg [Am]* 1977;2:441–451.
57. Pennington D. The locking loop tendon suture. *Plast Reconst Surg* 1979;63:648–52.
58. Urbaniak J, Cahill JD, Mortensen RA. Tendon suturing methods: analysis of tensile strengths. In *American Academy of Orthopaedic Surgeons: Symposium on Tendon Surgery of the Hand.* CV Mosby, St. Louis, MO, 1975, pp. 70–80.
59. Tsuge K, Ikuta Y, Matshuishi, Y. Intra-tendinous tendon suture in the hand. A new technique. *Hand* 1975;7:250–255.
60. Tsuge K, Ikuta Y, Matshuishi Y. Repair of flexor tendons by intratendinous suture. *J Hand Surg* 1977;2:436–440.
61. Becker H. Primary repair of flexor tendons in the hand without immobilization: preliminary report. *Hand* 1978;10:37–47.
62. Savage R. In vitro studies of a new method of flexor tendon repair. *J Hand Surg* 1985;10B: 135–141.
63. Wagner WF, Carroll IV C, Strickland JW, Heck DA, Toombs JP. A biomechanical comparison of techniques of flexor tendon repair. *J Hand Surg* 1994;19A:979–983.
64. Winters SC, Gelberman RH, Woo SL, Chan SS, Grewal R, Seiler JG III. The effects of multiple-strand suture methods on the strength and excursion of repaired intrasynovial flexor tendons: a biomechanical study in dogs. *J Hand Surg* 1988;23A:97–104.
65. Strickland JW. Biologic rationale, clinical application and results of early motion following flexor tendon repair. *J Hand Ther* 1989;2:71–83.
66. Strickland JW. Flexor tendon injuries: Foundations of treatment. *J Am Acad Orthop Surg* 1995;3:44–54.
67. Hotokezaka S, Manske PR. Differences between locking loops and grasping loops: effects on 2-strand core suture. *J Hand Surg* 1997;22A:995–1003.
68. Hatanaka H, Manske PR. Effect of suture size on locking and grasping flexor tendon repair techniques. *J Hand Surg* 2000;24A:267–274.
69. Su B, Solomons M, Barrow A, Rosenwasser M. A randomized double blind clinical trial of Teno Fix; a novel device for tendon repair. Unpublished data 2003.
70. Kyle J, Eyre-Brook A. Flexor tendon injuries in the hand. *Br J Surg* 1954;41:502–511.
71. Wade PJF, Muir IFK, Hutcheon, LL. Primary flexor tendon repair: the mechanical limitations of the modified Kessler technique. *J Hand Surg* 1986;11B:71–76.
72. Pruitt DL, Manske PR, Fink B. Cyclic stress analysis of flexor tendon repair. *J Hand Surg* 1991;16A:701–707.

73. Lindsay WK, Thomson HG, Walker FG. Digital flexor tendons: and experimental study. Part II. The significance of gap occuring at the line of suture. *Br J Plast Surg* 1960;13:1–9.
74. Seradge H. Elongation of the repair configuration following flexor tendon repair. *J Hand Surg* 1983;8A:182–185.
75. Gelberman RH, Boyer MI, Brodt MD. The effect of gap formation at the repair site on the strength and excursion of intrasynovial flexor tendons: an experimental study on the early stages of tendon healing in dogs. *J Bone Joint Surg* 1999;81A:1975–1982.
76. Lin GT, An KN, Amadio PC. Biomechanical studies of running suture for flexor tendon repair in dogs. *J Hand Surg* 1988;13A:553–558.
77. Wade PJF, Wetherell RG, Amis AA. Flexor tendon repair: Significant gain in strength from the Halstead peripheral suture technique. *J Hand Surg* 1989;14B:232–235.
78. Silfverskiold KL, Andersson CH. Two new methods of tendon repair: An in vitro evaluation of tensile strength and gap formation. *J Hand Surg* 1993;18A:58–65.
79. Strickland JW. Development of flexor tendon surgery: twenty-five years of progress. *J Hand Surg* 2000 25A:214–229.
80. Barrie KA, Wolfe SW, Shean C, Shenbagamurthi D, Slade lll JF, Panjabi MM. A biomechanical comparison of multistrand flexor tendon repairs using an in situ testing model. *J Hand Surg* 2000;25A:499–506.
81. Iselin M. "Delayed emergencies" in fresh wounds of the hand. *Proc Royal Soc Med* 1958; 51:713–714.
82. Madsen E. "Delayed emergency" treatment of open lesions of the extremities. *Acta Orthop Scand* 1963;33:380.
83. Madsen E. Delayed primary suture of flexor tendons cut in the digital sheath. *J Bone Joint Surg* 1970;52B:264–267.
84. Schneider LH, Hunter JM, Norris TR, Nadeau PO. Delayed flexor tendon repair in no man's land. *J Hand Surg [Am]* 1977;2:452–455.

5

Basic Science of the Shoulder Ligaments

Louis J. Soslowsky and Jeffrey S. Cartmell

INTRODUCTION

The joints of the shoulder enable a large range of motion, but because they are relatively unconstrained, they can be inherently unstable. These shoulder joints are supported by numerous ligaments, which contribute to the strength and stability of the system. Knowledge of the material and structural properties of the shoulder ligaments is important in understanding shoulder function and in determining approaches to develop improved methods for repair and reconstruction of injured shoulders.

This chapter outlines the anatomy, geometry, structure, histology, biomechanics and effects on stability of the shoulder ligaments. A thorough review is provided for each ligament. It should be noted that certain ligaments of the shoulder have been more extensively studied than others. Therefore, these ligaments are discussed in greater detail than other ligaments that have a paucity of available data in the literature. The ligaments are examined in anatomical order—medial to lateral—beginning with the sternoclavicular attachments and concluding with the glenohumeral ligaments. The chapter ends with a review of the minor ligaments and ligaments with only modest data available in the literature.

STERNOCLAVICULAR LIGAMENT

Anatomy

The sternoclavicular joint is a synovial joint—the only point of true articulation between the arm and upper body. This joint consists of the medial end of the clavicle and a notch in the superolateral aspect of the sternal manubrium. The oblique anterior and posterior sternoclavicular ligaments support the anterior and posterior aspects of the sternoclavicular joint, respectively. These ligaments pass downward and medially from the sternal end of the clavicle to the anterior and posterior surfaces of the manubrium. Of these ligaments, the anterior sternoclavicular ligament is stronger than the posterior sternoclavicular ligament *(1,2)*.

ACROMIOCLAVICULAR LIGAMENT

Anatomy

The acromioclavicular ligaments, including the coracoclavicular ligament (CCL), reinforce all aspects of the acromioclavicular joint capsule. In turn, the deltoid and

From: *Orthopedic Biology and Medicine: Repair and Regeneration of Ligaments, Tendons, and Joint Capsule*
Edited by: W. R. Walsh © Humana Press Inc., Totowa, NJ

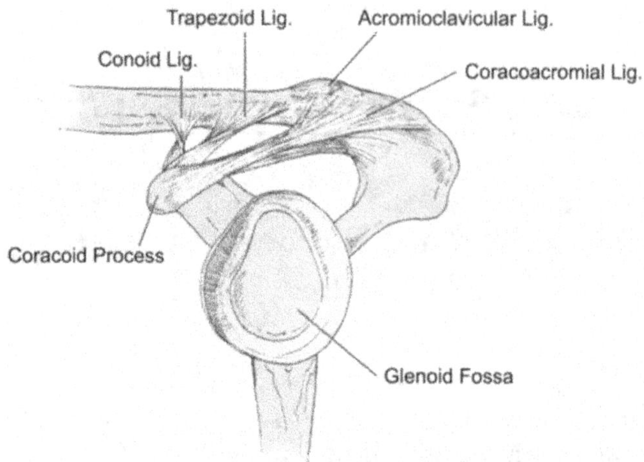

Fig. 1. Lateral view of the coracoacromial arch and glenoid fossa. Note the distinct insertions of the conoid and trapezoid ligaments on the clavicle and the close approximation of the CAL and acromioclavicular ligament. (Reprinted from ref. *4*).

trapezius muscles reinforce the superior acromioclavicular ligament. The deltoid insertion and trapezius origin also have a role in supporting the acromioclavicular joint. These ligaments act to limit movement of the clavicle relative to the scapula *(1)*. The low-threshold Ruffini neural receptor organs are commonly found in the acromioclavicular ligament in a similar quantity observed with acromioclavicular ligament and the CCL *(3)*.

CORACOCLAVICULAR LIGAMENT

Anatomy

A major support of the acromioclavicular joint is the CCL (*see* Fig. 1), which connects the clavicle and coracoid process (at the point where the clavicle passes just superior to the coracoid). The CCL is composed of two distinct components: the trapezoid and conoid ligaments. Each component connects to different aspects of the bony attachments *(1)*. It originates anterolaterally to the conoid attachment on the coracoid process and runs in an anterolateral-to-posteromedial direction to its attachment on the inferior aspect of the clavicle at the clavicle's trapezoidal line *(1,4)*.

The conoid ligament originates in a wide pattern at the base of the coracoid process. It then extends directly superior from the coracoid to its attachment on the inferior aspect of the clavicle, where its attachment appears as a tapered apex. In some cases (7.5%), the coracoid attachments of the trapezoid and conoid ligaments are confluent *(1,4–7)*.

Geometry

The trapezoid ligament is a horizontal ligament that is quadrilateral in shape, whereas the conoid ligament has the shape of a vertically oriented, inverted cone. The trapezoid ligament has a mean length of 15–19 mm and a mean width of 11–13 mm. At its clavicular attachment, the trapezoid ligament is 22 mm wide. The trapezoid ligament's

Table 1
Geometric Properties of the CCL Under Simulated In Vivo Loading (n = 24)

Geometric properties	Mean ± standard deviation
Medial conoid length	19.4 ± 4.8
Conoid clavicular width	20.6 ± 3.6
Conoid coracoid width	10.6 ± 2.0
Conoid thickness: superior	8.6 ± 1.6
Conoid thickness: medial	5.9 ± 1.1
Conoid thickness: inferior	4.4 ± 0.7
Anterior trapezoid length	19.3 ± 2.6
Trapezoid clavicular width	21.7 ± 4.0
Trapezoid coracoid width	14.0 ± 2.6
Trapezoid thickness: superior	16.0 ± 3.1
Trapezoid thickness: medial	5.5 ± 1.9
Trapezoid thickness: inferior	4.8 ± 0.6

Source: ref. *8*.

clavicular insertion is roughly three times as large as its coracoid insertion. Recent data on the dimensions of the trapezoid ligament under simulated in vivo loading conditions is presented in Table 1. The conoid ligament is slightly smaller than the trapezoid ligament with a mean length that ranges from 13 to 19 mm, and its midpoint width ranges from 5.5 to 11.5 mm. The insertion on the clavicle for the conoid ligament is approximately twice as large as its insertion on the coracoid. Data on the dimensions of the conoid ligament under simulated in vivo loading conditions is also presented in Table 1 *(1,4–8)*.

Harris et al. proposed a classification system for the three distinct types of conoid ligaments observed. In type 1 ligaments, the common conoid ligament origin is seen. In type 2 ligaments, a two-point attachment formed by the conoid ligament and transverse scapular ligament extends from the medial scapular notch, across the coracoid and to the clavicle. Type 3 attachments are a variation of type 2 ligaments, where an accessory conoid lateral fascicle arises inferomedially from the junction of the superior transverse scapular ligament and the conoid ligament. The prevalence of these ligaments types is varied: 52% show type 1 ligaments, 33% show type 2 cases, and 15% demonstrate type 3 conoid ligaments *(8)*.

Biomechanics

Elastic Response

Structural properties (peak load, stiffness, and elongation to failure) for the intact CCL are similar to those of the isolated trapezoid and conoid ligaments, demonstrating that division of one of the CCL bands has little effect on its overall strength. However, the energy absorbed at failure is significantly greater (by 73%) in the trapezoid ligament related to the conoid ligament. The structural properties for the differ-

Table 2
Structural Properties of the CCL

	Mean ± standard deviation			
	Peak load (N)	Stiffness (N/mm)	Failure elongation (mm)	Energy absorbed (Nm)^2
Intact CCL (n = 7)	500 ± 134	103 ± 30	7.7 ± 1.9	1.6 ± 0.62
Isolated conoid ligament (n = 6)	394 ± 170	105 ± 45	7.1 ± 2.1	1.1 ± 0.60
Isolated trapezoid ligament (n = 6)	440 ± 118	84 ± 19	9.2 ± 2.6	1.9 ± 0.53

Source: ref. *9*.

ent regions are shown in Table 2. During tensile testing, the intact CCL and the isolated conoid ligaments fail primarily in the ligament midsubstance or at the coracoid insertion; the isolated trapezoid ligament fails primarily at its coracoid insertion *(9)*. With decreases in mean specimen age (70–57 yr), stiffness values remain the same, but a slight increase in peak load is observed, showing age-related ligament degeneration. In these cases, sample rupture occurs mostly in the ligament midsubstance *(10)*.

In Situ Loads

With the exception of posterior loading, the conoid and trapezoid ligaments both bear similar *in situ* loads under all loading conditions. However, with posterior loading, the *in situ* loads of the trapezoid ligament are three times greater than the loads within the conoid ligament *(7)*.

Stability

The CCL is the major support of the acromioclavicular joint. However, the CCL alone cannot limit scapular rotation about the clavicle *(1,11)*. The acromioclavicular ligament helps to prevent inferior acromioclavicular joint displacement during posterior joint displacement *(7)*.

The conoid ligament limits scapular depression associated with the clavicle and inferior scapular rotation, and it also counteracts clavicle axial rotation. At large displacements, the conoid ligament is the dominant restraint to acromioclavicular joint rotation *(1,5,12)*. The trapezoid ligament provides scapular restraint during upward clavicle displacement, and helps to prevent shear forces from occurring in the acromioclavicular joint *(1,4,5)*.

CORACOACROMIAL LIGAMENT

Anatomy

The coracoacromial ligament (CAL) is a trapezoidal shaped ligament twisted into a helix between the coracoid and acromion *(13)*. As shown in Fig. 2, the CAL courses an oblique pattern over the rotator cuff and shoulder capsule, with which it has a close spatial relationship *(4)*. In fetal development, the CAL is visible by 13-wk gestation as a band that is continuous with the acromion's undersurface. By 36-wk gestation, fibers of the CAL are well organized *(14)*.

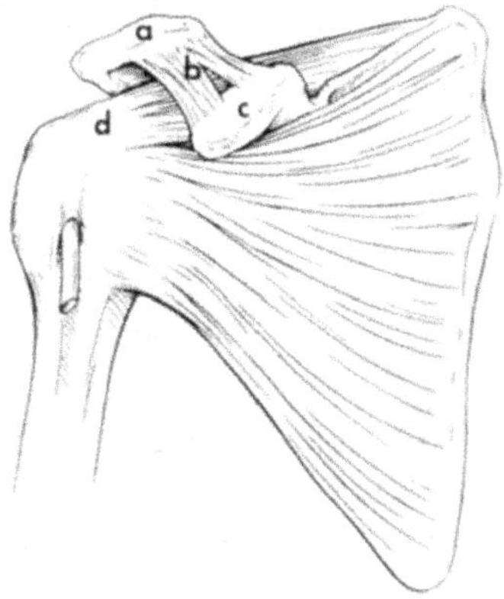

Fig. 2. Anterior view of the right shoulder, demonstrating the anatomical position of the CAL. The acromion (a) forms the origin of the CAL (b), which then attaches to the coracoid process (c). The supraspinatus tendon (d) passes through the arch formed by the CAL. (Reprinted from ref. *18*).

Table 3
Geometric Properties of the CAL

	Mean ± standard deviation)			
	Length (mm)	Thickness (mm)	Width (mm)	Area (mm^2)
Lateral Band (n = 10)	34 ± 4.2	0.96 ± 0.33	8.0 ± 2.1	8.0 ± 3.8
Medial Band (n = 10)	32.4 ± 3.1	0.99 ± 0.35	6.3 ± 1.6	6.2 ± 2.7

Source: ref. *18*.

The origin of the CAL is on the proximal third of the coracoid's lateral edge (stretching to the coracoid tip), where it attaches with the biceps tendon and coracobrachialis muscles *(4,13,15,16)*. The acromial attachment for the CAL is on the dorsal edge of the acromion, where it inserts in a Y-shaped pattern on the anterior and inferior acromial surfaces. The more superior fibers of the CAL blend with the deltoid attachments prior to entering the acromion. The medial fibers also blend into the inferior surface of the acromioclavicular joint. The more inferior fibers insert into the acromion via periosteum and fibrocartilage *(4,13,16)*.

Geometry

The CAL has a variable shape, but it is predominantly quadrangular (48%) or Y-shaped (42%), with the side of the ligaments curved, not straight. A small number of CALs (8%) display a broad band ligament, where a difference of no more than 2 mm is observed between the widths of the acromial and coracoid attachments. The broad band is primarily found in taller individuals, but the length and gap distance between the coracoid and acromion do not differ with CAL pattern *(17)*. Overall, the CAL averages 1.7 cm wide and 3.7 cm long *(4)*. However, the CAL can be divided into two anatomically distinct bands: the lateral and medial bands. Both bands show similar length and thickness, but the lateral band is wider and has a greater cross-sectional area (Table 3;

18). The CAL origin on the coracoid is approx 37 mm in length; its attachment on the acromion is 15 mm wide *(4,13,15,16)*.

Structure and Histology

The CAL consists of tightly packed parallel bundles of nearly equal-diameter collagen fibers. The structure is primarily acellular, but some elongated fibroblasts are present between the collagen fibers. A small number of parallel elastic fibers are also present *(17,19,20)*. The CAL contains mechanoreceptors, primarily the low-threshold Ruffini end organs with a lesser distribution of the fast-adapting Pacinian corpuscles *(3)*. Its vascularity includes arterial blood vessels on the posterior surface *(13)*.

The cells of the CAL have a fairly uniform appearance throughout the ligament. They are generally small and have an irregular shape owing to cytoplasmic protrusions. The cell interior is occupied mostly by the cell nuclei, and the remaining space is taken up by rough endoplasmic reticulum, mitochondria, and a few intermediate filaments *(19)*.

The CAL displays age-related histological degeneration. In younger specimens, closely packed collagen bundles, separated by thin strands of loose connective tissue with sparse vascularity and curvilinear-shaped cells, are present. With age, the collagen bundles become straightened out with a moderate increase in cellularity and a decreased vascularity in the ligament midsubstance. However, increased vascularity in periligamentous connective tissue is also observed with age *(21)*.

Biomechanics

Elastic Response

Structural and Material Properties

Mechanical testing demonstrates that the lateral CAL band is stronger than the medial band of the CAL. The stiffness of the CAL lateral band does not vary with age *(22)*. In shoulders with rotator cuff tears, the lateral band of the CAL is shorter in length with a decreased cross-sectional area relative to the lateral band from shoulders without rotator cuff tears. Decreases in material, but not structural properties, are observed in the CAL from rotator cuff–deficient shoulders associated with normal shoulders (Table 4). The differences in these observed properties may partly be a result of impingement seen in shoulders with rotator cuff tears subjecting the CAL to a more complex multidirectional loading regime *(18,23)*.

In Situ Loads

Measurable *in situ* loads of 18.3 ± 9.8 N (stress = 2.4 ± 1.8 MPa) are present in the CAL, which correspond to *in situ* strains of 4.9 ± 2.9% in the CAL. Similar values for *in situ* load and strain are observed in the CALs from shoulders with rotator cuff tears, which is interesting given the decreased CAL length in these shoulders *(23)*. This finding demonstrates that although the ligament is under significant *in situ* load, the anecdotal evidence of a "stiffer" or "tighter" CAL with rotator cuff tears is not supported.

Failure Properties

The failure loads, but not the failure stress, of the CAL lateral band decreases with age. During tensile testing, the mode of CAL failure varies between failure at the acromial insertion (68%), coracoid insertion (24%), and the ligament midsubstance (8%; 22).

Table 4
Structural and Material Properties of the Lateral Band of the CAL (n = 10)

	Mean ± standard deviation	
	Intact Rotator Cuff	Torn Rotator Cuff
Failure load (N)	311.7 ± 127.4	305.4 ± 154.8
Failure displacement (mm)	7.8 ± 2.0	7.5 ± 2.3
Stiffness (N/mm)	59.3 ± 26.3	57.5 ± 37.3
Failure stress (MPa)	46.9 ± 30.7	25.3 ± 8.7 [a]
Total failure strain (%)	23.7 ± 9.5	28.3 ± 8.6
Ligament failure strain (%)	5.6 ± 1.7	5.1 ± 1.2
Total modulus (MPa)	291.6 ± 154	120.3 ± 38.9 [a]
Ligament modulus (MPa)	1174.4 ± 437.7	658.4 ± 261.3 [a]

Source: ref. *18*.
[a] Statistical significance ($p < 0.05$)

Viscoelastic Response

Cyclic loading of the CAL for 15 cycles (between 1% and 5% strain) results in a 4% decrease in the peak load. In stress-relaxation experiments, the stress at equilibrium of the CAL is 71.2 ± 6.9% of the peak stress. With rotator cuff tears, larger decreases in the peak load (during cyclic loading) and the stress at equilibrium during relaxation are observed in the CAL relative to those seen from normal shoulders *(18,23)*.

Stability

The CAL stabilizes the superior lateral bony aspects of the shoulder and is a significant stabilizer of the glenohumeral joint at low abduction levels. Specifically, the CAL limits the anterior and inferior translation of both internally and externally rotated glenohumeral joints *(24,25)*. The CAL stabilizes the acromion and acromioclavicular joint and is the final restraint to superior subluxation of the humeral head. Lastly, the CAL reinforces the inferior capsular ligament. It may also act as a "soft tissue buffer" between the acromion and clavicle and rotator cuff *(4,16)*.

CORACOHUMERAL LIGAMENT

Anatomy

The coracohumeral ligament (CHL) is a trapezoidal ligament located in the superior part of the shoulder capsule (on its nonarticulating surface) and runs parallel to and is closely overlaid by the CAL. It is present in fetal development by 14-wk gestation as a small band of tissue between the CHL and the CAL.

The origin of the CHL is at the most posterior point on the lateral aspect of the coracoid process base (deep relative to the origin of the CAL). It appears as a broad band (2.5 cm wide) and stretches from the root of the coracoid to about 1 cm from the coracoid tip (covering approximately two thirds of the length of the coracoid process).

The superior portion of the CHL originates on the medioposterior portion of the coracoid, whereas the inferior portion of the CHL originates 1 cm medially of the coracoid tip *(4,14,20,26–30)*.

The CHL passes over the top of the shoulder and fans out laterally before joining the shoulder capsule. A small segment of the CHL blends with the rotator cuff attachments as it attaches to the anterior aspect of the greater humeral tuberosity. A larger segment extends posteriorly through the joint capsule (beneath the infraspinatus and over the bicep tendons) to attach to the lesser tuberosity of the humerus. By attaching on either side of the bicipital groove, the CHL provides a tunnel for the biceps tendon. Renditions of the CHL in the various layers of the rotator interval are shown in Fig. 3 *(20,26, 28,31,32)*.

The CHL displays distinct anterior and posterior borders *(32)*. On its lateral side, the CHL covers the interval between the anterior border of the supraspinatus muscle and superior border of the subscapularis muscle and tendon. At the lesser tuberosity, the CHL blends with the insertion of the subscapularis tendon. In its inferior direction, the CHL joins with the superior glenohumeral ligament (SGHL) *(28)*.

Geometry

The CHL has a variable thickness, which is demonstrated by the fanning of the cross-sectional area along its distal length (toward the humerus) with a midpoint value of 53.7 ± 3.2 mm^2. Additionally, the CHL displays a variable humeral insertion with 75% of CHL specimens inserting into the rotator interval between the supraspinatus and subscapularis tendons, rather than a direct bony insertion. An additional 25% of CHLs insert into the supraspinatus tendon. Cooper demonstrated some variability in CHL appearance, finding well-defined structures in only 76% of shoulders examined. In the remaining shoulders, the CHL appeared only as a fold in the anterosuperior glenohumeral capsule *(15,27,33,34)*.

Structure and Histology

Histologically, the deep layer of the CHL (on the articular side) forms a portion of the superior capsule. Conversely, the superficial layer partly covers the bursal side and is embedded in fatty tissue with only a few collagen fiber bundles present. There is only a clear demarcation between the CHL and other surrounding fiber bundles in 16.3% of observations *(35)*.

The superior portion of the CHL shows an irregular organization of collagen fibers that are interspersed with loose connective tissue and filled with fat and blood vessels. The inferior portion of the CHL has an anterior region of disorganized collagen fibers and a posterior region with distinct bundles of collagen fibers *(30)*.

Biomechanics

Elastic Response

Structural and Material Properties

During mechanical testing at a strain rate of 100 mm/min, all CHL specimens failed in the proximal ligament substance near the coracoid insertion. The ultimate load of the CHL is 359.8 ± 40.3 N, corresponding to a stress of 6.7 MPa. The stiffness of the CHL is 36.7 ± 5.9 N/mm. The CHL absorbs 2285 ± 378.2 N-m of energy and stretches 35.9

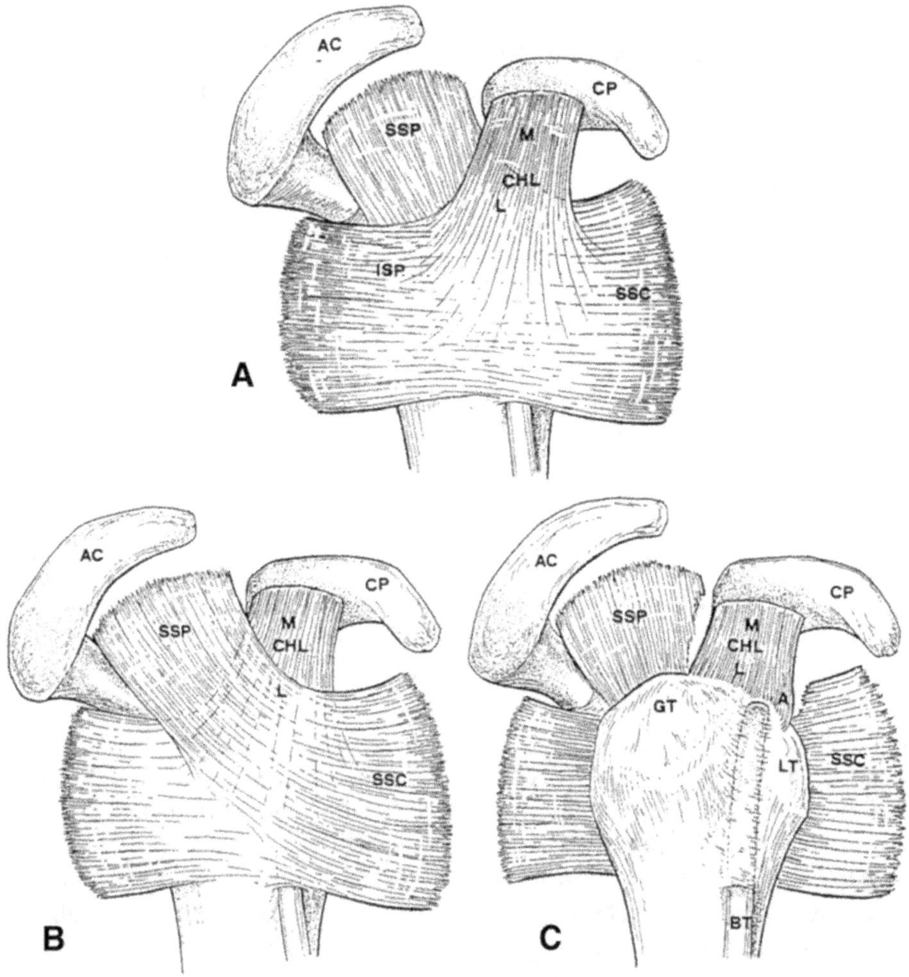

Fig. 3. **(A)** Anterolateral view of the right shoulder rotator interval that demonstrates the superior layer of the lateral rotator interval (L), which contains the superior layer of the CHL. These CHL fibers extend from the coracoid process (CP) to the insertions of the subscapularis (SSC) and supraspinatus (SSP) muscles. **(B)** Second layer of the rotator interval of the same shoulder. Fibers of the SSP and subscapularis blend with CHL fibers. **(C)** The third layer of the rotator interval from the same shoulder, showing deep CHL fibers inserting into the greater tuberosity (GT) and lesser tuberosity (LT). A, anterior covering band of long-head biceps tendon; M, medial rotator interval; ISP, infraspinatus muscle; AC, acromion. (Reprinted from ref. *33*).

± 11.9% prior to failure. This suggests that although the CHL is a capsular thickening, it displays similar biomechanical behavior to ligaments *(34)*.

In Situ Loads

With applied external anterior loading, the CHL carries internal loads at all angles of abduction. However, during posterior loading, the CHL's maximum *in situ* load is observed at 0° of abduction, and decreases with increasing abduction angles *(36)*.

Stability

The CHL resists anterior and posterior subluxation of the humeral head *(32)*. During internal rotation, the CHL contributes to the subluxation force; in neutral rotation, the CHL is a primary anterior constraint of the glenohumeral joint *(37,38)*. The CHL also limits external rotation and prevents inferior subluxation *(28)*. With the inferior glenohumeral ligament (IGHL), the CHL is the primary restraint to external rotation in abduction *(39)*. The CHL (with the SGHL) contributes to joint constraint in both anterior and posterior load application *(36)*. Inferior stabilization by the CHL may be proportional to compressive loads and displacements *(40)*.

The CHL becomes taut in flexion and external rotation of the shoulder, as well as in anterior and posterior translation of the humeral head. During lateral motion, CHL tightening occurs earlier than during medial rotation. Therefore, release of the CHL may aid in the treatment of frozen shoulders *(20,41)*.

INFERIOR GLENOHUMERAL LIGAMENT

Anatomy

In 1981, Turkel et al. described the IGHL as a structure attached to the inferior, anterior, and posterior margins of the glenoid labrum just below the epiphyseal line and the humeral neck *(42)*. In fetal development, the IGHL is present by 14-wk gestation and appears as several layers of poorly organized collagen fibers, which are better organized than their surrounding capsular structure. With gestational time, the amount of fibrous tissue increases while the cellularity decreases *(14,43)*.

The three glenohumeral ligaments are named for the location of their origins on the humeral head. The IGHL origin is just below the articular margin on the inferior humeral head *(15,44)*. Ticker et al. observed that the IGHL has an anterior and posterior insertion into the humerus. The anterior insertion is inferior to the lesser tuberosity, whereas the posterior insertion is inferior to the greater tuberosity, with an equal distribution between V-shaped (with the axillary pouch forming the apex of the V) and collar-like (entire IGHL attached inferior to the humeral head articular edge) attachments *(45)*.

The IGHL passes beneath the humeral head to insert primarily into the anterior inferior glenoid. But the IGHL also inserts posteriorly into the posterior labrum and capsule and has an axillary insertion directly into the bone. In the labrum attachment, transitional zones of fibrocartilage and mineralized fibrocartilage are present between the IGHL and glenoid bone. The fibrocartilage zone and glenoid attachments both have a variable thickness, which decreases in the inferior direction along the glenoid *(46,47)*.

The IGHL appears as a triangular structure that extends between the glenoid labrum, triceps tendon, and the subscapularis muscle *(48)*. As noted by Turkel, the anterosuperior edge of the ligament is significantly thickened and termed the superior band of the IGHL. There are also thickenings in the anteroinferior portion of the joint capsule, which Turkel termed the "axillary pouch." This pouch could be divided into two portions: the anterior and posterior axillary pouch. The anatomic locations of the three IGHL bands are demonstrated in Fig. 4 *(42)*.

In contrast, O'Brien noted the IGHL was comprised of a superior band, posterior band, and an axillary pouch in which both anterior and posterior bands of IGHL were

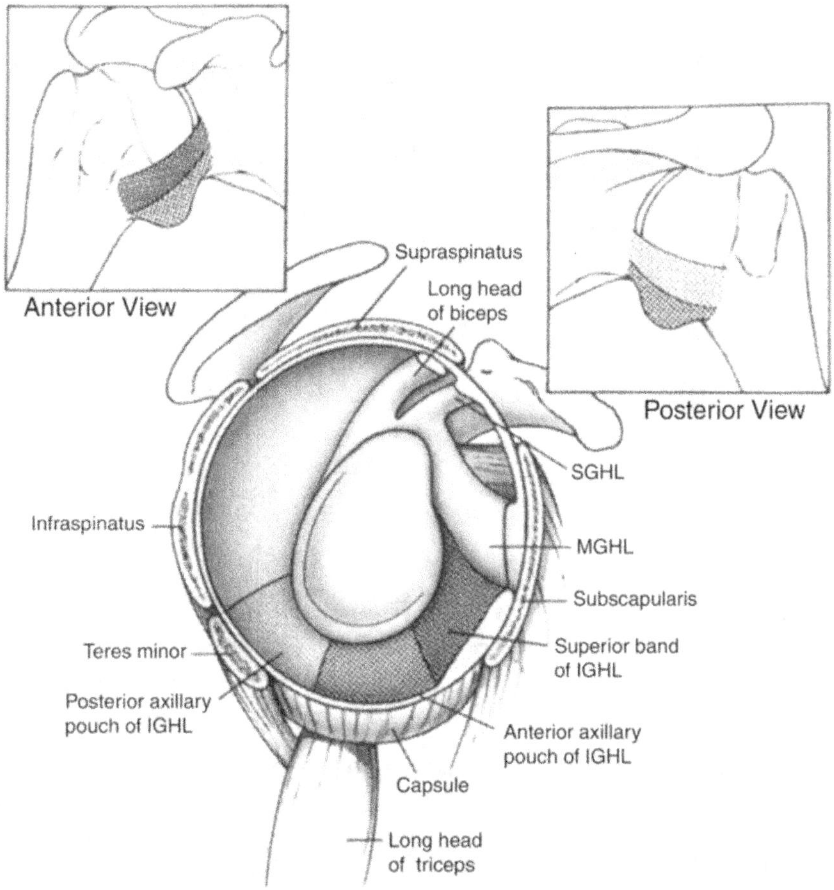

Fig. 4. Anatomy of the three distinct regions of the IGHL from both intracapsular and extra-capsular views. Also shown in the intracapsular view are the location of the MGHL and SGHL. (Reprinted from ref. *45*).

thickenings of the surrounding joint capsule. These bands showed well organized collagen bundles running in the coronal plane (from the humerus to the glenoid). In the axillary pouch, the bundles were thicker but less well-organized with intermingling of fibers from inner and middle capsular layers. The posterior capsule appeared thinner than the anterior capsule *(44)*. However, further studies by Ticker et al. identified a posterior band in only a small percentage (12.5%) of shoulders examined *(45)*. The difference between these observations may be a result of the external rotation of the upper arm. As the arm is externally rotated, the posterior axillary pouch folds on itself and appears to actually be a thickening of the joint capsule.

The IGHL helps to form the anterior border of the glenohumeral joint complex. In this area of the joint capsule, a predominantly radial orientation of the fiber bundles exists. Microscopic evaluation reveals crossing of superficial fiber bundles, oriented in a circular manner. Fibers of the middle glenohumeral ligament (MGHL) also have a role in this area of the joint capsule (Fig. 5; *35*).

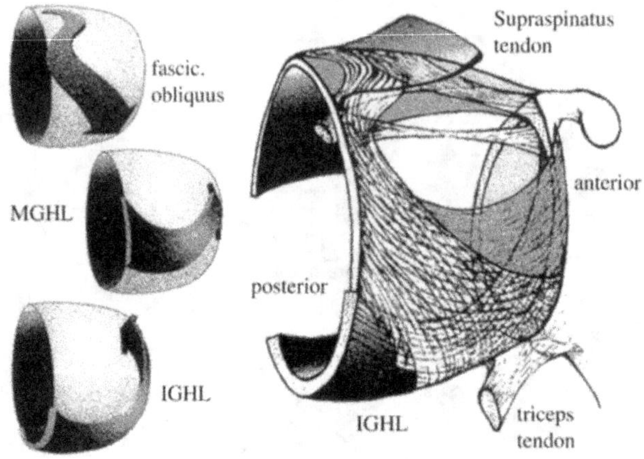

Fig. 5. Collagen fiber bundle orientation in ligamentous structures of the anterior glenohumeral joint capsule. The fibers of both the MGHL and the IGHL are oriented primarily in a radial manner. (Reprinted from ref. *35*).

Table 5
Geometric Properties of the IGHL

	Mean ± standard deviation		
IGHL region	Length (mm)	Thickness (mm)	Width (mm)
Superior band (n = 16)	41.3 ± 4.5	2.79 ± 0.49	13.33 ± 2.66
Anterior axillary pouch (n = 16)	39.8 ± 5.6	2.34 ± 0.43	12.61 ± 3.05
Posterior axillary pouch (n = 16)	41.0 ± 4.2	1.70 ± 0.55	10.86 ± 2.94
Mean (n = 48)	40.7 ± 4.7	2.28 ± 0.66	12.27 ± 2.88

Source: ref. *51*.

The IGHL is generally present, but its anatomy can be variable. Steinbeck found a clearly defined structure in only 72% of cases studied. In the remainder of the cases, only a thickening of the inferior glenohumeral joint capsule was seen *(48,49)*. When the glenohumeral joint capsule is viewed in a layered approach, the IGHL is present in the deepest layer (i.e., the layer closest to the joint; *15*). Generally, the superior band of the IGHL appears either band- or fan-like. However, in a few cases, cord-like ligament band patterns were present *(50)*.

Geometry

Bigliani et al. measured the average thickness of the IGHL as 2.28 ± 0.66 mm with a width of 12.27 ± 2.88 mm. Assuming a rectangular cross-section, this yields an average cross-sectional area of 40.7 ± 4.7 mm^2. The lengths and widths of individual bands are all comparable in size (Table 5). Ticker et al. showed similar results but also showed that the superior band is significantly thicker than both the anterior and posterior axillary pouches. Additionally, the anterior axillary pouch is thicker than the posterior axillary pouch. Within each region, the proximal portions of the IGHL bands (near the glenoid insertion) are notably more thick than the middle or distal portions (Table 6; *45,51*).

Table 6
Thickness (mm) of the IGHL Bands as Measured Along the Length of the Ligament

	Mean ± standard deviation		
IGHL region	Proximal	Middle	Distal
Superior band ($n = 8$)	2.63 ± 0.48 [a]	2.15 ± 0.41	1.91 ± 0.36
Anterior axillary pouch ($n = 8$)	2.30 ± 0.28 [a]	1.89 ± 0.46	1.65 ± 0.46
Posterior axillary pouch ($n = 8$)	1.97 ± 0.73 [a]	1.52 ± 0.65	1.27 ± 0.57
Mean ($n = 24$)	2.30 ± 0.57	1.85 ± 0.56	1.61 ± 0.52

Source: ref. *45*.
[a] Proximal more than middle and distal within each region ($p < 0.05$).

Table 7
Geometric Data of the IGHL Superior Band

	Mean ± standard deviation		
Region	XS_A (mm^2)	Thickness (mm)	Width (mm)
Glenoid insertion ($n = 16$)	73.5 ± 7.5	2.9 ± 0.2 [a]	24.8 ± 1.1
Midsubstance ($n = 12$)	61.7 ± 6.7 [a]	2.6 ± 0.2	23.3 ± 0.8
Humeral insertion ($n = 12$)	74.0 ± 7.0	2.6 ± 0.2	28.5 ± 0.9

Source: ref. *46*.
[a] One-way analysis of variance (ANOVA): Midsubstance XS_A significantly less; Glenoid insertion thickness significantly greater; all widths significantly different ($p < 0.05$).

McMahon demonstrated similar geometric properties for the superior band *(46)*; but in a different study, he showed a thicker superior band with a cross-sectional area significantly less in the midsubstance than near the insertion sites (Table 7; *52*). Lee et al. showed that the length of the superior band was 37.3 ± 0.9 mm and that width, thickness, and cross-sectional area do not change with age *(53)*.

Structure and Histology

Bigliani et al. observed longitudinally organized fibers in the ligamentous portion of the IGHL that has a consistent crimping pattern between regions (superior band and axillary pouches). The fiber bundles appeared uniform in the ligament midsubstance with increased fiber bundle interweaving near the bony insertion sites. The superior band had greater interweaving in the midsubstance relative to other regions, whereas the anterior axillary pouch had more crimping and less interweaving. This evidence suggests that some variability in IGHL microcomposition exists *(51,54)*.

Invariably, the IGHL displays closely packed collagen fiber bundles. These fibers generally follow a circular course through the joint cavity, but a percentage run at a 14° angle into the bony edge of the scapular neck *(55)*. Yet, Gohlke showed that there was a fairly even distribution between fibers that insert into the labrum at acute angles

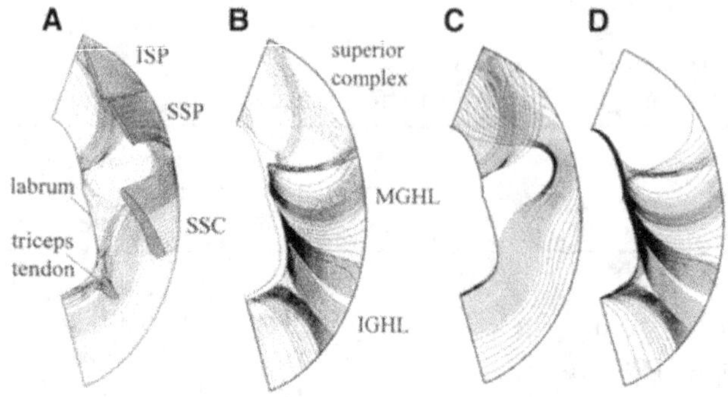

Fig. 6. Schematics of collagen fiber bundles of the glenohumeral joint capsule as viewed using polarized light microscopy. **(A)** External and **(B)** articular side surfaces of flat capsule specimens that show fibers systems with predominately **(C)** circular and **(D)** radial orientations. ISP, infraspinatus muscle; SSP, supraspinatus muscle; SSC, subscapularis muscle. (Reprinted from ref. *35*).

(53%) and those that are radially oriented (46%). Although a gross simplification, the fibers with mostly a circular orientation are predominately in the superficial layer and course around the joint to enter the labrum at acute angles (Fig. 6). The fiber bundles with a radial orientation are located in the deeper joint layer on the articular side, where they run from the glenoid to the humerus. These deeper fibers are believed to be stronger *(35)*. The fibers in the anterior axillary pouch run caudally and curve posteriorly from the glenoid to their attachment on the anatomic neck of the humerus. In contrast, the fibers in the posterior portion of the IGHL curve cranially and anteriorly from the glenoid to their attachment on the humeral surgical neck *(42)*.

Innervation of the glenohumeral ligaments comes from the axillary, suprascapular, subscapular, and musculocutaneous nerves *(43)*. All glenohumeral ligaments also display fast-adapting Pacinian corpuscles but not the low-threshold Ruffini end organs *(3)*.

Biochemistry

The content of water, collagen, and the hydroxylysyl pyridinoline crosslink do not significantly vary by region (Table 8). However, sulfated glycosaminoglycan (GAG) content (a measure of the proteoglycan content) is much greater in the superior band than in the anterior and posterior axillary pouches. Given the viscoelastic properties present in this region the higher sulfated-GAG content in the superior band is noteworthy *(54,56)*.

Biomechanics

Elastic Response

Structural and Material Properties

The Young's modulus in the anterior axillary pouch was observed to be slightly lower than the moduli values for the posterior axillary pouch and superior band at a slow strain rate (0.01–0.1 % strain/s) that minimizes viscoelastic effects. Additionally, in the posterior axillary pouch, the toe region modulus is greater than that of either the anterior axillary pouch or the superior band. The decreased modulus in the anterior axillary pouch may be a result of increased crimping in this region. (Table 9; *51*).

Table 8
Biochemical Properties of Individual Bands of the IGHLs

	Mean ± standard deviation			
IGHL region	Water content (%)	Collagen content (g/g dry wt)	HP content [a] (mole/mole collagen)	S-GAG content [b] (mg/g dry wt)
Superior band ($n = 8$)	82.1 ± 2.2	0.81 ± 0.09	0.71 ± 0.13	0.19 ± 0.14
Anterior axillary pouch ($n = 8$)	80.0 ± 2.7	0.85 ± 0.08	0.61 ± 0.23	0.37 ± 0.20
Posterior axillary pouch ($n = 8$)	80.5 ± 2.0	0.75 ± 0.06	0.73 ± 0.16	0.29 ± 0.07

Source: ref. *56*
[a] HP: hydroxylysyl pyridonoline.
[b] S-GAG in superior band greater than in anterior or posterior axillary pouches ($p < 0.05$).

Table 9
Stress-Strain Failure Data for the IGHL Bands at Both Slow (0.01–0.1 %/s) and Fast (10%/s) Strain Rates

	Mean ± standard deviation				
Slow Strain Rate	Stress (MPa)	Total Specimen Strain (%)	Ligament Strain (%)	Total specimen modulus (MPa)	Stiffness (MPa)
Superior band ($n = 16$)	5.2 ± 2.7	24.0 ± 6.2	8.3 ± 3.2	38.74 ± 18.09	5.50 ± 2.73
Anterior axillary pouch ($n = 16$)	5.5 ± 2.0	34.0 ± 10.5 [a]	15.1 ± 5.7 [a]	30.33 ± 10.58	4.38 ± 3.32
Posterior axillary pouch ($n = 16$)	5.6 ± 1.9	23.1 ± 4.6	9.9 ± 5.3	41.91 ± 12.50 [d]	8.42 ± 3.88 [d]
Avg ($n = 48$)	5.5 ± 2.2	27.0 ± 8.9	10.9 ± 5.5	36.92 ± 14.55	6.11 ± 3.72
Fast Strain Rate	Stress (MPa)	Total Specimen Strain (%)	Ligament Strain (%)	Total specimen modulus (MPa)	Stiffness (MPa)
Superior band ($n = 8$)	8.4 ± 2.2 [c]	20.8 ± 3.8	9.1 ± 2.8	62.63 ± 9.78 [e]	15.09 ± 4.92 [f]
Anterior axillary pouch ($n = 8$)	7.8 ± 3.1 [c]	30.4 ± 4.3 [a]	10.8 ± 2.4 [b]	47.75 ± 17.89	7.97 ± 3.76
Posterior axillary pouch ($n = 8$)	5.9 ± 1.7	25.2 ± 5.8	7.8 ± 3.6	39.97 ± 13.29	10.70 ± 5.39
Avg ($n = 32$)	7.4 ± 2.5	25.4 ± 6.0	9.3 ± 3.1	50.19 ± 16.50	11.25 ± 5.43

Source: refs. *45,51,54*.
Slow strain rates minimize viscoelastic effects during loading while increased strain rates simulate physiologic loading conditions.
[a] Anterior axillary pouch greater than superior band and posterior axillary pouch ($p < 0.05$).
[b] Anterior axillary pouch greater than posterior axillary pouch ($p < 0.05$).
[c] Superior band and anterior axillary pouch greater than posterior ($p < 0.05$).
[d] Posterior axillary pouch greater than anterior axillary pouch and superior band ($p < 0.05$).
[e] Superior band greater than anterior and posterior axillary pouches ($p < 0.05$).
[f] Superior band greater than anterior axillary pouch ($p < 0.05$).

At a higher strain rate (10% strain/s), the modulus of the superior band (calculated using the total specimen strain) is significantly greater than that of both the posterior and anterior axillary pouches at this increased strain rate. Application of the exponential stress–strain association also indicates that the stiffness of the superior band in the toe region is more than that of the axillary pouch. Ligament modulus at the faster strain rate is generally double the total specimen modulus for each band *(45)*.

Repetitive subfailure loading of the IGHL induces ligament laxity, as measured by decreased peak loads and irrecoverable ligament elongation, where the axillary pouch shows the greatest laxity. This laxity may be from microdamage (owing to nonrecoverable deformation) and viscoelastic stress-relaxation effects. The micro-damage likely occurs early in the loading regime as the crimped collagen fibers are cyclically stretched. These microdamage effects are also cumulative, because increased cycling frequency results in greater drops in peak loads. Presumably, some fiber recruitment occurs during this microdamage process; more highly crimped fibers are recruited to bear load as less crimped fibers are broken. Regional variations in microdamage may be caused by variable collagen fiber micro-orientation between regions *(52,57)*.

Collagen shortening via laser induction results in decreased energy absorption during cyclic testing for the posterior band. This effect is not seen in other regions and may be a consequence of increased collagen crosslinking or other extracellular matrix changes from the laser-heating process (i.e., decreased water content). Additionally, laser-treated specimens revealed greater yield strain and greater strain prior to plastic deformation, both of which are suggestive of some matrix modification process *(58)*.

Lee et al. illustrated that both material and structural properties of the IGHL superior band tested with the shoulder in the position of apprehension differ with age. For structural properties, decreases in ultimate load (38.8%) and energy absorbed to failure (38.1%) occur with the aging process. For material properties, decreases in modulus (45.9%), failure stress (53.2%), and failure strain (39.4%) are observed with older specimens *(53)*.

The use of an exponential stress-strain law demonstrates that the stress-strain response in the toe regions for each band is also different. Specifically, the anterior pouch shows more strain than the other regions for the same applied stress. A possible explanation is that the anterior pouch is composed of more highly crimped fibers in relationship to the other regions and therefore requires greater elongation (corresponding to fiber recruitment) before reaching the same stress level as other regions. However, increased proteoglycan content in the superior band may decrease the viscous component and thus cause an increased strain response *(51)*.

Bigliani et al. found strain variations along the IGHL length, and significant strain was present near the insertions of the IGHL into the glenoid and humerus. This may account for the greater viscoelastic effect seen in the IGHL insertion regions associated with the ligament midsubstance. Specifically, the insertion site for the IGHL superior band appears stiffer than those of the other regions *(51)*.

In Situ Loads

Debski et al. measured the *in situ* IGHL loads during the application of an external force. During anterior loading, the IGHL superior band carries increasing *in situ* forces with increases in abduction, and a maximum *in situ* force occurs at 90° abduction.

During posterior loading, the *in situ* force for the IGHL superior band is negligible, and the posterior band carries only minimal loads during anterior loading. With posterior loading, the IGHL posterior band forces increase with abduction, and a maximum force is observed at 60° abduction *(36)*.

FAILURE LOADS

When tested at a slow strain rate (0.01-0.1% strain/s), the IGHL failure stress (5.5 ± 2.2 MPa) does not vary by region. However, the IGHL total midsubstance failure strain is region-specific, and the anterior pouch fails at a remarkably higher strain (15.1 ± 5.7%) than either the posterior pouch (9.9 ± 5.3%) or superior band (8.3 ± 3.2%). Because the midsubstance failure strain represents only a percentage (35–45%) of the total specimen strain, some strain variations must exist along the length of the IGHL and may be indicative of regional differences in IGHL matrix organization and microcomposition *(51)*.

When measuring the mechanical properties of the isolated IGHL regions at a faster constant strain rate (10% strain/s), the tensile stress of both the superior band and anterior axillary pouch are each much greater than the tensile stress of the posterior axillary pouch with no differences in strain energy density. Additionally, the faster strain rate yields a midsubstance strain greater in the anterior axillary pouch relative to the other regions, whereas the total specimen strain is only different between the anterior and posterior axillary pouches *(45)*.

Ligament failure location is dependent upon the strain rate used during testing. An increase from a slow strain rate (0.01–0.1% strain/s) to a fast strain rate (10% strain/s) results in a higher incidence of ligament midsubstance failures (35% slow, 54% fast). Humeral insertion site failures also decrease with elevations in strain rate (25% slow, 8% fast), but the frequency of glenoid insertion failure does not change appreciably (40% slow; 38% fast; *45,51,56*).

When preconditioned before failure testing (at a fast strain rate), the mode of failure becomes more evenly distributed: 25% failing at the glenoid, 33% failing in the midsubstance, and 42% failing at the humerus *(58)*. The failure mode of the isolated IGHL superior band varies with age. In younger specimens mechanically tested with the shoulder in apprehension, the failure modes were fairly evenly distributed among the midsubstance and insertion regions. However, older specimens tested in the same manner failed predominantly near the glenoid insertion site *(53)*.

McMahon et al. analyzed material and structural properties regarding to failure location of the IGHL superior band and showed that ultimate elongation and yield strain for glenoid insertion failures were significantly greater than for samples that failed elsewhere. No other structural or material property exhibited variation with failure location. Failure location statistics were 64% glenoid insertion, 18% humeral insertion, and 18% ligament midsubstance *(52)*.

Viscoelastic Response

Mechanical properties vary by strain rate and IGHL region studied. Because slow strain rates lessen the viscoelastic effect in biologic tissues, and faster strain rates are more clinically relevant, the comparisons of mechanical data at slow (0.01 and 0.1% strain/s) and fast (10% strain/s) strain rates enable the evaluation of viscoelastic influences. As seen in Table 9, failure stress and modulus rise significantly in the superior band and anterior pouch with increased strain rate. The anterior pouch also demonstrates decreased failure strain at the higher strain rates.

The implication of this data is that the IGHL superior band has greater stiffness during the fiber recruitment phase and that collagen microcomposition in the IGHL may differ based on region. Also, the higher proteoglycan content in the superior band may cause viscoelastic stiffening because of collagen fibers uncrimping during loading, which then compresses proteoglycan molecules, thus causing interstitial fluid flow *(45,51,54,56)*.

Stability

The IGHL is the primary static stabilizer to subluxation, especially at large displacements *(37,54)*. It is also an important passive stabilizer in external rotation, providing increasing stabilizing effects as the displacement increases, and it is the dominant restraint to anterior dislocation *(40,42,59)*. During external rotation, the anterior components of the IGHL limit rotation; with internal rotation, posterior IGHL components restrain rotation *(60)*. Urayama et al. indicated that the superior band and anterior axillary pouch are anterior stabilizers, whereas the posterior axillary pouch is a posterior stabilizer *(61)*. The IGHL is the leading joint constraint during anterior loading *(62,63)*.

With the CHL, the IGHL is the primary restraint to external rotation in abduction *(39)*. In all abduction positions, the IGHL maintains a cruciate orientation in the antero-posterior plane (The cruciate orientation is a result of varying locations of the attachments for each band.) During abduction, the IGHL provides the dominant constraint to joint translation and limits humeral abduction *(38,41)*. Increasing shoulder abduction increases the impact of the IGHL in limiting anterior translation. At 45° of abduction, all the glenohumeral ligaments are at their loosest, resulting in the greatest amount of total superior–inferior translation.

At increased anterior abduction angles, the anterior band takes over the duty to stabilize the joint. At 90° of abduction, both the anterior and posterior portions of the IGHL are parallel to the antero-posterior plane. These bands cradle the humeral head, and internal or external rotation of the humeral head causes reciprocal tightening or loosening of the anterior and posterior portions of the IGHL. This motion rolls the humeral head back into place upon movement of the glenoid. As the IGHL tightens with external rotation and abduction, it is the major limit to anterior and posterior instability at 90° abduction *(29,49,64–66)*.

MIDDLE GLENOHUMERAL LIGAMENT

Anatomy

The MGHL is the second of three glenohumeral ligaments and is attached to the non-articulating surface of the glenohumeral joint capsule *(31)*. In fetal development, the MGHL is present by 14-wk gestation as a distinct thickening of the joint capsule *(14)*.

The MGHL originates on the lesser tuberosity of the humerus along the anatomic neck and blends with the insertion of the subscapularis tendon into the humerus *(28,42,47)*. The MGHL then passes across the subscapularis tendon in an oblique manner, appearing as a chisel-shaped band that widens laterally *(47,67)*. The average width of the MGHL is 1–1.5 cm, but width can range between 0.4 and 5 cm *(35)*.

The MGHL attaches proximally to the anterosuperior glenoid labrum (above the epiphyseal line), and its attachment extends along the glenoid anterior aspect *(42)*. Gohlke showed that the MGHL glenoid insertion was at the labrum in 86% of cases and at the glenoid rim in the remaining 14% *(28,35,48)*. The fibers of the MGHL are oriented primarily in a radial fashion *(35)*.

The MGHL is the most anatomically variable of the three glenohumeral ligaments. Steinbeck et al. observed the MGHL in 84.6% cases with an average diameter of 3.6 mm (range 2–5 mm) and an average width of 18 mm (range 6–25 mm). However, in 11.5% of cases studied, only a rudimentary MGHL was observed *(48)*. Warner found that a missing or rudimentary MGHL was present in eight of 11 shoulders studied *(29)*.

Structure

The MGHL usually appears as a large fibrous band that blends into the labrum. However, the it can also present as a cord-like structure, which may be attached to the base of the biceps tendon and is contiguous with the anterior superior labrum, giving the appearance of a sublabral hole *(47)*.

Superiorly, the MGHL appears as an intra-articular band that becomes part of the joint capsule as it descends to the humeral attachment. When the free intra-articular band is short or absent, the MGHL presents only as a focal thickening or folding of the joint capsule. The attachments of the MGHL are less than 1 cm in width on both the glenoid and humerus *(50)*.

Biomechanics

Elastic Response

IN SITU LOADS

The MGHL is a factor in the passive and dynamic restraint of the glenohumeral joint. In this role, the MGHL experiences *in situ* forces only during anterior loading, coupled with a shoulder abduction of at least 30°, and reaches a maximum *in situ* force at 60° abduction. When a 22 N compressive load is applied to the medial side of the humerus, and an anterior load of 89 N is applied in the orthogonal directions, the MGHL carries approx 35 N of load at 60° of abduction. In contrast, when an 89 N posterior load (but not anterior load) is applied to the same circumstance, the MGHL carries a maximum load of 5 N at 0° abduction. For 89 N of anterior loading, the angle of the *in situ* force in the MGHL relative to the transverse plane decreases from –12° to –18° as abduction increases from 30° to 90°. At the same time, the direction of force relative to the scapular plane increases from 76° to 102° *(36)*.

Stability

The MGHL (with the CHL) resists external rotation and prevents inferior subluxation *(28,37,63)*. As displacement increases during external rotation, the MGHL provides an increasing stabilizing force *(59)*. During abduction, it shortens as the glenohumeral joint rotates from 0° to 90°. This phenomenon is functionally important in the adducted shoulder during neutral and external rotation *(29,49)*. The MGHL limits translation in neutral abduction and in abduction combined with external rotation *(38)*. It also offers anterior stability at low and medium abduction levels. The contribution of the MGHL decreases with high levels of abduction (>60°) but provides support in concert with the IGHL *(42,63,65,66)*.

SUPERIOR GLENOHUMERAL LIGAMENT

Anatomy

The SGHL is the third of the glenohumeral ligaments and is attached to the non-articulating edge of the glenohumeral joint capsule. The origin of the SGHL is near the top of the lesser tuberosity of the humerus, and it blends with the anterior edge of the CHL (beneath the superior edge of the subscapularis tendon) to insert into the fovea capitas *(28,31,47)*. In fetal development, the SGHL is present as thickenings of the joint capsule by 14-wk gestation *(14)*.

The SGHL faces the glenohumeral joint cavity just ventral to the ligament of the biceps tendon and running parallel to the cranial margin of the subscapularis muscle. With the CHL, the SGHL forms the anterior covering band around the long head of the biceps tendon. In 18.6% of cases, the SGHL branches in a cranial manner and crosses under the biceps tendon, forming a part of the tendon's fibrous canal *(33,35,67)*.

The SGHL attaches to the glenoid labrum above the glenoid's epiphyseal line near the coracoid's base and anterior to the long head of the biceps tendon. It blends with the long head of the biceps prior to its bony insertion *(28,42,47)*. The attachments of the SGHL are small—less than 1 cm in width on both the glenoid and humerus *(50)*.

Some variability in SGHL anatomy exists. Steinbeck et al. demonstrated that the SGHL is present in 94% of shoulders examined. However, only a rudimentary structure exists in 29%, whereas the SGHL diameter in the remaining shoulders is in excess of 2 mm. A significant number (73%) of SGHL's come into contact with the long head of the biceps tendon, and a much smaller number (17%) share an insertion with the MGHL *(48)*.

Geometry

The midpoint cross-sectional area of the SGHL is 11.3 ± 1.6 mm^2, but the ligament tapers significantly from 20.4 ± 3.0 mm^2 near its glenoid attachment to 9.0 ± 1.2 mm^2 at its humeral insertion. However, the SGHL's midpoint cross-sectional area is significantly less (by a factor of 5) than that of the CHL, with which it is closely associated *(34)*.

Structure

The SGHL band appears equally as either a cord-like or fold-like structure *(50)*. Warner et al. observed that the SGHL was well developed in only half of the shoulders observed *(49)*. Although the thickness of the SGHL varies, it does so without any relationship to the age of the specimen *(28)*. The majority of SGHL fibers insert directly into the bone of the superior glenoid tubercle at a mean 20° angle. The remaining fibers run in a curve to join the long head of the biceps tendon and insert near its origin *(55)*.

Biomechanics

Elastic Response

In Situ Loads

With applied external anterior loading, the SGHL carries *in situ* loads at all angles of abduction. However, with posterior loading, the SGHL maximum *in situ* load is observed at 0° of abduction and decreases with increasing abduction angles *(36)*.

Failure Loads

When mechanically tested at an extension rate of 100 mm/min, the SGHL elongates 20.3 ± 4.5 % prior to failure, which occurs near the humeral insertion. It has a stiffness of 17.4 ± 1.5 N/mm and an ultimate load of 101.9 ± 11.5 N, corresponding to a modulus of 9.0 MPa at the ligament's midpoint. Also, the SGHL absorbs 384.4 ± 77.7 N-m of energy prior to failure. In comparison to the CHL, SGHL stiffness is half that of the CHL, and the ultimate load is one third that of the CHL. However, the SGHL midpoint stress is greater than the CHL's owing to its smaller midpoint cross-sectional area *(34)*.

Stability

With the CHL, the SGHL limits posterior dislocation and anterior translation, contributing to the posterior subluxation force. At low abduction levels, the SGHL provides anterior stability. It shortens as the glenohumeral joint rotates and becomes one of the primary stabilizers of inferior dislocation with increased arm abduction *(36,37,49,63,65,66)*. Inferior stabilization by the SGHL may be proportional to compressive loads and displacements *(40)*.

During inferior neutral laxity tests, the SGHL provides motion constraint *(38)*. It also offers an increasing stabilizing force with increased displacement during external rotation *(59)*.

OTHER LIGAMENTS

The coracoglenoid ligament has been described as a bundle of dense, parallel-oriented collagen fibers with good vascularity that stretches between the coracoid and superior glenoid tubercle. Its origin is in the middle of the posterior surface of the coracoid process, between the two limbs of the acromioclavicular ligament. Its glenoid insertion separates the inferior portion of the CHL and base of the coracoid process. The existence of this ligament is controversial and is not recognized by the Terminologica Anatomica *(30)*.

The costoclavicular ligament is a bilaminar structure attached to the inferior surface of the medial clavicle and the first rib. Its posterior component passes upward and medially *(2)*. The anterior portion of the costoclavicular ligament crosses medially from the clavicle to the rib and is stronger than the posterior portion. Its length has been reported to be from 10 mm to almost 30 mm during humeral abduction. The costoclavicular ligament limits the elevation and stabilizes the lateral clavicle end *(1,5)*.

The interclavicular ligament crosses the superior aspect of the sternoclavicular joint and joins the two clavicle ends. It is believed to provide stability to the superior aspect of the joint capsule *(1,2)*.

The spinoglenoid (or inferior transverse) ligament travels from the lateral base of the scapular spine to the superior margin of the glenoid, fixing neurovascular bundles within the spinoglenoid notch. It is composed of type I collagen fibers and has Sharpey's fibers present at the insertion site into the spine of the scapula. A direct insertion into the periosteum of the scapular spine also exists. In up to 20% of cases, the spinoglenoid ligament is missing *(68,69)*. A superior transverse ligament also exists. It arches the scapular incisures *(69)*.

The transverse humeral ligament is composed of a few densely arranged layers of the joint capsule extended between the greater and lesser tuberosities of the humerus. Its function is to keep the long head of the biceps tendon in its groove. Some free neurofilament endings are present in this ligament *(43,70)*.

CONCLUSION

The shoulder is composed of several joints, including the acromioclavicular joint, sternoclavicular joint, and the glenohumeral joint. The shoulder ligaments are an integral part of the shoulder's system because they provide stability and strength to these joints.

Although a significant body of work has been developed on some shoulder ligaments as revealed in this chapter, some gaps remain in the literature. Further understanding of the basic science of these ligamentous structures will aid in the treatment of shoulder injuries. For example, given the role that the MGHL has in stability, little is known about its basic mechanical properties and how these properties relate to its stabilizing function. Similarly, the SGHL has an impact in anterior stability at low levels of abduction, but not much is known about the viscoelastic response of this ligament. An important question is whether the stability provided by the SGHL is related to the application rate of the external force. Additionally, the anatomy of the acromioclavicular and sternoclavicular ligaments has been well developed. However, knowledge of the mechanics of these ligaments is lacking. Investigations into these areas may help in understanding the underlying stabilizing effect that these ligaments provide to the acromioclavicular and sternoclavicular joints.

One essential area for future research is how the structure and function of the shoulder ligaments are altered in various disease or pathologic states. This may be the first step developing various treatment modalities. Some data has been presented here on the changes in ligament mechanical properties in shoulders with rotator cuff tears or impingement syndrome. Other pathologic conditions of interest include bursitis and shoulder dislocations. Questions that need to be answered include: Are the properties of shoulder ligaments altered in these conditions? How do alterations in pathologic shoulders differ from the normal course of alterations observed with age? Based on the answers to these questions, can treatment approaches be developed that alleviate pathologic conditions or slow down age-related degeneration of the shoulder ligaments? These are just a few of the questions that should be answered to fully understand the function of the shoulder ligaments and the effects that ligament degeneration has upon the function and stability of the shoulder.

REFERENCES

1. Pratt NE. Anatomy and biomechanics of the shoulder. *J Hand Ther* 1994;7:65–76.
2. Peat M. Functional anatomy of the shoulder complex. *Phys Ther* 1986;66:1855-65.
3. Vangsness Jr CT, Ennis M, Taylor JG, Atkinson R. Neural anatomy of the glenohumeral ligaments, labrum, and subacromial bursa. *Arthroscopy* 1995;11:180–184.
4. Salter EG, Nasca RJ, Shelley BS. Anatomical observations on the acromioclavicular joint and supporting ligaments. *Am J Sports Med* 1987;15:199–206.
5. Pronk GM, van der Helm FC, Rozendaal LA. Interaction between the joints in the shoulder mechanism: the function of the costoclavicular, conoid and trapezoid ligaments. Proceedings of the Institution of Mechanical Engineers. Part H. *J Eng Med* 1993;207:219–229.
6. Kiefer H, Claes L, Burri C, et al. The stabilizing effect of various implants on the torn acromioclavicular joint. A biomechanical study. *Arch Orthop Trauma Surg* 1996;106: 42–46.
7. Lee KW, Debski RE, Chen CH, et al. Functional evaluation of the ligaments at the acromioclavicular joint during anteroposterior and superoinferior translation. *Am J Sports Med* 1997;25:858–862.

8. Harris RI, et al. Anatomic variance of the coracoclavicular ligaments. *J Shoulder Elbow Surg* 2001;10:585–588.
9. Harris RI, et al. Structural properties of the intact and the reconstructed coracoclavicular ligament complex. *Am J Sports Med* 2000;28:103–108.
10. Motamedi AR, et al. Biomechanics of the coracoclavicular ligament complex and augmentations used in its repair and reconstruction. *Am J Sports Med* 2000;28:380–384.
11. Branch TP, et al. The role of the acromioclavicular ligaments and the effect of distal clavicle resection. *Am J Sports Med* 1996;24:293–297.
12. Fukuda K, et al. Biomechanical study of the ligamentous system of the acromioclavicular joint. *J Bone Joint Surg Am* 1986;68:434–440.
13. Gallino M, et al. Coracoacromial ligament: a comparative arthroscopic and anatomic study. *Arthroscopy* 1995;11:564–567.
14. Fealy S, et al. The developmental anatomy of the neonatal glenohumeral joint. *J Shoulder Elbow Surg* 2000;9:217–222.
15. Cooper DE, O'Brien SJ, Warren RF. Supporting layers of the glenohumeral joint. An anatomic study. *Clin Orthop* 1993;289:144–155.
16. Hunt JL, Moore RJ, Krishnan J. The fate of the coracoacromial ligament in arthroscopic acromioplasty: an anatomical study. *J Shoulder Elbow Surg* 2000;9:491–494.
17. Holt EM, Allibone RO. Anatomic variants of the coracoacromial ligament. *J Shoulder Elbow Surg* 1995;4:370–375.
18. Soslowsky LJ, et al. Geometric and mechanical properties of the coracoacromial ligament and their relationship to rotator cuff disease. *Clin Orthop* 1994;304:10–17.
19. Sarkar K, Taine W, Uhthoff HK, The ultrastructure of the coracoacromial ligament in patients with chronic impingement syndrome. *Clin Orthop* 1990;254:49–54.
20. Edelson JG, Taitz C, Grishkan A. The coracohumeral ligament. Anatomy of a substantial but neglected structure. *J Bone Joint Surg Br* 1991;73:150–153.
21. Uhthoff HK, et al. The role of the coracoacromial ligament in the impingement syndrome. A clinical, radiological and histological study. *Int Orthop* 1988;12:97–104.
22. Fremerey R, Bastian L, Siebert WE. The coracoacromial ligament: anatomical and biomechanical properties with respect to age and rotator cuff disease. *Knee Surg Sports Traumatol Arthroscopy* 2000;8:309–313.
23. Soslowsky LJ, et al. Coracoacromial ligament: in situ load and viscoelastic properties in rotator cuff disease. *Clin Orthop* 1996;330:40–44.
24. Lee TQ, et al. Release of the coracoacromial ligament can lead to glenohumeral laxity: a biomechanical study. *J Shoulder Elbow Surg* 2001;10:68–72.
25. Kummer FJ, Blank K, Zuckerman JD. Coracoacromial ligament function: a phylomorphic analysis. *Bull Hosp Jt Dis* 1996;55:72–74.
26. Clark J, Sidles JA, Matsen FA. The relationship of the glenohumeral joint capsule to the rotator cuff. *Clin Orthop* 1990;254:29–34.
27. Neer 2nd CS, et al. The anatomy and potential effects of contracture of the coracohumeral ligament. *Clin Orthop* 1992;280:182–185.
28. Ferrari DA. Capsular ligaments of the shoulder. Anatomical and functional study of the anterior superior capsule. *Am J Sports Med* 1990;18:20–24.
29. Warner JJ, et al. Static capsuloligamentous restraints to superior-inferior translation of the glenohumeral joint. *Am J Sports Med* 1992;20:675–685.
30. Kolts I, et al. Anatomy of the coracohumeral and coracoglenoidal ligaments. *Ann Anat* 2000;182:563–566.
31. Clark JM, Harryman 2nd DT. Tendons, ligaments, and capsule of the rotator cuff. Gross and microscopic anatomy. *J Bone Joint Surg Am* 1992;74:713–725.
32. Arnoczky S, Soslowsky LJ. Anatomy of the shoulder: form reflecting function. In McGinty JB, et al. eds., *Operative Arthroscopy*. Lippincott-Raven, Philadelphia, PA, 1996, pp. 603–624.

33. Jost B, Koch PP, Gerber C. Anatomy and functional aspects of the rotator interval. *J Shoulder Elbow Surg* 2000;9:336–341.
34. Boardman ND, et al. Tensile properties of the superior glenohumeral and coracohumeral ligaments. *J Shoulder Elbow Surg* 1996;5:249–254.
35. Gohlke F, Essigkrug B, Schmitz F. The pattern of the collagen fiber bundles of the capsule of the glenohumeral joint. *J Shoulder Elbow Surg* 1994;3:111–128.
36. Debski RE, et al. In situ force distribution in the glenohumeral joint capsule during anterior-posterior loading. *J Orthop Res* 1999;17:769–776.
37. Blasier RB, et al. Posterior glenohumeral subluxation: active and passive stabilization in a biomechanical model. *J Bone Joint Surg Am* 1997;79:433–440.
38. Brenneke SL, et al. Glenohumeral kinematics and capsulo-ligamentous strain resulting from laxity exams. *Clin Biomech* 2000;15:735–742.
39. Kuhn JE, et al. Ligamentous restraints to external rotation of the humerus in the late-cocking phase of throwing. A cadaveric biomechanical investigation. *Am J Sports Med* 2000;28:200–205.
40. Soslowsky LJ, Malicky DM, Blasier RB. Active and passive factors in inferior glenohumeral stabilization: a biomechanical model. *J Shoulder Elbow Surg* 1997;6:371–39.
41. Gagey O, et al. Anatomic basis of ligamentous control of elevation of the shoulder (reference position of the shoulder joint). *Surg Radiol Anat* 1987;9:19–26.
42. Turkel SJ, et al. Stabilizing mechanisms preventing anterior dislocation of the glenohumeral joint. *J Bone Joint Surg Am* 1981;63:1208–1217.
43. O'Brien SJ, et al. Developmental anatomy of the shoulder and anatomy of the glenohumeral joint. In Rockwood CA, et al., eds., *The Shoulder*. Saunders, Philadelphia, PA, 1998, pp. 1–33.
44. O'Brien SJ, et al. The anatomy and histology of the inferior glenohumeral ligament complex of the shoulder. *Am J Sports Med* 1990;18:449–456.
45. Ticker JB, et al. Inferior glenohumeral ligament: geometric and strain-rate dependent properties. *J Shoulder Elbow Surg* 1996;5:269–279.
46. McMahon PJ, et al. The anterior band of the inferior glenohumeral ligament. Assessment of its permanent deformation and the anatomy of its glenoid attachment. *J Bone Joint Surg Br* 1999;81:406–413.
47. Nottage WM. Arthroscopic anatomy of the glenohumeral joint and subacromial bursa. *Orthop Clin North Am* 1993;24:27–32.
48. Steinbeck J, Liljenqvist U, Jerosch J. The anatomy of the glenohumeral ligamentous complex and its contribution to anterior shoulder stability. *J Shoulder Elbow Surg* 1998;7:122–126.
49. Warner JJ, et al. Dynamic capsuloligamentous anatomy of the glenohumeral joint. *J Shoulder Elbow Surg* 1993;2:115–133.
50. Yeh L, et al. Anterior labroligamentous structures of the glenohumeral joint: correlation of MR arthrography and anatomic dissection in cadavers. AJR. *Am J Roentgenol* 1998;171: 1229–1236.
51. Bigliani LU, et al. Tensile properties of the inferior glenohumeral ligament. *J Orthop Res* 1992;10:187–197.
52. McMahon PJ, et al. The anterior band of the inferior glenohumeral ligament: biomechanical properties from tensile testing in the position of apprehension. *J Shoulder Elbow Surg* 1998;7:467–471.
53. Lee TQ, et al. Age related biomechanical properties of the glenoid-anterior band of the inferior glenohumeral ligament-humerus complex. *Clin Biomech* 1999;14:471–476.
54. Bigliani LU, et al. Glenohumeral stability. Biomechanical properties of passive and active stabilizers. *Clin Orthop* 1996;330:13–30.
55. Huber WP, Putz RV. Periarticular fiber system of the shoulder joint. *Arthroscopy* 1997;13: 680–691.

56. Mow VC, et al. Material properties of the inferior glenohumeral ligament and the glenohumeral articular cartilage. In: Matsen FA, Fu FH, Hawkins RS, eds., *The Shoulder: A Balance of Mobility and Stability*. American Academy of Orthopaedic Surgeons, Rosemont, IL, 1993, pp. 29–67.
57. Pollock RG, et al. Effects of repetitive subfailure strains on the mechanical behavior of the inferior glenohumeral ligament. *J Shoulder Elbow Surg* 2000;9:427–435.
58. Selecky MT, et al. The effects of laser-induced collagen shortening on the biomechanical properties of the inferior glenohumeral ligament complex. *Am J Sports Med* 1999;27:168–172.
59. Malicky DM, et al. Anterior glenohumeral stabilization factors: progressive effects in a biomechanical model. *J Orthop Res* 1996;14:282–288.
60. Branch TP, et al. The role of glenohumeral capsular ligaments in internal and external rotation of the humerus. *Am J Sports Med* 1995;23:632–637.
61. Urayama M, et al. Function of the 3 portions of the inferior glenohumeral joint ligament: A cadaveric study. *J Shoulder Elbow Surg* 2001;10:589–594.
62. Debski RE, et al. Contribution of the passive properties of the rotator cuff to glenohumeral stability during anterior-posterior loading. *J Shoulder Elbow Surg* 1999;8:324–329.
63. Itoi E, Hsu HC, An KN. Biomechanical investigation of the glenohumeral joint. *J Shoulder Elbow Surg* 1996;5:407–424.
64. O'Brien SJ, et al. Capsular restraints to anterior-posterior motion of the abducted shoulder: a biomechanical study. *J Shoulder Elbow Surg* 1995;4:298–308.
65. O'Connell PW, et al. The contribution of the glenohumeral ligaments to anterior stability of the shoulder joint. *Am J Sports Med* 1990;18:579–584.
66. Pagnani MJ, Warren RF. Stabilizers of the glenohumeral joint. *J Sholder Elbow Surg* 1994;3:173–190.
67. Kolts I, et al. Anatomical composition of the anterior shoulder joint capsule. A cadaver study on 12 glenohumeral joints. *Ann Anat* 2001;183:53–59.
68. Cummins CA, et al. Anatomy and histological characteristics of the spinoglenoid ligament. *J Bone Joint Surg Am* 1998;80:1622–1625.
69. Prescher A. Anatomical basics, variations, and degenerative changes of the shoulder joint and shoulder girdle. *Eur J Radiol* 2000;35:88–102.
70. Soifer TB, et al. Neurohistology of the subacromial space. *Arthroscopy* 1996;12:182–186.

Part III

Current Clinical Status

6

History of Cruciate Ligament Repair

Development of Repair and Reconstruction

Jon Karlsson

INTRODUCTION

The first known description of the cruciate ligaments is approx 5000 yr old. The anatomy of the knee was mentioned in the Smith Papyrus (3000 BC). Hippocrates (460–377 BC) described subluxation of the knee and correlated this to ligament injury. Almost 200 yr later, Galen (200–130 BC) was the first to thoroughly describe the anatomy of the soft tissue structures stabilizing the knee. Galen recognized the importance of the ligaments to stabilize the joint and to restrict abnormal motion.

INTERNAL DERANGEMENT OF THE KNEE

The term "internal derangement of the knee" was used by Hey in 1782 *(1)*, usually to describe problems associated with knee motion. Surgical interventions were limited prior to the introduction of anesthesia and Hey advocated prolonged immobilization. "Internal derangement of the knee" was subsequently used to specify the functional insufficiency linked to cruciate ligament injuries for more than 200 yr, despite that his publications were more concerned with meniscal pathology than cruciate ligament injury. In 1836, the Weber brothers from Germany *(2)* provided a detailed description of the mechanics of joint motion and clarified the function of the intra-articular structures, as well as the importance of the periarticular components. They performed biomechanical investigations and researched the abnormal movement of the tibia in the cruciate deficient knee *(2)*, which is the first description of the abnormal kinematics correlated with cruciate ligament injury. The Weber brothers were also the first to elaborate on the different anatomical bundles of the anterior cruciate ligament, i.e., the anteromedial and posterolateral bundles. It has become evident that faulty kinematics is partly a cause in the development of osteoarthrosis, which is found in approx 50% of patients, 10–15 yr after a cruciate ligament injury. Only recently has the same anatomical phenomenon been for the posterior cruciate ligament. Presumably, the different anatomical bundles may be functionally important, but it has been questioned.

The French surgeon Bonnet from Lyon published extensive anatomical studies on the mechanism of knee ligament injuries based on cadaveric dissections *(3,4)*. He made

From: *Orthopedic Biology and Medicine: Repair and Regeneration of Ligaments, Tendons, and Joint Capsule*
Edited by: W. R. Walsh © Humana Press Inc., Totowa, NJ

several important observations that still hold true, such as the correlation of hemarthrosis and cruciate ligament rupture and the fact that the anterior cruciate ligament most often ruptures from its femoral insertion, not the tibial insertion. He also stated the cruciate ligament injuries were more frequent than previously reported.

Subluxation of the knee has been repeatedly related to cruciate ligament injury; today, this is described as "giving-way" and the pivot shift test is used to grade this phenomenon. Bonnet *(3)* described the subluxation of the knee in detail along with the functional consequences. Furthermore, he reviewed the combination of medical collateral ligament (MCL) rupture and cruciate ligament rupture. Interestingly, it took more than 100 yr to fully appreciate the importance of combined MCL and cruciate ligament ruptures (i.e., combined injuries), often believed to produce inferior functional results. The treatment of combined injuries has been only recently understood.

In a later publication, Bonnet *(4)* evaluated the treatment of unstable knees using a knee brace, which included a hinge for both the knee and hip. In the same publication, he also mentioned the negative effects of prolonged immobilization and proposed a machine to promote active and passive motion of the knee. The scientific background of passive active motion was thoroughly described more than 100 yr later by Salter et al. *(5)*. Bonnet's recommendations *(4)* of acute treatment of extremity injuries were far ahead of his time. Some of these treatment modalities, e.g., early range of motion and the use of cold packs, are often still the first line of defense in cases of sports injuries.

Nearly simultaneously in 1850, Stark *(6)* mentioned two cases of anterior cruciate ligament ruptures that were successfully treated using a cast. More importantly, Stark emphasized several important clinical signs associated with cruciate ligament injury, such as giving-way, subluxation, and audible snapping *(6)*. Clinical signs became more apparent; in 1875, Noulis *(7)* described the clinical sign of the Lachman test for the first time. Since then, this test has been the mainstay of the clinical evaluation of anterior cruciate ligament rupture. Noulis reviewed both the anterior translation of the tibia with the knee only minimally flexed and when the femur was firmly fixed with one hand and the tibia was moved forward and backward with the other. He also noted a backward movement of the tibia in 70° flexion in the case of posterior cruciate ligament injury *(7)*. It is interesting to note that the last decade has shown that 70° is the best position to test posterior cruciate ligament insufficiency, and this is also the position that the final fixation of reconstructed posterior cruciate ligament should be performed. The "screw movement" of the knee joint was recognized and described by Meyer in 1873, which has later been described as the "screw-home mechanism." This important concept introduced the understanding of the rotational aspect, which is produced by the inequality of the femoral condyles.

A NEW UNDERSTANDING

Segond *(8)*, a French surgeon, was the first to publish a thorough description of knee ligament injuries in 1879—both clinical signs and functional impairment. He explained the pain reaction accompanied with rupture of the cruciate ligaments. He also described the frequently heard "pop" and the importance of the rapidly evolving joint effusion, which he presumed was because of hemarthrosis. Furthermore, he performed a detailed clinical examination, including anterior-posterior shift of the tibia upon femur with anterior cruciate ligament rupture. He also described the "Segond-fracture" *(8)*. This small fracture is the tubercle of Gerdy and is thought to be pathognomonic of anterior cruciate ligament rupture and is well recognized today as an important radiological sign.

EARLY TREATMENT

Conservative and Repair

Early descriptions of surgical treatment of knee disorders are focused on infectious conditions—in most cases, tuberculosis. Paré performed the first known surgical correction of a knee dysfunction. He reported removal of a loose body from the knee joint in 1558. The first surgical removal of a torn and displaced medial meniscus was performed by Brodhurst in 1866. Annandale *(9)* introduced the antiseptic surgical technique; until then, surgical treatment of the knee joint had mainly been confined to drainage of septic joints. Annandale founded arthrotomy of the knee joint, and he studied the removal of loose cartilages in the joint in 1879, likely a part of the torn meniscus *(9)*. Allingham described several modifications of the arthrotomy technique. In 1889, he performed a successful suture of a torn medial meniscus for the first time. Katzenstein noted poor results after resection of the meniscus; therefore, he strongly advocated suture of the torn meniscus rather than than total meniscectomy. To gain the best access to the meniscus, he divided and subsequently reinserted the MCL. However, his postoperative rehabilitation protocol was more interesting. He advocated early mobilization without a cast using vigorous quadricep exercises and suggested the patient should also learn the exercises before the surgery was performed. Synovectomy was used for the treatment of chronic arthritis, introduced by Volkmann for tuberculosis of the joint. Arthrodesis of the knee joint was first evaluated by Albert in 1878 and further described by Hibbs, who fused a knee joint destroyed by tuberculosis in 1911.

The recognition of the treatment of anterior cruciate ligament injury was probably first reported by Stark in 1850 *(6)*. However, he advocated conservative treatment using cast immobilization. It was not until 50 yr later that Battle *(10)* published a report of a successful repair of the anterior cruciate ligament with a 2-yr follow-up. Robson *(11)* reported an 8-yr follow-up of a repair of the anterior and posterior cruciate ligaments in 1903. This is likely the first description of knee dislocation and involved a patient who was a miner and injured his knee in an earthfall. The functional recovery was complete, and the miner returned to heavy labor after the successful surgical repair. Robson reported full extension, normal stability (no signs of increased laxity), and only a minor limitation of flexion *(11)*—a result most knee surgeons would be very proud of today.

The first publication that included several cases was by Goetjes in 1913 *(12)*. He reported the results of 30 patients (he had operated on seven himself) and strongly advocated repair (suture) of acute anterior cruciate ligament ruptures. He also reviewed examination under anesthesia to establish a more exact diagnosis of the extent of ligament injury, especially in difficult cases. The publication by Goetjes was very detailed and featured a thorough description of the mechanism of injury based on cadaver studies. He not only advocated surgical repair of acute injuries but also the reduction of tibial spine injuries and cast immobilization in chronic cases. At this time, only "repair" had been described, but later, "reconstruction" was advocated because it was shown that the results after repair were unsuccessful, at least in the medium and long term. In 1916, Jones *(13)* reported poor results after suture of acute ligament rupture. Thus, repositioning the torn ligaments at the anatomical origin did not lead to a functionally stable knee in the long term, which has been repeatedly shown during the last 10–20 yr. This led to a wave of conservative therapy, followed by the next step in knee surgery: reconstruction of the torn anterior cruciate ligament.

CRUCIATE LIGAMENT RECONSTRUCTION

It is often reported that the concept of "reconstruction" was first introduced by Hey Groves in 1917 *(14)*. He used a part of the iliotibial tract, which was proximally based and detached from the tibial insertion. Thereafter, it was rerouted through drill holes in the femur and tibia to mimic the course and attachment sites of the normal anterior cruciate ligament. It was, however, 5 yr earlier that Giertz *(15)* from Sweden performed an operation on a young girl who suffered from a unstable knee after severe intra-articular infection at 1 yr of age. A staged operation was performed: initially an osteotomy to compensate for the fixed flexion deformity, and then 2 wk later, he reconstructed the knee using two strips of fascia lata, one on each side, sutured to the medial and lateral femoral epicondyles proximally and the tibial tubercle and fibular head distally. The functional result was reported as very satisfactory, and the knee was stable. In 1914, Hesse *(16)* studied reconstruction of both the anterior and posterior cruciate ligaments using free fascia lata grafts, rerouted through drill holes in the femur and tibia. A technique using a resected (and torn) meniscus to replace the torn cruciate ligament was performed by zur Verth in 1914 and reported by Hölzel in 1917 *(17)*. The initial result was satisfactory, but failure occurred after 9 mo. This evidence shows that several surgeons had innovative solutions for reconstruction of unstable knees before Hey Groves reported his technique using the free fascia lata graft in 1917 *(14)*. However, it took 20 yr until the extra-articular technique was well described by Bosworth and Bosworth in 1936 *(18)*. They used free fascia lata grafts, woven in a cruciate ligament manner on both the medial and lateral side of the knee. Mattj described a similar technique in 1918 *(19)* also using a free fascia lata strip.

COMBINED INJURIES

The significance of combined injuries, e.g., cruciate ligament ruptures, collateral ligament ruptures and meniscal ruptures, was usually not recognized. In 1936, Campbell *(20)* found a frequent correlation of combined ruptures of the medial meniscus, medial collateral ligament, and anterior cruciate ligament. This was later called "the unhappy triad", owing to the fact that the results were often described as unsatisfactory in patients with combined injuries. Campbell also introduced a reconstruction of the anterior cruciate ligament with a strip of patellar tendon routed through drill holes in the femur and tibia *(20)*, but this technique was not new. In 1932, zur Verth reported for the first time the use of a patellar tendon strip, which was distally attached to treat patients with chronic anterior cruciate ligament injuries. In 1935, Wittek reported a "modified zur Verth-technique", in which he sutured the proximal end of the patellar tendon strip to the posterior cruciate ligament *(21–24)*.

MODERN ERA OF CRUCIATE LIGAMENT INJURIES AND THEIR TREATMENT

The modern era in treating cruciate ligament injuries began in 1938 with the publication by Ivan Palmer on the injuries to the knee ligaments *(25)*. His publication was a comprehensive treatise, including detailed descriptions of the anatomy and pathophysiology. He also reviewed the current therapeutic options and proposed new concepts of biomechanics correlated to injury and treatment. His work was a monumental step forward to a better understanding of ligamentous injuries of the knee. Without doubt, his studies opened a new field of cruciate ligament surgery, but it took decades until his work was fully appreciated. O'Donoghue published his well-known study in 1950, which stimulated researchers to reevaluate the treatment of cruciate ligament injuries *(24)*. He advocated treatment of the triad of torn meniscus, torn medial collateral ligament and torn anterior cruciate ligament. His studies also negated the concept that these injuries were devastating and could only be treated conservatively.

Another important description of a new surgical technique was by Jones in 1963 *(26,27)*. In his own publication, this technique was considered simpler and more physiological than previously described techniques. This procedure was called the "Kenneth Jones technique" for several years *(27)*. However, his approach was not anatomically correct. He did not use a drill hole in the tibia but routed the patellar tendon strip with a full-length bone block from the patella beneath the fat pad at the anterior aspect of the tibia. The femoral drill hole was placed anteriorly in the intercondylar notch, just posterior to the margin of the articular cartilage. This meant that the placement of the reconstructed ligament was far too anterior in the knee. This incorrect (nonisometric) placement has later been shown to be one of the most common reasons for failure of the graft. Yet, Jones published very favorable results, e.g., maximal weight-bearing, full extension, and completely stable knees. In 1966, the German surgeon Brückner described another new method for anterior cruciate ligament reconstruction *(28,29)*, which was later called "Brückner plastic." He advocated the use of the medial one third of the patellar tendon (whereas Jones used the central part) that was distally attached and routed through a tibial tunnel. On the femoral side, he used an inside-out tunnel. This appears to be the first anterior cruciate ligament reconstruction that closely resembles the modern principles. Brückner also discussed harvesting a free contralateral patellar tendon graft using a conical bone block to fit in the tibial drill hole if the ipsilateral patellar tendon was not available because of an old injury or any other reason. It is interesting to note that the results of most techniques were reported as good or excellent in the majority of patients.

ARTIFICIAL LIGAMENTS AND PROSTHESES

During the last decades, several attempts have been proposed to use artificial ligaments or even ligament prostheses. In 1933, Bircher published his experience of using kangaroo tendons for the replacement of both anterior and posterior cruciate ligaments *(30)*. He recommended early postoperative range of motion training, and the results were reported as satisfactory in many cases. During the 1980s and 1990s, an increased interest in using allografts was noted, and several publications have reported the results as good. However, owing to problems of availability and the possible risk of disease transmission (HIV and/or hepatitits), the use of allografts has probably diminished.

In 1903, Lange *(31,32)* proposed the use of silk sutures as prosthetic ligaments. He reported four cases of flail knee joints, which were successfully stabilized using artificial silk ligament and combined with hamstrings (semitendinosus and semimembranosus) plasty. Lange stated that silk was surrounded with fibrous tissue with time and that it had an effective ability to produce solid and strong fibrous tissue, especially under functional stress *(31,32)*. The same idea was mentioned by Ludloff in 1927 *(33)*, who used a rather wide fascia lata strip and wrapped it around a strong silk suture as a kind of an augmentation, an idea which later was popularized by Kennedy (ligament augmentation device [LAD]; *30)* and others *(34–36)*. However, the success of silk sutures was very limited. During the last two to three decades, several ligament augmentation devices, as well as synthetic ligaments and ligament prostheses, were introduced (e.g., carbon fiber, polypropylene, and several others). These devices were either used as ligament prostheses or load-shearing scaffolds. The use of scaffolds should theoretically reduce the load on the new ligament, at least during the immediate postoperative period. This should also facilitate the early rehabilitation process and possibly encourage the in-growth of new collagen fibers. Regretably, it has been shown in several publications that the functional results, including the restoration of knee laxity, were either equivocal or inferior to traditional treatment methods. The complication rate has also been markedly higher, such as the risk of particle wear. Artificial ligaments are therefore hardly used today.

TODAY AND THE FUTURE

Approximately 20 yr ago, the first reports on arthroscopic treatment of cruciate ligaments were published. The first known arthroscopically-assisted anterior cruciate ligament reconstruction was performed by Dandy in 1980 *(28)*. He used a carbon-fiber artificial ligament, which was supplemented by an extra-articular lateral augmentation. During the last two decades, a rapid evolution of new methods has made cruciate ligament repair a well-defined science. Today, almost all cruciate ligament reconstructions are arthroscopically assisted using minimally invasive methods to minimize the surgical morbidity. The most common method is likely the use of a free central-third patellar tendon graft, which has been used for almost 20 yr, producing predictably good results. However, during the last 5–7 yr, use of hamstring tendons (semitendinosus/gracilis) has gained popularity. However, it must be kept in mind that there are several unanswered questions concerning the optimal treatment of cruciate ligament injuries. Hopefully, the future will answer these questions, such as how to determine which patients should be operated on, whether the risk of meniscal injuries can be reduced *(37)*, whether the risk of development of osteoarthrosis can be reduced, and if it is possible to reduce the number of cruciate ligament injuries by some kind of prophylactic measures.

REFERENCES

1. Hey W. On internal derangement of the knee. In *Practical Observations in Surgery*. Hansard, London, UK, 1803.
2. Weber W, Weber E. *Mechanik der Menischlichen Gehwerkzeuge*. Göttingen, Germany, 1836.

3. Bonnet A. *Traité des Maladies des Articulations*. Balliére, Paris, France, 1845.
4. Bonnet A. *Traité de Therapeutique des Maladies des Articularies*. Balliére, Paris, France, 1853.
5. Salter RB, Simmonds DF, Malcoms BW. The biological effect of continuous passive motion on the healing effect of full thickness defects in articular cartilage: an experimental investigation in the rabbit. *J Bone Joint Surg* 1980;63A:1232–1251.
6. Stark J. Two cases of ruptured cucial ligaments of the knee joint. *Edinburgh Med Surg* 1850;5:267–271.
7. Noulis G. Entorse de genou. In: *Faculté de Medicine Paris*. Paris, France: 1875.
8. Segond P. Recherches cliniques et expérimentales sur les épanchements sanguins du genou par entrose. *Prog Med* 16:295–422.
9. Annandale T. An operation for displaced semilunar cartilage. *Brit Med J* 1885;1462: 779.
10. Battle WH. A case after open section of the knee joint for irreducible traumatic dislocation. *Clin Soc London Trans* 1900;33:232–233.
11. Robson MAW. Ruptured crucial ligaments and their repair by operations. *Ann Surg* 1903; 37:716–720.
12. Goetjes H. Über Verletzungen der Ligaments cruciata des Kniegelenks. *Dtsch Zeitschrift für Chirugie* 1913;123:221–289.
13. Jones R. Disabilities of the knee joint. *Brit Med J* 1916;2:169–173.
14. Hey Groves EW. Operation for the repair of the crucial ligaments. *Lancet* 1917;11:674–676.
15. Giertz K. Über freie Transplantation der fascia lata als Ersatz für Sehnen und Bânder. *Dtsch Zeitschrift für Chirugie* 1913;125:480–496.
16. Hesse E. Über den Ersatz der Kreutzbänder des Kniegelenkes durch freie Fascientransplantation. *Verh Drsch Ges Chir* 1914;43:188–189.
17. Hölzel A. Fall von Zerreisung beider Kreutzbänder geheilt durch Ersatz aus dem luxierten äuseren Meniskus. *Münch Med Wochenschr* 1917;64:928–930.
18. Bosworth D, Bosworth B. Use of fascia lata to stabilize the knee in cases of ruptured crucial ligaments. *J Bone Joint Surg* 1936;18A:178–179.
19. Mattj H. Ersatz der gerissenen vorderen Kreutzbandes durch extraarticuläre freie Fazientreanplantation. *Münch Med Wochenschr* 1918;65:451–452.
20. Campbell WC. Repair of ligaments of the knee. *Surg Gynecol Obstet* 1936;62:964–968.
21. Snook GA. A short history of the anterior cruciate ligament and the treatment of tears. *Clin Orthop* 1983;172:11–13.
22. Snook GA. The ACL: a historical review. In Feagin JA, ed., *The Crucial Ligaments*. Churchill-Livingstone, New York, NY, 1988, pp. 157–160.
23. Paessler HH. The history of cruciate ligaments. *Sports Exercise and Injury* 1988;1:166–171.
24. O'Donoghue DH. Surgical treatment of fresh injuries to the major ligaments of the knee. *J Bone Joint Surg* 1950;32–A:721–738.
25. Palmer I. On the injuries to the knee joint—a clinical study. *Acta Ort Chir* 1938;81(Suppl 53): 2–282.
26. Jones K. Reconstruction of the anterior cruciate ligament. *J Bone Joint Surg* 1963;45A: 925–932.
27. Jones KG. Reconstruction of the anterior cruciate ligament usign the central one-third of the patellar ligament: A follow-up report. *J Bone Joint Surg* 1970;52A:1302–1308.
28. Dandy DJ. *Arthroscopic Surgery of the Knee*. Churchill-Livingstone, Edinburgh, London, UK, 1981, pp. 67–68.
29. Kennedy JC, Roth JH, Schmidt AA. The ligament augmentation device (LAD) in the anterior cruciate ligament deficient knee. *Orthop Trans* 1980;4:403–404.
30. Bircher E. Über Binnenverletzungen des Knigelenkes. *Arch Klin Chir* 1933;177:290–359.
31. Lange F. Über die Sehnenplastik. *Verh Dtsch Orthop Ges* 1903;2:10–12.
32. Lange F. Künstliche Bänder aus Seide. *Münch Med Wochenschr* 1907;52:834–836.

33. Larson RL. Introduction and historical perspective. In Larson RL, Grana WA, eds., *The Knee: Form, Function, Pathology and Treatment.* WB Saunders Company, London, UK, 1993, pp. 3–10.
34. Ludloff K. Der operative Ersatz des vorderen Kreutzbandes am Knie. *Zentralbl Chir* 1927; 54:3162–3166.
35. Olson EJ, Kang JD, Fu FH. The biochemical and histological effects of artificial ligament wear particles: in vitro and in vivo studies. *Am J Sports Med* 1988;16:558–570.
36. Shino K, Tamura T, Hirose H. Reconstruction of the anterior cruciate ligament by allogenic tendon graft. *J Bone Joint Surg* 1986;68B:739–746.
37. Brantigan OC, Voshell AF. The mechanics of the ligaments and menisci of the knee joint. *J Bone Joint Surg* 1941;23A:44–66.

7
Rotator Cuff

Richard O. Evans, Peter J. Hughes, and David H. Sonnabend

INTRODUCTION

Over the last 20 yr, the frequency of surgical intervention for rotator cuff tears has risen dramatically. The surgery and postoperative rehabilitation has been mostly empirical with little scientific foundation. There is a wide range of pathology found in the rotator cuff, particularly the horizontal cleavage tear or delamination, which is frequently observed but rarely studied.

The rotator cuff is a complex tendon and is formed by the joining of the supraspinatus, infraspinatus, and teres minor tendons. The separate tendon of the subscapularis muscle is sometimes included in the definition of the rotator cuff. It is a large flat tendon that inserts along the greater tuberosity of the proximal humerus. The cuff functions by holding the humeral head apposed to the glenoid. The musculotendinous cuff is firmly adherent to the underlying glenohumeral capsule and provides circumferential reinforcement, except at the rotator interval and axillary recess. Recognition of the cuff as being unique to animal species capable of bipedal locomotion and overhead arm activity enhances the appreciation of its significance.

INCIDENCE

The precise incidence of rotator cuff pathology is not known; until recently, estimates were based on postmortem studies *(1–3)*. Some studies do not report age distribution and correlation, some do not distinguish between partial and full thickness of cuff tears, and others only report findings from the examination of the dorsal surface. Many partial thickness tears are confined to the articular (deep) surface and are not visible from the dorsal surface.

Human rotator cuff pathology is not uncommon. It includes full and partial thickness tears, macroscopic visibility, and interstial cuff disease that can be identified by numerous imaging techniques and histopathology. Cadaver studies indicate that partial thickness tears, especially those on the deep (articular) side of the cuff, occur in the 40–60 yr range, earlier in life, and more frequently than full thickness tears. The incidence of interstitial tears is difficult to determine from clinical or cadaver studies. Tears of partial thickness may propagate within the substance of the cuff producing lamination.

The cuff is composed of multiple orthogonally aligned fiber layers, where the thicker layers run in the direction of the muscle origin *(4)*. A great deal of the pathology in the

From: *Orthopedic Biology and Medicine: Repair and Regeneration of Ligaments, Tendons, and Joint Capsule*
Edited by: W. R. Walsh © Humana Press Inc., Totowa, NJ

rotator cuff reflects this microstructure. Healing of these defects, even after surgical repair, is believed to be complex, unpredictable, and frequently incomplete.

By the seventh decade, the incidence of partial and full thickness tears combined is reported to range from 30% to 50% *(1,5)*. Although most series also report nearly equal frequencies between right and left sides, other series disagree, and some authors report significantly higher incidence in women than in men *(5)*.

AETIOLOGY

There is no universal agreement regarding the etiology of cuff degeneration and disruption. In most cases, the pathology is probably multifactorial. Mechanisms include relative hypovascularity, age-related connective tissue changes, mechanical impingement beneath the coracoacromial arch, single episodes of major trauma, and repeated episodes of microtrauma *(6–10)*.

Tears of the rotator cuff typically involve the supraspinatus tendon, and they will often include the posterior cuff to a variable degree. The subscapularis tendon, although less frequently involved, may be easily overlooked if not considered during diagnostic evaluation. The torn rotator cuff can demonstrate variably shaped defects that should be noted with surgical reconstruction. A vertical tear, in line with the course of the tendon, can often be repaired with a side-to-side closure. Horizontal tears run transverse to the normal course of the tendon and demonstrate variability in size and the extent of retraction. Typically, closure of such defects requires a transosseous repair to the greater tuberosity. Complex tears that contain both horizontal and vertical components also occur and may require a combination of the techniques.

CLASSIFICATION

There is no universally accepted classification scheme for rotator cuff disease, making studies difficult to compare. Aspects to consider when reviewing rotator cuff lesions include the duration, depth, and size of a tear, as well as the condition of the muscle and tendon. Tears can be acute or chronic and may be associated with a variable degree of weakness and discomfort. Gradation of partial-thickness lesions has been described; however, difficulty lies in the definition and accurate assessment of such lesions. For example, fraying of the tendon observed during an operation may be considered as a partial tear by some surgeons and not by others. Moreover, the incidence of such lesions in relation to symptoms and the treatment results are not easily determined because of variability in imaging capabilities, interpretation, and lack of uniformity in classification.

Full-thickness tears may be described as small (<2 cm in diameter), medium (2–4 cm), large (4–5 cm), or massive (>5 cm). Additionally, a torn rotator cuff may be retracted, deficient, attenuated, or friable at the time of surgical assessment.

An arthroscopic classification has been developed by the Southern California Orthopaedic Institute *(11)*. This is a simple descriptive scheme that uses letters and numbers to designate the pathological condition of the tendon, incorporating partial- and full-thickness pathology.

IMAGING

Plain radiographs are important to eliminate other sources of shoulder pain, such as calcific tendinitis, glenohumeral osteoarthritis, or destructive bone lesions. They provide clinical help in diagnosing large rotator cuff tears but are not sufficient for scientific studies *(12)*. Cuff arthrography is accurate for the detection of full-thickness rotator cuff tears, but it is invasive and does not give precise information on tear size or the condition of the rotator cuff muscles. The high-resolution real-time ultrasound has also been used to evaluate the integrity of the rotator cuff *(13)*. Accuracy is operator-dependent *(13,14)*. A recent study in asymptomatic adults *(5)* has provided valuable information, but this and other studies show that the ultrasound is not reliable *(15,16)*. Therefore, the ultrasound has not become a commonly employed method to assess the rotator cuff. However, it retains the advantages of being quick, inexpensive, and noninvasive.

The muscle can be best assessed with the aid of quality magnetic resorance imaging (MRI) scans on which cross-sectional area, degree of fatty infiltration, and alterations in overall muscle signal intensity can be determined *(17–19)*. MRI is therefore the investigation of choice because it shows the correlation of supraspinatus muscle atrophy in association with rotator cuff tears and partial thickness pathology *(20)*.

CLINICAL SIGNIFICANCE

Postmortem studies suggest that degeneration of the rotator cuff is progressive with age, but controversy continues to exist concerning the pathogenesis of rotator cuff disease. The heterogeneity of the disorder and the notion that rotator cuff disease may not actually represent a continuum of the same process, but instead, is a compilation of independent disorders, may partly explain the differing viewpoints on its origin. Epidemiological studies imply that the prevalence of symptomatic shoulder disorders may decrease in years beyond middle age *(21)*. It is not always possible to determine precisely what proportion of shoulder discomfort is caused by rotator cuff pathology, but several studies *(21,22)* support the widespread clinical impression that most shoulder discomfort in middle and old age is because of rotator cuff pathology. Chard et al. *(21)* and Chakravarty and Webley *(23)*, studying apparently healthy people, suggested a prevalence of identifiable symptomatic shoulder disorders of approx 20%, and indicated that approx 70% of those cases involved the rotator cuff. These studies confirm that an appreciable number of elderly people (≥65 yr) are disabled by shoulder pain. Interestingly, the annual incidence of a painful shoulder has been reported as the highest, and more than 2% per annum in the middle-aged group of 42–46 yr *(22)*.

In addition to age, symptomatic shoulder pathology is also associated with heavy manual labor. Biomechanical studies show that shoulder muscles are heavily loaded when the arm is elevated and that the weight of hand-held tools increases the strain, particularly in the spinati *(24)*.

PATHOLOGY

Two contrasting pathogenetic mechanisms have been extensively described and include vascular (intrinsic) causes and impingement (extrinsic) factors. But other etiologies have also been reported that include trauma, congenital or developmental factors, and instability.

Vascular

The relationship between the microvascular blood supply of the rotator cuff and tendon degeneration remains a subject of debate. Conflicting reports about the vascularity of the supraspinatus tendon exist; however, in many investigations, the methods employed were limited. Moreover, although vascular-mediated mechanisms have been suggested as an important factor in the genesis of rotator cuff disease, studies have been unable to sufficiently attribute hypovascularity as a direct cause for observed tears of the rotator cuff.

An early physiological study suggested that tendons received a vascular supply from three sources: muscular, osseous, and direct tendinous sites *(25)*. Subsequently, it was proposed that a critical portion existed within the distal rotator cuff tendon, predisposing it to degeneration and calcification *(26)*. A vascular or ischemic mechanism was recommended, which in association with trauma, leads to tearing of the rotator cuff. This concept was reinforced when normal musculotendinous specimens were placed under mechanical loads; the muscle became the initial point of failure *(27)*. However, if the tendon was compromised secondary to an interrupted blood supply and repeated stress, it then became the first site of failure, while the muscle integrity was preserved.

Various cadaveric studies also confirmed a region of relative hypovascularity within the distal rotator cuff tendon after arterial latex injection *(28,29)*. They noted consistent vascular patterns in their specimens which were independent of age, but they felt that their methods were not entirely accurate to reflect age-related changes. Furthermore, a study of cadaveric histology of the rotator cuff showed a decrease in vessel number, size, and percentage of tendon occupied by vessels in both the distal supraspinatus and infraspinatus tendons *(30)*.

However, other researchers have failed to show similar reduction in vascularity of the rotator cuff tendon. Research using both microangiographic and histologic techniques to evaluate the tendon vascularity of the rotator cuff in cadavers showed adequate vascularity when injections were performed on the abducted arm, but the vessels were "wrung out" and no longer perfused in the adducted arm. They hypothesized that the critical zone was subject to a transient hypovascularity that was mediated by arm position *(31)*.

Another cadaveric study revealed differential vascularity between the bursal and articular surfaces of the rotator cuff. The bursal surface was observed to be well vascularized, whereas the articular surface demonstrated a sparse arteriolar pattern *(32)*. The authors found that deficient tendon vascularity differentially predisposed the articular surface of the rotator cuff to degenerative changes and failure.

Intraoperative laser Doppler flowtometry has also been used to assess rotator cuff tendon vascularity in symptomatic patients. One investigation was aimed at clarifying the discrepancy between surgical findings of increased vascularity in patients with impingement within the supraspinatus tendon. The patients with tendinitis and intact tendons always showed increased vascularity in the area of greatest mechanical impingement—the critical zone. Increased vascularity was also observed at the tendon margins of those patients with partial-thickness tears. Patients with complete tendon tears had differing degrees of vascularity at the tendon edges. The investigators concluded that impingement generates a hypervascular response that results in the resorption of injured tendon fibers by neovascular tissue and mediates the progression of rotator cuff disease *(33)*.

Impingement

Neer *(8,34)* initially popularized the concept of impingement syndrome, noting that the rotator cuff was potentially subject to repeated mechanical insult by the coracoacromial arch during arm elevation. He described three stages of the impingement syndrome that exist as a continuum, ultimately leading to tears of the rotator cuff: stage 1, characterized by subacromial edema and hemorrhage; stage 2 included fibrosis and tendonitis; and stage 3, rotator cuff failure that was characterized by partial or complete tendon tears. He attributed 95% of all rotator cuff lesions to primary mechanical impingement.

Acromion morphology has been implicated in the etiology of impingement syndrome and rotator cuff disease. A cadaveric study evaluating 140 anatomic specimens *(35)* identified three predominant acromial forms. The acromion undersurface was categorized as flat (type 1), curved (type 2), or hooked (type 3). Of observed rotator cuff tears, 70% were associated with hooked anterior acromions. Since this, the same group *(36)* has verified these observations in a clinical setting in patients with various shoulder complaints.

Despite the strong association between degenerative subacromial hypertrophic spur formation and full-thickness tears of the rotator cuff, a causal relationship remains difficult to prove *(26,35,37)*. The contribution of scapulothoracic movement is also unclear.

Subacromial spurs have been thought to represent secondary changes that occur as a result of the rotator cuff's existing tears *(38)*. Conversely, others have suggested that observed lesions of the rotator cuff occur because of mechanical insult by inferiorly projecting subacromial bony excrescences *(34)*. The formation of such spurs has been indicated to be owing to repeated tension exerted on the coracoacromial ligament *(39)*. Despite controversy over the initial lesion, subacromial spurs appear to have a role in the development and progression of commonly observed rotator cuff tears. One histologic evaluation of bursal side rotator cuff tears in surgical specimens revealed variable-thickness tears of the supraspinatus, corresponding with areas of impingement of the overlying acromion and coracoacromial ligaments. Avascular regions of the proximal edge of the torn tendon were also seen. The combined findings led the authors to conclude that multiple etiologies, including both intrinsic and extrinsic causes, were responsible for the observed abnormalities *(40)*. The question of pathogenesis will likely remain unanswered until controlled studies are conducted. Retrospective clinical and cadaveric investigations remain limited in their ability to sufficiently address this issue.

Alternative sources of impingement have been implicated in the development of rotator cuff disease. In certain patients, distally pointing acromioclavicular osteophytes, the coracoid process, and the posterosuperior aspect of the glenoid can contribute to shoulder pain and rotator cuff lesions *(41–43)*.

The impingement syndrome represents a specific diagnosis with characteristic findings; however, clinical observation has suggested an overdiagnosis of this entity, which may partly explain why some patients do not improve with accepted treatment methods. Despite the underlying etiology, the heterogeneity of rotator cuff disease, impingement syndrome, and other abnormalities that can mimic impingement disorders should all be thoroughly considered to avoid potential pitfalls in diagnosis and treatment.

LAMINATION

Many full-thickness tears of the rotator cuff are associated with tendon lamination *(37)*. The deeper layer is generally thinner; at surgery, the deeper layer is often found to be retracted further that the dorsal layer (DS, personal observation). The multilaminar structure of the rotator cuff has been well described *(4)*, but the mechanism is not understood. It may be multifactorial. It is not uncommon to find a "rim rent" of the deep surface in the critical zone of Codman *(6)*, representing a partial-thickness tear. A combination of effects, e.g., critical vascularity *(9,37,44,45)* and arteriolar intimal hyperplasia *(10)*, all render this zone of the supraspinatus prone to initial degeneration and tearing. The layered nature of the cuff tendons lends itself to delamination. The general principles of the histological structure are well described *(4,46,47)*. The dorsal surface consists largely of longitudinally arranged larger diameter collagen fibers, and the articular surface has an increasing number of transversally arranged collagen fibers. Five histological layers describe this arrangement *(4)*.

Nakajima et al. *(47)* studied the relationship between histology and biomechanics of the supraspinatus. They showed differing mechanical properties between the two surfaces, where the bursal side generally has greater tensile strength, which again explains why many cuff tears arise on the distal part of the joint surface of the cuff insertion.

The role of other mechanical factors, such as subacromial impingement and the curved course of the rotator cuff over the humeral head, is difficult to define. Cuff impingement *(34)* might add to the differential shear on the rotator cuff, exacerbating interlaminar seperation. The passage of the supraspinatus tendon around the curve of the humerus might also produce recurring deep surface pressures and a shearing effect.

The glenohumeral capsule's impact in the production or exacerbation of lamination tears is also difficult to assess. The "capsular cable" described by Burkhart *(48)* as shielding the cuff insertion from stress, is not fully understood. The capsule of the shoulder joint is certainly thinner within the crescent outlined by that cable. As the cuff and capsule are effectively fused in that area, this may suggest a relative weakness in that part of the cuff. As the capsular fibers in that area are largely transverse *(46)*, the capsular support to the cuff is relatively weaker than elsewhere, further predisposing the cuff to the deep surface disruption. Burkhart describes a spectrum of cables and crescents with "cable-dominant" and "crescent-dominant" rotator cuffs, emphasizing the multifactorial etiology of delamination.

In an experimental study by the senior author (DS) reviewing the histology and immunochemistry of 17 rotator cuff tears, five of the samples had synovial-like cells in between the laminated layers. If the laminated layers of a rotator cuff are repaired to each other, their surfaces should be curetted prior to suture, to remove any synovial lining and to fecilitate the healing of the layers to each other. The continued presence of synovial layers might prevent healing as synovial B type cells produce hyaluronate—a recognized "joint lubricant." Therefore, it may be advisable that all laminated tears be curetted before suture repair.

Most rotator cuff tears occur at the tendon bone junction, and their repair involves reattachment of tendon to bone at that site. Although tendon-to-tendon repair has been studied in many species *(49–51)*, tendon-to-bone repair is less well understood, and the repair of the flat tendon to bone is only partially understood *(52)*.

Tendons attach to bone via four sequential tissue zones: pure tendon, uncalcified fibrocartilage, mineralized fibrocartilage, and bone *(53,54)*. In first describing these layers, Cooper and Misol *(53)* studied the patella tendon in adult dogs and noted that the collagen fibers were closely parallel. In contrast, they found that the collagen fibers ran in numerous directions in the medial collateral ligament.

Most research of bone–tendon junctions and bone healing has involved tendons in which the collagen fibers are oriented along the axis of the particular tendon being studied. Considerable differences exist between the insertions of different tendons, where collagen fibers are oriented longitudinally *(54)*. As noted previously, the human rotator cuff is multilayered with numerous orthogonal layers *(4)*. Histologically, the different layers (uncalcified fibrocartilage, calcified fibrocartilage and bone) appeared very similar to the corresponding layers in other tendon bone junctions, but the multiple directions of the collagen fibers and the multiple potential lines of pull of the human rotator cuff suggested that differences might exist in both rates and natures of tendon bone healing.

The few reported studies of experimental bone tendon healing in animal shoulders may not be entirely relevant to humans. The only reported study of shoulder tendon repair in a primate model is that of Paulos and Franklin *(55)*. This study recognized the difference between the anatomy and function of primate and quadruped shoulders. Unfortunately, few histological details are provided.

Rehabilitation following rotator cuff repair in the human is a gradual process. Most surgeons begin with passive mobilization, proceeding to active assisted exercises and closed chain exercises, and finally to active resisted exercises. The timing of these is largely empirical. Paulos and Franklin *(55)* found that the adult monkey supraspinatus regained 36% of projected strength recovery by 1 mo; 55% by 2 mo; 64% by 4 mo; 73% by 5 mo; 79% by 12 mo; and 100% by 30 mo. Miyahara et al. *(56)* found that the adult dog supraspinatus regained 30% of projected strength by 2 wk; 62.5% by 6 wk; and 82.5% by 24 wk. The rotator cuff repair in the adult dog never reached the tensile strength of the normal shoulder. In a more detailed study of goat infraspinatus healing to bone, Rodeo et al. *(57)* assessed load to failure, energy to failure, and stiffness with two different repair techniques. The repair types did not significantly affect the outcomes. Load to failure and energy to failure were both approx 20% of the control group at 6 wk and 35% at 12 wk.

PATIENT CHOICE

Patients with rotator cuff problems will typically complain of pain, weakness, or both. Many patients cannot recall an injury; in others, symptoms may have begun after a trivial trauma. McLaughlin *(58)* noted about 25% of cadavers studied had a rotator cuff tear and hypothesized that not all of these had been symptomatic in life. Hence, if not all rotator cuff tears are symptomatic, the aim of nonoperative treatment is to help a patient with symptomatic rotator cuff disease become asymptomatic. This may involve activity modification, corticosteroid injections, and physical therapy. The physiotherapy is primarily based on scapula stabilization, capsular stretching, and rotator cuff strengthening.

Data suggests that nonoperative treatment of rotator cuff tears is successful in 33–92% of cases, with most studies reporting a satisfactory result in approx 50% of patients. Bokor et al. *(59)* reported on 53 patients with documented rotator cuff tears undergoing nonoperative treatment at an average follow-up of longer than 7 yr. Of patients, 75% had satisfactory pain relief, particularly those presenting after an acute injury. Patients with long-standing pain (>6 mo) did not respond well to nonoperative therapy.

In our experience, nonoperative treatment for patients with rotator cuff disease who present with pain works very well. All patients receive a trial of this treatment, unless an acute traumatic tear is suspected from the history and examination. Furthermore, if weakness is a major or progressive symptom, then investigation and often surgical intervention is expedited. Bassett and Cofield *(60)* reported that in patients who have an acute injury and a full-thickness rotator cuff tear, repair within the first 3 wk resulted in the best surgical outcome.

The presence of a rotator cuff tear is not necessarily an indication for surgery—both MRI *(61)* and cadaver studies *(58)* have shown asymptomatic patients with cuff tears. The indications for surgical repair are the presence of pain or functional deficits that interfere with activities and have not responded to conservative measures. Most surgeons would continue nonoperative treatment for at least 3–4 mo before considering repair; when weakness is significant or progressive, more timely repair may be considered.

SURGICAL TECHNIQUE

Since Codman's first description of rotator cuff repair in 1911, techniques for this operation have evolved. Early reports *(6)* described various approaches, some crossing the acromioclavicular joint and others splitting the anterior deltoid more laterally. Acromium-splitting approaches have been popularized in the past *(62,63)*. In 1972, Neer *(34)* described combined acromioplasty and cuff repair through an anterosuperior incision. Since then, the reported outcomes of surgical rotator cuff repair have considerably improved. A number of studies since that time have described successful repair of full-thickness tears with a high degree of satisfactory results, reduced pain and improved shoulder function *(64–66)*. Some debate remains as to whether or not all cuff repairs should be accompanied by acromioplasty and a limited subdeltoid bursectomy *(67,68)*. Other contentious issues in rotator cuff repair include the necessary extent, if any, of distal clavicular excision.

Arthroscopic repair is now widely described and is performed once the glenohumeral joint arthroscopy is completed, and the posterior portal may be redirected into the subacromial space. A lateral or anterolateral portal is then created for instrumentation. An arthroscopic bursectomy, anterior acromioplasty, and coracoacromial ligament resection may then be performed as needed. If there is a full-thickness tear, the cuff may be mobilized with traction sutures. The most commonly used techniques of tendon repair utilize the anterior, lateral, and posterior portals to place suture anchors in the tuberosity, pass the sutures through the cuff tendon edge, and tie down the knots arthroscopically.

Various techniques have been described for suturing rotator cuffs. One important study suggested that modified Mason-Allen sutures provided the best holding power in a weak tendon while minimizing strangulation *(66)*. However, simple sutures elongate least under load and thus gap less in a strong tendon. The most accepted arthroscopic techniques are placing suture anchors, threading the sutures through the edge of the torn tendon, and then arthroscopically tying knots. Alternatively, a transfixing implant (e.g., a tack or staple) may be used, or a suture anchor with attached suture may be threaded directly through the tendon edge. Attempts to place transosseous tunnels have been made *(69)*, but the risk of injury to the circumflex branch of the axillary nerve has kept most surgeons to suture-anchor techniques. These approaches are still in rapid evolution but do appear to reproduce the steps of the open repair well. The major advantage of arthroscopic repair is believed to be the preservation of the deltoid origin. However, Rockwood and Lyons *(70)* suggested that subperiosteal elevation of the deltoid, as is performed with arthroscopic acromioplasty, may detach a large proportion of the Sharpey fibers of the deltoid origin, causing substantial weakening.

In an arthroscopic-assisted approach, the initial procedure is the same as with an arthroscopic repair, usually with an arthroscopic subacromial decompression. A small incision is then used to directly repair the tear through a deltoid split without detachment. This approach is especially useful for small- and medium-cuff tears. Although some authors have made quite large skin incisions and still called it a "mini-open" approach, if only a deltoid split is used, most surgeons have kept the incision small and in the skin creases. This is the "portal-extension" approach, in which the anterolateral portal is extended to a length of 3 cm *(71)*. This approach provides good exposure of the supraspinatus and infraspinatus tendons, but access to the subscapularis and teres minor is difficult.

Several authors have described extensive tendon mobilization to repair large defects. Cofield *(72)* transposed subscapularis, and 25 out of 26 patients were satisfied with their outcome. Debeeyre et al. *(62)* described supraspinatus advancement again with satisfactory results. Latissimus dorsi transfers have been used to manage large defects and patient pain *(52)*, relief satisfaction was high (94%), and 80% of normal shoulder function was achieved.

Massive irrepairable cuffs have also been treated with an anterior deltoid inlay flap *(73)*. In this study, 17 out of 20 patients were satisfied, and active forward flexion had improved in 17 patients. Burkhart et al. *(48)* described a technique of partial repair of the margins of a large tear to restore force transmission, and only one patient reported unsatisfactory results.

Biologic and prosthetic grafts have been used by many authors with varying outcomes. Heikel *(74)* used fascia lata to close cuff defects. Nevaiser et al. *(75)* reported using freeze-dried cadaveric rotator cuff in chronic large tears. All 16 patients reported a decrease in nocturnal pain. Synthetic cuff prostheses in the form of Teflon and Marlex have also been indicated *(38,76)* in 23 of 25 patients with improved range of movement and absence of pain in 23 of patients. More recently, a porcine small-intestine graft, Restore (Depuy), has become commercially available. Although initial animal work shows improved healing *(77)*, no human results are available yet.

PARTIAL-THICKNESS TEARS

Surgical management of partial thickness tears remains controversial; a wide range of options exist, from conservative therapy to open rotator cuff debridement and repair. Prior to arthroscopic surgery, excision and repair of significant partial-cuff tears was common. However, since the advent of arthroscopic techniques, recommendations for the operative management of partial tears vary between investigators. Essentially, there are three surgical options: debridement alone, decompression and debridement, and excision of damaged tendon with primary repair.

Andrews et al. *(78)* reported good success with debridement in a young and athletic group of patients. Snyder et al. *(79)* reported their results on arthroscopic cuff debridement with or without subacromial decompression. They had 85% satisfactory results, with similar results between those patients who had and did not have a decompression. Arroyo et al. *(80)* noted that young overhead athletes frequently develop subacromial scarring and bursitis owing to overuse and instability and that soft-tissue cleanout of the subacromial space may be helpful. Altchek and Carson *(81)* studied 50 throwing athletes with anterior shoulder pain, which was refractory to nonoperative treatment, and found that most had fraying of the articular surface of the cuff. Debridement of this area, combined with debridement of bursitis and coracoacromial ligament hypertrophy when noted, was associated with favorable results in 80% of cases.

When deep-surface partial-cuff tears are associated with internal impingement, most surgeons have employed simple debridement *(82)*, but results are not well described in the literature. However, this group are usually younger patients, who are often involved in throwing sports and are therefore a different group from older patients with degenerative tendon failure.

In older patients, simple debridement has been shown as much less successful *(83)*. Investigators treated 57 partial-cuff tears with arthroscopic debridement alone and found that only half achieved satisfactory results. In this more elderly group, subacromial decompression appears to improve results *(84,85)*. Gartsman *(86)* noted that 83% of 40 patients with partial-thickness tears had major improvements in their shoulders at an average of 29 mo after arthroscopic acromioplasty. However, others *(87)* observed that the results of debridement and decompression of partial tears were not as favorable as those from decompression in shoulders with intact cuffs.

PATIENT SATISFACTION

Not all repairs of the rotator cuff are associated with satisfactory pain relief or the return of shoulder function. Realistic assessment of the likelihood of patient satisfaction is an essential component of preoperative counseling. The surgeons are interested in the precise range of motion and return to strength, whereas the patient's interests are in pain relief and restored ability to undertake activities of daily living, employment, and recreation.

Many structural factors, such as tear shape and size, tissue quality, biceps integrity, and degree of muscular atrophy may affect the outcome of rotator cuff repairs. However, several nonstructural variables may also be important, including patient age, gender, workers' compensation status, and revision surgery. In a major review of the senior author's patients (DS) in 667 repairs, the overall subjective patient satisfaction with the outcome was 88%. This level of satisfaction is comparable to several other studies evaluating rotator cuff outcomes based on both subjective and objective criteria *(85,88–92)*. Slightly fewer patients (83.5%) reported willingness to have surgery again.

Given that pain was the most common indication for surgery, with 95.6% of patients reporting pain preoperatively, pain reduction is an important goal of surgery. In this series rotator cuff repair was highly successful in reducing pain, where 79% of patients reported improvement in daytime pain and 81% in nighttime pain. These results are similar to those seen by several other series *(12,62,88,93)*. Nonetheless, there was a subset of patients who reported that their pain was worse after surgery (3–5%). Results were also consistent with previous literature, showing that patients suffering compensable work-related injuries are less likely to do well following shoulder surgery than noncompensable patients undergoing similar operations *(65,88,94)*.

Several authors have reported that rotator cuff surgery is more effective for pain relief than for improvement in strength and function *(65,88,93)*. In our study, the findings were similar; however, nearly 70% of patients did report that activities of daily living were improved and that abilities to play sports or to return to work was improved. For primary surgery, less than 3% of patients thought that they were worse after surgery with these activities. Patient satisfaction in revision surgery has again been reported as 76% *(95)*, despite less improvement in activities of daily living. Bigliani et al. *(93)* found similar results—52% satisfactory results—based on pain and motion, but 81% of patients had satisfactory relief of pain. Both studies concluded that the primary indication for repeat surgery was pain.

The reasons for poor functional outcome after revision surgery may be poor or deficient cuff tissue, larger tears, persistent subacromial impingement, deltoid and cuff muscle atrophy, deltoid detachment, prior lateral acromionectomy, persistent acromioclavicular (AC) joint tenderness, inadequacy or noncompliance of physical therapy, and inadequate postoperative immobilization *(76,91,93,96)*.

REFERENCES:

1. Jerosch J, Muller T, Castro W. The incidence of rotator cuff rupture, an anatomic study. *Acta Orthop Bel* 1991;57:124–129.
2. Petersson CJ. Ruptures of the supraspinatus tendon: cadaver dissection. *Acta Orthop Scand* 1984;55:52.
3. DePalma AF. In DePalma AF, ed. *Surgery of the Shoulder*, 3rd Ed. JB Lippincott, Philadelphia, PA, 1983, pp. 211–241.
4. Clark JM, Harryman DT. Tendons, ligaments and capsule of the rotator cuff—gross and microscopic anatomy. *J Bone Joint Surg* 1992;74A:713–725.
5. Milgrom C, Schaffler M, Gilbert S. Rotator cuff changes in symptomatic adults. *J Bone Joint Surg* 1985;77B:296–298.
6. Codman EA. *The Shoulder: Rupture of the Supraspinatus Tendon and Other Lesions In or About the Subacromial Bursa.* Thomas Todd, Boston, MA, 1934.
7. Macnab I. Rotator cuff tendinitis. *Ann R Coll Surg Engl* 1973;53:271–287.
8. Neer CS. Impingement lesions. *Clin Orthop* 1983;173:70–77.
9. Wilson CL, Duff GL. Pathologic study of degeneration and rupture of the supraspinatus tendon. *Arch Surg* 1943;47:121–135.
10. Yamanaka K, Fukuda H. Ageing process of the supraspinatous tendon with reference to rotator cuff tears. In Watson MS, ed., *Surgical Disorders of the Shoulder*, 1991, pp. 247–258.
11. Snyder SJ. In *Shoulder Arthroscopy*. 2nd Ed. Lippincott, Williams & Wilkins, New York, NY, 2003, p. 204.
12. Weiner DS, Macnab I. Superior migration of the humeral head. *J Bone Joint Surg Br* 1970;52:524–527.
13. Mack LA, Matsen FR, Kilcoyne JF, et al. Ultrasound evaluation of the rotator cuff. *Radiology* 1985;157:205–209.
14. Miniaci A, Salonen D. Rotator cuff evaluation: imaging and diagnosis. *Orthop Clin North Am* 1997;28:43–58.
15. Sonnabend DH, Hughes JS, Giuffre BM, Farrell R. The clinical role of shoulder ultrasound. *ANZJ Surg* 1997;67:630–633.

16. Teefey SA, Hasa AS, Middleton WD, Patel M, Yamaguchi K. Ultrasound of the rotator cuff: A comparison of ultrasonographic and arthroscopic findings in one hundred consecutive cases. *Clin Orthop* 2000;194:159–163.
17. Maurer K, Schmidt D, Refior HJ. Diagnosis of rotator cuff tears: Prospective comparison of arthrography, non-enhanced MR imaging and MR arthrography in 22 surgically proven cases. *Orthopaedics International Edition* 1997;5:193–200.
18. Van Moppes F, Veldcamp O, Roorda J. Role of shoulder ultrasonography in the evaluation of the painful shoulder. *Eur J Radiol* 1995;19:142–146.
19. Zanetti M, Hodler J. Imaging of degenerative and post-traumatic disease in the shoulder joint with ultrasound. *Eur J Radiol* 2000;35:119–125.
20. Guckel C, Nidecker A. Diagnosis of tears in rotator cuff injuries. *Eur J Radiol* 1997;25: 168–176.
21. Chard MD, Hazelman R, King RH, Reiss BB. Shoulder disorders in the elderly: a community survey. *Arthritis Rheum* 1991;10:807–822.
22. Allander E. Prevalence, incidence and remission rates of some common rheumatic diseases or syndromes. *Scand J Rheum* 1974;3:145–153.
23. Chakravarty KK, Webley M. Disorders of the shoulder: an often unrecognised cause of disability in elderly people. *BMJ* 1990;300:848–849.
24. Herberts P, Kadefors R, Hogfors C, Sihholm G. Shoulder pain and heavy manual labour. *Clin Orthop* 1984;191:166–178.
25. Mayer L. The physiologic method of tendon transplantation. *Surg Gynecol Obstet* 1915; 22:182.
26. Codman EA, Akerson TB. The pathology associated with rupture of the supraspinatus tendon. *Ann Surg* 1931;93:348–359.
27. McMaster P. Tendon and muscle ruptures. *J Bone Joint Surg* 1933;15:705.
28. Lindblom K. On the pathogenesis of ruptures of the tendon aponeurosis of the shoulder joint. *Acta Radiol* 1939;20:563.
29. Rothman RH, Parke WW. The vascular anatomy of the rotator cuff. *Clin Orthop* 1965;41: 176–186.
30. Brooks CH, Revell WJ, Heatley FW. A quantitative histological study of the vascularity of the rotator cuff tendon. *J Bone Joint Surg* 1992;74B:151–153.
31. Rathbun JB, Macnab I. The microvascular pattern of the rotator cuff. *J Bone Joint Surg Br* 1970;52:540–553.
32. Lohr JF, Uhthoff HK. The microvascular pattern of the supraspinatus tendon. *Clin Orthop* 1990;254:35–38.
33. Swiontowski MF, Iannotti JP, Boulas HJ, et al. Intraoperative assessment of rotator cuff vascularity using laser doppler flowtometry. In Post M, Morrey BF, Hawkins RJ, eds., *Surgery of the Shoulder*. Mosby–Year Book, St. Louis, MO, 1990, pp. 208–212.
34. Neer CS. Anterior acromioplasty for the chronic impingement syndrome. A preliminary report.. *J Bone Joint Surg Am* 1972;54:41–50.
35. Bigliani LU, Morrison DS, April EW. The morphology of the acromion and rotator cuff impingement. *Orthop Trans* 1986;10:288.
36. Morrison DS, Bigliani LU. The clinical significance of variations in acromial morphology. *Orthop Trans* 1987;11:234.
37. Fukuda H, Hamada K, Yamanaka K. Pathology and pathogenesis of bursal-side rotator cuff tears viewed from en bloc histologic sections. *Clin Orthop* 1990;254:75–80.
38. Ozaki J, Fujuimoto S, Masuhara K, et al. Reconstruction of chronic massive rotator cuff tears with synthetic materials. *Clin Orthop* 1986;202:173–183.
39. Harris JE, Blackney M. The anatomy and function of the coracoacromial ligament (abstr). *J Shoulder Elbow Surg* 1993;2:S6.
40. Fukuda H. Shoulder impingement and rotator cuff disease. *Curr Orthop* 1990;4:225–232.

41. Walch G, Boileau P, Noel E, et al. Impingement of the deep surface of the supraspinatus tendon on the posterosuperior glenoid rim: an arthroscopic study. *J Shoulder Elbow Surg* 1992;1:238–245.
42. Taylor GM, Tooke M. Degeneration of the acromioclavicular joint as a cause of shoulder pain. *J Bone Joint Surg* 1977;59:507.
43. Tirman PF, Bost FW, Garvin GJ, et al. Posterosuperior glenoid impingement of the shoulder: findings at MR imaging and MR arthrography with arthroscopic correlation. *Radiology* 1994;193:431–436.
44. Brewer BJ. Aging of the rotator cuff. *Am J Sports Med* 1979;7:102–110.
45. Uhtoff HK, Loehr J, Sarkar K. *The Pathogenesis of Rotator Cuff Tears*. Proceedings of the 3rd International Conference on Shoulder Surgery, Fukuoka, Japan, 1986, pp. 211–212.
46. Gohlke F, Barthel T, Gandorfer A. The influence of variations of the coracoacromial arch on the development of rotator cuff tears. *Arch Orthop Trauma Surg* 1994;113:28–32.
47. Nakajima T, Rokuuma N, Hamada K, Tomatsu T, Fukuda H. Histologic and biomechanical characteristics of the supraspinatus tendon: reference to rotator cuff tearing. *J Shoulder Elbow Surg* 1994;3:79–87.
48. Burkhart SS. Reconciling the paradox of rotator cuff repair versus debridement: a unified biomechanical rationale for the treatment of rotator cuff tears. *Arthroscopy* 1994;10:4–19.
49. Lane JM, Black J, Bora WJ. Gliding function following flexor tendon injury: a biomechanical of rat tendon function. *J Bone Joint Surg* 1976;58A:985–990.
50. Manske PR, Lesker PA, Gelberman RH. Intrinsic restriction of the flexot tendon surface in the non human primate. *J Hand Surg* 1985;10A:632–637.
51. Gelberman R, Khabie V, Cahill CJ. The revasularization of healing flexor tendons in digital sheath: a vascular study in dogs. *J Bone Joint Surg* 1991;73A:868–881.
52. Gerber C, Schneeberger AG, Beck M, Schlegel U. Mechanical strength of repairs of the rotator cuff. *J Bone Joint Surg Br* 1994;76:371–380.
53. Cooper RR, Misol S Tendon and Ligament insertion. A light and electron microscopy study. *J Bone Joint Surg* 1970;52A:1–20.
54. Benjamin M, Evans EJ, Corp L. The histology of tendon attachments to bone in man. *J Anat* 1986;149:895100.
55. Paulos IF, Franklin JL. Arthroscopic subacromial decompression development and application: a five year experience. *Am J Sports Med* 1990;18:235–244.
56. Miyahara H, Takagishi K, Arita C, Aria K. A morphologic and biomechanical study on the healing of the repaired rotator cuff insertion in dogs. In Post M, Morrey BF, Hawkins RJ, eds., *Surgery of the Shoulder*. Mosby, St. Louis, MO, 1990, p. 224.
57. Rodeo SA, Arnoczky SP, Torzilli PA, Hidaka C, Warren RF. Tendon healing in a bone tunnel. A biomechanical and histological study in the dog. *J Bone Joint Surg* 1993;75A: 1795–1803.
58. McLaughlin HL. Ruptures of the rotator cuff. *J Bone Joint Surg* 1962;44:979–983.
59. Bokor DJ, Hawkins RJ, Huckell GH, Angelo RL, Schickendantz MS. Results of nonoperative management of full-thickness tears of the rotator cuff. *Clin Orthop* 1993;294: 103–110.
60. Bassett RW, Cofield RH. Acute tears of the rotator cuff. The timing of surgical repairs. *Clin Orthop* 1983;175:18–24.
61. Sher JS, Uribe JW, Posada A, Murphy BJ, Zlatkin MB. Abnormal findings on magnetic resonance images of asymptomatic shoulders. *J Bone Joint Surg Am* 1995;77:10–15.
62. Debeyre J, Patte D, Elmelik E. Repairs of rupture of the rotator cuff of the shoulder: with a note on advancement of the supraspinatus muscle. *J Bone Joint Surg Br* 1965;47:36–42.
63. Kessel L, Watson M. The painful arc syndrome: Clinical classification as a guide to management. *J Bone Joint Surg* 1964;59B:166–172.
64. Neer CS, Flatow EL, Lech O. Tears of the rotator cuff. long term results of anterior acromioplasty and repair. *Orthop Trans* 1988;12:735.

65. Iannotti JP, Bernot MP, Kuhlman JR, Kelley MJ, Williams GR. Postoperative assessment of shoulder function: a prospective study of full-thickness rotator cuff tears. *J Shoulder Elbow Surg* 1996;5:449–457.
66. Gerber C, Fuchs B, Hodler J. The results of repair of massive tears of the rotator cuff. *J Bone Joint Surg* 2000;82A:505–515.
67. Iannotti JP, ed. *Rotator Cuff Disorders—Evaluation and Treatment*. American Academy Orthopaedic Surgeons, Park Ridge, IL, 1991.
68. Uhthoff HK, Sarkar K. The surgical repair of the rotator cuff: The importance of the subacromial bursa. *J Bone Joint Surg* 1991;73B:399–401.
69. Flatow EL, Soslowski LJ, Ticker JB. Excursion of the rotator cuff under the acromion. Patterns of subacromial contact. *Am J Sports Med* 1994;22:779–788.
70. Rockwood CA, Lyons FR. Shoulder impingement syndrome: diagnosis, radiographic evaluation, and treatment with a modified Neer acromioplasty. *J Bone Joint Surg Am* 1993;75:409–424.
71. Pollock RG, Flatow EL. Full-thickness tears: mini-open repair. *Orthop Clin North Am* 1997;28:169–178.
72. Cofield RH. Subscapular muscle transposition for repair of chronic rotator cuff tears. *Surg Gynecol Obstet* 1982;154:667–672.
73. Dierickx C, Vanhoof H. Massive rotator cuff tears treated by a deltoid muscular inlay flap. *Acta Orthop Belg* 1994;60, 94–100.
74. Heikel HVA. Rupture of the rotator cuff of the shoulder. Experiences of surgical treatment. *Acta Orthop Scand* 1968;39:499–502.
75. Nevaiser JS, Nevaiser RJ, Nevaiser TJ. Thr repair of chronic massive ruptures of the rotator cuff. *J Bone Joint Surg Am* 1978;60:681–684.
76. Post M. Complications of rotator cuff surgery. *Clin Orthop* 1990;254:97–104.
77. Dejardin LC, Arnoczky SP, Ewers BJ, Haut RC, Clarke RB. Tissue engineered rotator cuff tendon using porcine small intestine submucosa. *Am J Sports Med* 2001;29:175–184.
78. Andrews JR, Broussard TS, Carson WG. Arthroscopy of the shoulder in the management of partial tears of the rotator cuff: a preliminary report. *Arthroscopy* 1985;1:117–122.
79. Snyder SJ, Pachelli AF, Del Pizzo W, Friedman MJ, Ferkel RD, Pattee G. Partial thickness rotator cuff tears: results of arthroscopic treatment. *Arthroscopy* 1991;7:1–7.
80. Arroyo JS, Hershon SJ, Bigliani LU. Special considerations in the athletic throwing shoulder. *Orthop Clin North Am* 1997;28:69–78.
81. Altchek DW, Carson EW. Arthroscopic acromioplasty: current status. *Orthop Clin North Am* 1997;28:157–168.
82. Flatow EL, Altchek DW, Gartsman GM. Commentary. *Orthop Clin North Am* 1997;28: 277–294.
83. Ogilvie-Harris DJ, Demaziere A. Arthroscopic debridement versus open repair for rotator cuff tears: a prospective cohort study. *J Bone Joint Surg Br* 1986;75:416–420.
84. Braezeale NM, Craig EV. Partial-thickness rotator cuff tears: pathogenesis and treatment. *Orthop Clin North Am* 1997;28:145–156.
85. Ellman H. Diagnosis and treatment of incomplete rotator cuff tears. *Clin Orthop* 1990;254: 64–74.
86. Gartsman GM. Arthroscopic acromioplasty for lesions of the rotator cuff. *J Bone Joint Surg* 1990;72:169–180.
87. Altchek DW, Warren RF, Wickiewicz TL, Skyhar MJ, Ortiz G, Schwartz E. Arthroscopic acromioplasty. *J Bone Joint Surg Am* 1990;72:1198–1207.
88. Hawkins RJ, Misamore GW, Hobeika PE. Surgery for full-thickness rotator-cuff tears. *J Bone Joint Surg Am* 1985;67:1349–1355.
89. Bjorkenheim JM, Paavolainen P, Ahovuo J, Slatis P. Surgical repair of the rotator cuff and surrounding tissues. Factors influencing results. *Clin Orthop* 1988;236:148–153.

90. Essman J, Bell R, Askew M. Full thickness rotator cuff tears. *Clin Orthop* 1991;265: 170–177.
91. Cofield RH. Rotator cuff disease of the shoulder. *J Bone Joint Surg Am* 1985;67:974–979.
92. Packer NP, Calvert PT, Bayley JIL, Kessel L. Operative treatment of chronic ruptures of the rotator cuff of the shoulder. *J Bone Joint Surg Br* 1983;65:171–175.
93. Bigliani LU, Cordasco FA, McIlveen SJ, Musso ES. Operative treatment of massive rotator cuff tears: long-term results. *J Shoulder Elbow Surg* 1992;1:120–130.
94. Misamore GW, Ziebler DW, Rushton JL. Repair of the rotator cuff. A comparison of results in two populations of patients. *J Bone Joint Surg* 1995;77A:1335–1339.
95. DeOrio JK, Cofield RH. Results of a second attempt at surgical repair of a failed initial rotator cuff repair. *J Bone Joint Surg Am* 1984;66:563–567.
96. Wolfgang G. Rupture of the musculotendinous cuff of the shoulder. *Clin Orthop* 1978;134: 230–243.

8

Frozen Shoulder

Peter J. Hughes, Richard O. Evans, and Jerome A. Goldberg

INTRODUCTION

Idiopathic frozen shoulder, or adhesive capsulitis, is a common condition characterized by a capsular pathology that is associated with pain and the progressive loss of passive and active movement. Its incidence in the general population is approx 2% *(1)*; of these, 20–30% will develop the condition bilaterally. It is more common in females *(1)*, over 40 yr of age *(2)*, and in the nondominant arm *(3)*. A strong association exists with diabetes mellitus *(4)* and, to a lesser extent, with thyroid disease *(5)*.

Frozen shoulder syndrome was first described by Duplay in 1872 *(6)*. He felt that the pain and stiffness noted in these patients was not because of arthritis but was from the soft-tissue pathology of the periarticular structures. In 1934, Codman *(7)* first proposed the term "frozen shoulder." He described a slow onset of pain felt near the deltoid insertion, inability to sleep on the affected side, and painful and restricted elevation and external rotation with a normal radiological appearance. The loss of passive range of movement, particularly related to external rotation, has remained pivotal to the diagnosis of frozen shoulder. However, Codman was unable to explain the pathology. Only recently, the pathogenesis has become more clear but as yet, it is not fully understood.

Matsen *(8)* has defined the condition experienced by patients with stiff shoulder syndrome occurring *de novo* as an idiopathic global limitation of humeroscapular motion that results from contracture and loss of compliance of the glenohumeral joint capsule. These patients with primary idiopathic frozen shoulder comprise up to 5% of all patients with stiff shoulder syndrome *(9)*. Harryman *(10)* has emphasized the importance of recognizing any previous history of trauma to categorize patients with stiff shoulders. With a history of trauma or other preceding stimulus, another group can be defined as having a limitation in humeroscapular motion after an injury, low-level trauma, or part of an accompanying condition, which results in a contracture of structures in the glenohumeral or humeroscapular motion interfaces. This second group can be further subdivided by the injury or disease process and is analogous to secondary adhesive capsulitis, as proposed by Lundberg *(11)*, in which a known intrinsic, extrinsic, or systemic precursor can be identified. Cuomo *(12)* believes it is inappropriate to include all various etiologies within secondary frozen shoulder. Frozen shoulders because of systemic disorders, such as diabetes mellitus or hypothyroidism,

From: *Orthopedic Biology and Medicine: Repair and Regeneration of Ligaments, Tendons, and Joint Capsule*
Edited by: W. R. Walsh © Humana Press Inc., Totowa, NJ

only differ from the idiopathic group in their resistance to treatment and can be easily included as part of this primary group. Intrinsic disorders, e.g., rotator cuff pathology, merit their own subdivision, and treatment must be directed at the initial pathology and the shoulder stiffness.

A multitude of pathologies can predispose to the frozen shoulder *(13)*. It can follow fractures or dislocations about the shoulder, cervical or thoracic surgery, or immobilization after any upper limb surgery. It can occur in association with soft-tissue pathologies, such as rotator cuff and biceps tendonitis and can follow any degenerative shoulder joint disease process. It has also been seen with cervical spine disorders, intrathoracic pathology, and abdominal pathology. Clearly, as noted by Kozin *(14)*, many of these conditions link the patient with a period of pain, immobility, or both.

Frozen shoulder research has been limited by the heterogeneous nature of the patient groups presenting with shoulder stiffness, as represented by these various definitions. Wiley *(15)* has reported on a series of 150 patients with presumed diagnosis of frozen shoulder. After arthroscopic examination, only 37 patients were found to have primary frozen shoulder. Other studies have confirmed the importance of arthroscopy in accurately selecting patients for study *(16)*. Research performed without the control of arthroscopy to exclude other pathologies must therefore be questioned. Improved identification of homogeneous patient groups will simplify treatment decisions and make outcomes more predictable *(13)*.

NATURAL HISTORY

The Pathological Stages of Primary Frozen Shoulder

One of the most contentious issues regarding the frozen shoulder is defining the exact natural history. It has traditionally been regarded as a self-limiting condition, which universally settles over a variable time course *(17)*. Codman believed even the most protracted cases recover with or without treatment in about 2 yr. Reeves *(18)* has performed a prospective longitudinal study of the natural history in 41 patients, and three sequential stages were noted. An early painful stage was described as lasting between 10 and 36 wk, followed by an intermediate stiff or frozen stage from 4 to 12 mo. Finally, a recovery stage was described that lasted from 5 to over 24 mo. Reeves noted all but three of the patients ultimately obtained useful function in the affected limb, but 25 patients showed some residual signs of mild range of motion limitation. The overall impression of the frozen shoulder was that it was a self-limiting disorder and that most patients would be expected to recover within 2.5 yr. Another important observation of Reeves was that the length of the painful period could be directly related to the length of the recovery period.

This self-limiting nature of the frozen shoulder has been challenged by others *(19,20)*. Shaffer and coworkers *(61)* have followed up a cohort of 62 patients with frozen shoulder for a mean time period of 7 yr. They found that 50% of patients still had either stiffness or mild pain affecting the shoulder, and 60% of patients demonstrated some loss of expected range of movement, particularly in external rotation. Thus, although producing little functional disability, half of the patients remained symptomatic. This evidence has led them to question whether the frozen shoulder should be regarded as a self-limiting condition.

The stages of adhesive capsulitis have been further investigated by Hannafin et al. *(21)*. They have correlated the clinical appearance and histology of patients with their arthroscopic stage, as defined by Neviaser and Neviaser *(3)*. Using this information, they have produced a comprehensive classification of adhesive capsulitis divided into four stages, which are summarized here.

In stage 1, symptoms have been present for less than 3 mo and consist of an aching pain exacerbated at extremes of range of movement. Patients demonstrate a mild loss of forward flexion, abduction, and internal and external rotation that invariably resolves upon administration of local anesthetic, as most of the loss of motion is owing to synovitis, not capsular contraction. Arthroscopy shows a hypertrophic vascular synovitis, and biopsy confirms the hypervascular nature of the synovium and normal morphological structure of the underlying capsule.

In stage 2, "the freezing stage," symptoms have been present for 3–9 mo. Significant loss of all movement is present and is persistent even under anesthesia. At arthroscopy, it is frequently difficult to introduce the arthroscope because of a loss in capsular volume, and a diffuse, pedunculated, hypervascular synovitis is often seen. Again, biopsy shows dense, proliferative, hypervascular synovitis, but there is also perivascular scar formation and capsular fibroplasias with the deposition of disorganized collagen fibrils and a hypercellular appearance. Inflammatory infiltrates are not seen.

In stage 3, "the frozen stage," symptoms have been present from 9 to 14 mo. Patients often report a previous painful phase that has substantially settled, leaving a relatively painless but stiffened glenohumeral joint. Arthroscopic appearance illustrates patchy synovial thickening without hypervascularity, and biopsy shows dense, hypercellular collagenous tissue.

In stage 4, "the thawing stage," gradual improvement occurs between 15 and 24 mo. There is little pain, and as capsular remodeling occurs, there is a progressive increase in range of movement. Arthroscopic and histological correlations have not been investigated because surgery is unusual at this phase.

Other researchers have reported on the pathological appearance of frozen shoulder, principally during open surgery for stage 3 disease. The macroscopic observations by Neviaser *(22)* described "a thickened contracted capsule peeled from the humeral head like an adhesive plaster from skin." These observations, which led him to coin the term "adhesive capsulitis," remain true today. DePalma *(19)* observed that the corocohumeral ligament is converted into a tough inelastic band of fibrous tissue, spanning the interval between the corocoid process and the tuberosities of the humerus. He felt this structure is thus converted into a powerful check rein. Therefore, he described the division of this abnormal ligament to allow early restoration of movement.

Lundberg *(11)* was first to find the similarity in pathology between frozen shoulder and Dupuytren's disease, observing the prominence of fibroblast-type cells in both tissues. This link has been confirmed in a study by Bunker, who identified a highly vascular, cellular, collagenous tissue as the principle lesion. However, they were unable to show any significant inflammatory component in their histological investigations. They also commented that the synovium appeared inactive, but the presence of an initial inflammatory stage cannot be excluded, as none of the specimens were taken from patients in the early stage of disease.

Etiology of Primary Frozen Shoulder

A number of mechanisms have been proposed to explain the etiology of the primary frozen shoulder. Early suggestions localizing the pathology to the rotator cuff–bursa interface have been dismissed *(6,7)*. Most agree that the defining pathology is a capsular fibrosis, but the exact cause of this fibrosis is not clearly understood. An inflammatory process has been suggested based on the histological observations of synovial or subsynovial inflammatory reactions *(11,20)*. This, in turn, has led investigators to attempt to identify a particular inflammatory stimulus in the frozen primary shoulder. Bulgen and coworkers have found increased levels of circulating immune complexes together with an elevation of serum C-reactive protein level. This is suggestive of an autoimmune type IV reaction *(23)*. Reduced serum immunoglobulin A levels have also been noted in patients with frozen shoulder, which have persisted after recovery *(24)*. Unfortunately, further studies have failed to confirm this data *(25)*. The absence of identified autoantibodies and lack of polyarthropathy in association with the frozen shoulder mostly negates an autoimmune basis. An infective stimulus—whether viral, bacterial, or fungal—is unlikely *(26)*, as patients do not report a prodromal illness or systemic symptoms. There is also no evidence to link frozen shoulder causally with crystal arthropathy, reactive arthropathy, or hemarthrosis *(26)*. Bunker and coauthors *(15)* have recently investigated the link between frozen shoulder and fibromatoses, such as Dupuytren's disease. Clonal chromosomal abnormalities have been found in many of these conditions. Bunker has detected chromosomal abnormalities in some patients with frozen shoulder, similar to those found in Dupuytren's disease, i.e., trisomy 7 and trisomy 8 *(9)*. Both these conditions appear to be linked to each other and to a high prevalence of diabetes mellitus. In addition, these investigators have found an association between elevated serum lipid levels and frozen shoulder *(27)*. Serum lipid levels are also elevated in patients with Dupuytren's disease *(28)*. These facts add further weight to the hypothesis that idiopathic frozen shoulder is a variant of the fibromatoses.

Further work by Rodeo et al. *(29)* investigated the role of cytokines in the development of the frozen shoulder. They identified a rise of both the platelet-derived growth factor (PDGF) and transforming growth factor β (TGF-β) in the early stages of frozen shoulder. PDGF has been shown to stimulate fibroblast proliferation, and TGF-β promotes extracellular matrix production, leading to fibrosis. The stages of frozen shoulder, as already described, can be linked to the development of fibrosis. Hannafin and coworkers *(21)* have hypothesised that the initial hypervascular synovitis provokes a progressive fibroblastic response in the underlying capsule, which causes progressive fibroplasias, thickening, and contracture. These stages are modulated by the action of TGF-β and PDGF by both paracrine and autocrine abnormal upregulation.

A recent link between protease inhibitors and the genesis of frozen shoulders has also been proposed. In the work by Grasland et al., eight patients with HIV were identified as developing frozen shoulder (bilateral in four patients) after treatment with the protease inhibitor, indinavir *(30)*. This may suggest a link between the inhibition of metalloproteinases and development of abnormal fibrosis within the joint.

ABNORMAL BIOMECHANICS

Differences Between Primary Frozen Shoulder and Posttraumatic Stiff Shoulder

Movement at the shoulder occurs between the two articular surfaces of the glenohumeral joint and between the scapula and thoracic wall in a ratio of 2:1 *(31)*. Movement at the glenohumeral joint is facilitated by the mutual sliding of a set of bursal-lined surfaces, including the deep sides of the deltoid, acromion, corocoid process, and its tendons against the proximal humerus, rotator cuff, and long biceps head. Matsen et al. *(8)* and Romeo have coined the term "humeroscapular motion interface" (HSMI) to describe this articulation. Another term, the "scapulothoracic motion interface" has also been proposed to describe the bursal-lined surface between the scapula blade and thoracic wall. In a glenohumeral joint with healthy articular surfaces, stiffness can occur with three scenarios: (1) contractures that produce shortening of capsule, ligament or muscle-tendon units; (2) adhesions between gliding structures, e.g., the cuff and biceps tendon; and (3) adhesions crossing the HSMI. Clearly, the first scenario can explain primary frozen shoulder pathology with its recognized capsular contractures. The capsule is known to be essentially lax during motion in mid-range *(32)*. The capsule's distinct ligamentous structures become significantly tense only at the end-range extremes of motion. Different regions of the joint capsule have specific functions in limiting particular end-range motions. It is well recognized that the inferior glenohumeral ligament functions as a check rein for external rotation in abduction. In contrast, ligamentous structures within the rotator interval are more important in restraining external rotation in the adducted arm. Thus, we can link the findings of rotation loss in neutral with the observation of tight, contracted structures in the rotator interval.

However, contractures are not limited to the rotator interval. Isolated contractures of other capsulo-ligamentous structures can occur, leading to unusual patterns of motion loss *(26,33)*. Isolated posterior capsular contracture has been related to abnormal glenohumeral motion. With a significant posterior contracture, the humeral head can be translated antero-superiorly during motion, leading to compression of the rotator cuff beneath the coracoacromial arch and thus impingement *(32)*. Therefore, in the stiff shoulder associated with capsular contracture, potential exists to perform a limited release of tight structures. Clearly, if the procedure is to be successful, the correct structures limiting movement must be clarified.

The pathomechanics of some secondary frozen shoulders or posttraumatic stiff shoulders may require a different explanation. Neviaser and Neviaser *(3)* have identified a group of patients with stiff shoulders that occur after trauma, who appear to not have any capsular contracture. To explain these findings, we can look to the HSMI. If adhesions secondary to trauma or surgery cross the HSMI, then movement will be limited depending on the position and extent of the involvement. It is not known whether these patients settle with gradual improvement, as is the case with most patients with primary frozen shoulder. Treatments aimed at the capsular structures are obviously misplaced in this patient group and are likely to fail. In practice, however, it can be difficult to distinguish between the various groups of patients. There is clearly a considerable overlap between the conditions and potential for progression from one to the other.

DIAGNOSIS AND INVESTIGATIONS

History

Primary or idiopathic frozen shoulder is diagnosed from the history and investigation. As has been stated, it is a diagnosis of exclusion after other causes of painful shoulder stiffness are precluded. As part of the assessment, an attempt should be made to define the particular stage that the disease is presenting. This designation is invaluable in informing the patient about their individual prognosis and their best treatment. Codman's original description of the condition is still valid *(7)*. Pain, in the early stages, can be severe and usually radiates to the deltoid insertion. It is worse when the affected shoulder attempts movement but can also be present at rest, invariably interfering with sleep. The patient often notices a gradual loss of motion; specifically, movements overhead and behind the back become difficult. Patients with rotator cuff pathology can also present with these complaints, which can lead to difficulties in diagnosis. Enquiries should be directed at identifying any coexistent pathology that might allow a diagnosis of secondary frozen shoulder. Patients should be questioned about their past injuries. A history of major injury or surgery is easy to define. However, most patients can associate only minor trauma with the onset of symptoms, and the ability to identify the relevance of this can be difficult. Previous surgery predisposing to frozen shoulder is not limited to operations on the shoulder. Axillary node dissections and neck dissections are often seen to predispose to frozen shoulder, particularly when associated with radiotherapy *(34,35)*. Cardiac surgery and neurosurgery are also regarded as being a high risk regarding development of the frozen shoulder *(36,37)*. An incidence of adhesive capsulitis of 3.3% has been estimated in male postcardiac surgery patients *(38)*. The link between all these stimuli may be a period of immobility that is associated with pain. A prospective study of frozen shoulder development in neurosurgical patients has been performed. The condition occurred in 25% of patients and was related particularly to impaired consciousness and hemiparesis. Other neurological conditions have been linked to frozen shoulder and include Parkinson's disease and Brachial neuritis. In addition, the cervical spine should always be considered. Patients with cervical spine intervertebral disc degeneration have been shown to be at a greater risk of developing frozen shoulder *(11)*. Clearly, the importance of therapist guided rehabilitative mobilization in all these high-risk groups cannot be over emphasized. Enquiries should also be made concerning diabetes and thyroid disorders. Bridgman has found an incidence of almost 11% in diabetic patients contrasting to an incidence of 2% in a nondiabetic control group *(4)*. Abnormal glucose tolerance tests have also been observed in 28% of patients presenting with frozen shoulder *(39)*.

Examination

To exclude pathology, examination should commence with an assessment of the cervical spine. Both upper limbs should be properly exposed and formally examined. Reviewing the passive and active shoulder range of movement and defining the relative contributions from both the glenohumeral and scapulothoracic articulations is pivotal to grade the severity of the condition and also to analyze the future response to treatment. Movements examined to a firm end point should include forward flexion, abduction, and internal and external rotation both in neutral and abduction. It is possible to fix the scapula by holding the inferior pole of the scapular with the examiner's index finger and thumb. The examiner's other arm then can be used to evaluate gleno-humeral motion with the scapulothoracic articulation excluded. Most researchers in this area have suggested a decrease in motion range of about 50% as a criterion for the diagnosis of frozen shoulder *(10)*. If motion loss is not global, then the exact planes of movement should be defined. Loss of external rotation in abduction suggests a contracture in the antero-inferior capsule, whereas loss of external rotation in adduction is more indicative of a contracture in the rotator interval. Loss of internal rotation in either adduction or abduction suggests posterior capsule contracture. Movements within the examined range of motion should be smooth and free from crepitus. As an addition, a lignocaine injection can be performed to distinguish the loss of movement associated with pain seen in impingement from the fixed decrease in movement noted in frozen shoulder. Such injections can also be useful in helping to define disease stage *(21)*.

Investigations

No specific hematological tests are diagnostic for frozen shoulder. Although usually normal, routine hematological and biochemistry tests should be performed. A fasting blood glucose assessment is a sensible screening test useful in identifying patients with impaired glucose tolerance who are presenting with shoulder stiffness *(39)*. It is also effective to perform an erythrocyte sedimentation rate, which may be elevated in up to 20% of patients *(1)*.

A full series of shoulder radiographs should be obtained, including true antero-posterior, scapular lateral, and axillary views. These images should show, by definition, a normal joint appearance. Loss of bone density associated with disuse can be observed, but a diagnosis of idiopathic frozen shoulder is excluded if any other pathology is identified. Bone and soft-tissue tumors can occasionally mimic the presentation of frozen shoulder, and plain radiographs are useful for their identification. A bone scan is also useful to establish reflex sympathetic dystrophy. If there is any suspicion of the presence of an unusual pathology, then a bone scan should supplement the plain radiography. Diphosphonate bone scans have demonstrated an increased uptake in 90% of patients with frozen shoulder *(40)*. Scans have also shown a 50% increased activity on the contralateral-unaffected side. Yet, bone scan activity does not help to predict disease severity or prognosis. Dynamic ultrasonography has been used in the frozen shoulder *(41)* to illustrate a constant limitation in the sliding movement of the supraspinatus tendon against the scapula. Magnetic resonance imaging has been used to demonstrate an increase in the capsule thickness in patients with frozen shoulder *(42)*. Neither of these modalities are useful in the routine management of frozen shoulder, but they are useful in the investigation of those patients suspected of having a shoulder frozen secondarily to some other intrinsic pathology.

Arthrography has also been a method in the assessment of frozen shoulder. Neviaser pioneered its use in the evaluation of the frozen joint *(43)*. The joint's volume typically decreases between 10 and 12 mL with obliteration of the axillary recess and subscapularis bursa. Although useful for diagnosing frozen shoulder, arthrography cannot be used to differentiate between the primary and secondary forms of the disease *(40)*. It also cannot predict the extent and rate of recovery.

TREATMENT

The natural history of the frozen shoulder has already been presented. Typically, it is divided into four stages, lasting at least 18 mo and often with incomplete symptom resolution. Treatment should be aimed at pain relief, improving the quality of the recovery and reducing the time taken to achieve this recovery. High-risk groups include patients undergoing shoulder, arm, and cardio-thoracic surgery and neurosurgery. Early mobilization is of great importance in the prevention of shoulder stiffness symptoms. However, most patients present well into the second stage with a significantly stiffened shoulder. The first priority in treating patients is to control the pain. Without good pain relief, rehabilitation will be inadequate and poorly tolerated. Patients should be commenced on a nonsteroidal anti-inflammatory medication provided there is no contraindication to its use. Other analgesics can be added in for use in patients with severe resistant pain. Opiate analgesics should be avoided, as dependency is a risk associated with their use.

Conservative Therapy

Injections

Hannafin and Chiaia have presented a rationale for the use of an injection of steroid and local anesthetic into the glenohumeral joint *(44)*. If, after administration pain and range of motion are both improved, then a diagnosis of stage 1 disease can be made. However, if pain is improved, but motion is unimproved, then a diagnosis of stage 2 disease is made. It has been suggested that intra-articular steroid injections are more effective if administered in the early stage of the disease. Neviaser suggested that the presence of steroids can have little effect on established scar or contracture *(45)*. This view is supported by Hazelman *(46)*, who has reviewed the effect of intra-articular steroids using duration of symptoms at injection as the major variable. It appears that patients injected within 3 mo of symptom onset have a significantly accelerated improvement when compared with those patients injected more than 5 mo after symptom commencement. If this is the case, then staging the patients is important in studies analyzing outcomes posttreatment with intra-articular steroids. Intra-articular steroid therapy is not benign. Detrimental effects on tendon structure and function have been reported following their use *(47)*. There is also a small, but substantial, risk of infection associated with steroid injection. These factors have prompted several studies to determine their efficacy. Bulgen et al. *(48)* have performed a randomized study of steroids, physiotherapy, ice, and benign neglect. Initially, the steroid group had the best response to treatment, but no significant difference was found at final long-term review. In another prospective randomized study with observer blinding, local steroid injections were found to be as effective as physiotherapy alone or in combination *(49)*. Such injections were considered to accelerate recovery in the most cost-effective manner. Thus, the use of steroids in the early disease stages does seem to have a role in speeding recovery. However, the use of multiple steroid injections over a protracted time period cannot be supported. It should also be noted that the intra-articular injection of steroids without imaging control is at best unpredictable *(50)*. In our unit, we routinely use ultrasound control to ensure correct positioning of injections both above and beneath the cuff.

Physiotherapy

The importance and effectiveness of physical therapies as applied to the frozen shoulder has been highlighted *(44)*. Miller, Wirth, and Rockwood have presented a review of 50 patients treated with home therapy, moist heat, and anti-inflammatory medications under close supervision by a physician *(51)*. At review, all patients regained significant range of motion and returned to activities of daily living without pain. The objective of such physical therapies is to restore function by reducing inflammation and pain, thus allowing the reestablishment of normal shoulder mechanics. Historically, they have taken the form of simple repetitive stretching exercises and have been shown to be effective in the vast majority of cases *(52)*. In the early stage, gentle pain-free mobilization using the opposite arm can be used to decrease nociceptive input to break the cycle of pain and muscle spasm. Exercises should progress to include ROM and pendulum movements to increase the pain-free range of forward elevation, external rotation, internal rotation, and cross-body adduction. Wherever possible, this should be home-based and self-directed after a single instructional session and occasional reviews with a physiotherapist. In the resistant case, the therapist can adopt a more active role, possibly involving the use of hydrotherapy, which provides an environment for passive-assisted exercises. Other modalities can also be introduced, including transcutaneous electrical nerve stimulation (TENS), cryotherapy, and ultrasound—all of which may act to decrease pain perception. The effectiveness of a stretching-exercise program was investigated *(53)*. In a recent study, 64 patients (90%) reported a satisfactory outcome, and only five patients (7%) proceeded to either manipulation under anesthesia (MUA) or arthroscopic release. Patients with more severe pain and functional limitations before treatment had relatively worse outcomes, but the early use of more interventional therapies could not be supported. Most patients will have significant improvement by 12–16 wk *(44)*. If this is not apparent, or there is deterioration, then consideration should be given to more interventional modalities.

Distension Arthrography

Distension arthrography or brisement is a hydrostatic technique where fluid is insufflated into the glenohumeral joint to produce a stretching or rupture of the capsule *(11)*. During the procedure, incremental injections of fluid lead to a progressive increase in the intra-articular pressure to greater than 800 mmHg up to a maximum of 1500 mmHg *(10)*. Disruption of the capsule occurs at either the biceps tendon sheath or the subcoracoid bursa. Investigators have reported distension arthrography to be a reliable, safe and effective technique for treating frozen shoulder *(54)*. Others have not found such effective results. Harryman and coworkers found that treating a disease that affects the whole capsule by simply rupturing a small area of the anterior capsule, without specifically reducing inflammation or lengthening the contracted capsule, is unlikely to be effective in severe frozen shoulder *(10)*.

Interventional Therapies

Manipulation Under Anesthesia

The most difficult decision with frozen shoulder management is if and when to progress to operative treatment in what is regarded by some as a self-limiting condition. Neviaser and Neviaser have stated that operative intervention should be avoided while a patient is still experiencing severe pain and stiffness *(3)*. They believe that this circumstance is indicative of ongoing inflammation and that surgery at this stage is likely to worsen the condition. In contrast to this view, Harrymann has indicated to perform a gentle manipulation under anesthesia if the patient is unable to perform exercises owing to severe pain, usually following a failed intra-articular steroid and local anesthetic injection *(10)*. This discordance remains and will only be resolved by future prospective studies of the management of patients with painful and stiff shoulders. In addition, Harryman suggested manipulation in patients with increasing stiffness after 12 wk of physiotherapy or no improvement following 18–24 wk of physiotherapy.

The contraindications to closed manipulation have been summarized by Hannafin *(44)* and include patients with osteopenia or, in the presence of fractures, neurological injury, reflex sympathetic dystrophy, and instability. Manipulation is also relatively contraindicated following recent surgical repair of soft tissues around the shoulder because of the risk of disruption of the repair. The technique of closed manipulation for frozen shoulder treatment has been previously described by Haines and Hargadon *(55)*. In our unit, we perform manipulation under a general anesthetic with a scalene block. The block is advantageous in allowing immediate physiotherapy or continuous passive motion to be performed in the first few hours after manipulation. Prime importance during MUA is given to holding the humerus as near to the proximal end as possible to reduce the lever arm acting through the bone and thus limiting the risk of fracture. The scapula is stabilized with one hand cupped over the point of the shoulder. Return of motion is achieved by the use of steady controlled force addressing first the flexion, then adduction to stretch the posterior capsule, followed by abduction with both internal and external rotation. There is usually an audible release of soft tissues, particularly with the return of flexion, and force should not be increased if such an audible release is absent *(11)*.

A review of the literature reports results of shoulder manipulation alone or in combination with steroid injection to be extremely variable *(10)*. Those showing significant improvement at 3 mo ranged from 25 to 90% with a mean of 70% improvement at 6 mo. In a randomized study of 30 patients, manipulation and steroid injection significantly improved movement and pain in comparison to patients treated with steroid alone *(56)*. In addition, Hill and Bogumill have observed that MUA is a safe means to treat frozen shoulder and significantly shorten the course of the disease. Opponents of the use of MUA mainly do not question effectiveness but are more critical of the associated damage that they feel can occur during the procedure. If the clinician is aware of the contraindications to the use of MUA, it can be an effective therapy for the frozen shoulder not responding to physiotherapy. As has been stated, MUA has a limited role in the treatment of postsurgical shoulder stiffness.

Arthroscopic Release

As it has been described *(3,43)*, arthroscopy has a role in the staging of frozen shoulder. The arthroscopic stages have been correlated to clinical examination and histological appearance by Hannafin et al. *(21)*. The best clinical research with the frozen shoulder has included arthroscopy to stage the disease, which allows a more effective comparison of data from different studies. The lack of appropriate staging of the disease in previous studies has limited the value of such comparison *(44)*. Arthroscopy performed prior to MUA can yield useful diagnostic information, allowing identification of associated pathology, such as labral or cuff tears. The treatment of some associated pathology can also be addressed through the arthroscope. Arthroscopy performed immediately after MUA has identified intra-articular hemarthrosis, avulsion of the inferior capsule adjacent to or peripheral to the labrum, tears in the rotator interval capsule with occasional labral avulsions, or capsular tears anterosuperiorly or anteroinferiorly *(10,57)*. Such extensive, but variable, damage may explain the sometimes poor results seen with MUA *(58)*.

The best indication for the use of arthroscopy in the treatment of frozen shoulder is for the small group of patients who continue to have motion loss even after MUA. The advantages of this technique are its ability to perform precise selective capsular releases, which can allow further MUA (if it is required) in a very controlled manner. It also has a role in the postoperative stiff shoulder, lessening the risk of fracture or retearing of repaired soft tissues. However, patients with extensive extra-articular adhesions are probably better suited to open release. This technique, performed in either the lateral decubitus or beach chair positions, is invariably accompanied by difficulty with inserting the arthroscope into the joint, which is the result of the capsular contracture and decrease in joint volume. A gentle MUA can facilitate entry but will compromise the view because of the inevitable associated bleeding that ensues. The biceps is identified, and a second working portal is sited just beneath this laterally. A release is performed from the axilla of the biceps tendon to the upper border of the subscapularis tendon, thus freeing the rotator interval. This release normally reverses the loss in external rotation and can be completed by a gentle MUA. Further isolated releases of anterior or posterior capsule can be performed if more specific isolated contractures are apparent. Release of a posterior contracture in patients with limited cross-adduction is a specific example of this circumstance. To complete the procedure, the subacromial space is visualized, and any further adhesions identified here are released.

Warner and coworkers have reviewed their experience with arthroscopic capsular release in 23 patients with resistant frozen shoulder *(59)*. The procedure was followed by 48 h of physical therapy using an in-dwelling scalene block. All movements increased significantly and were within a mean of 7° of the values for the contralateral normal shoulder. These improvements were obtained without complications. Ogilvie-Harris and Wiley have reviewed manipulation vs arthroscopic release in 40 patients with resistant frozen shoulder *(58)*. All patients had experienced symptoms and functional loss despite 1 yr of nonoperative treatment. In the first group of 20 patients, MUA was performed in association with arthroscopy. In the second set of 20 patients, arthroscopic division of contracted structures was performed. At independent assessment between 2- and 5-yr follow-up, there was no difference in ROM, but there was notably improved pain relief and restoration of function in the arthroscopically released group. These coworkers have observed that following 1 yr of adequate nonoperative treatment with patients still having significant stiffness, arthroscopic release offers the best option for excellent long-term results, especially in patients with diabetes mellitus. (This has been our experience with regard to our own practice.) Clearly, in some circumstances, a simple MUA appears overly aggressive, leading to disruption of normal and pathological tissue. The ultimate result is thus less than optimal, but some patients have positive results following MUA. The answer as to which patients can be treated just with an MUA and which patients require an arthroscopic release remains unclear.

Open Release

As with arthroscopic release, the objective with open release is to free up any adhesions present. It gives the surgeon the ability to easily free up both intra- and extra-articular structures. Open release is especially useful in treating patients after unsuccessful arthroscopic release and after previous surgical repairs where manipulation might lead to disruption. It is also particularly effective in circumstances where adhesions are predominantly in the HSMI; thus, it is often indicated in the posttraumatic surgical stiff shoulder. Unfortunately, open release is associated with increased postoperative pain when compared with either MUA or arthroscopic release and this can inhibit early mobilization. The procedure is normally performed through a deltopectoral approach. Structures released usually include subacromial and subdeltoid bursal adhesions, the corocohumeral ligament, and the rotator interval *(19,60)*, but a complete perilabral capsular release around some or all of the glenoid can be performed *(58)*. Ozaki and coworkers have used open release to treat 17 patients with resistant frozen shoulder. They identified the major tethering structure as a contracture of the corocohumeral ligament and release of this restored motion in all patients. Therefore, open release can be recommended as an effective therapy in the most resistant forms of frozen shoulder. Such cases are fortunately rare. This technique is also very valuable in the management of postsurgical shoulder stiffness unresponsive to simple physiotherapy.

REFERENCES

1. Binder AI, Bulgen DY, Hazleman BL, Roberts S. Frozen shoulder: a long-term prospective study. *Ann Rheum Dis* 1984;43:361–364.
2. Lloyd-Roberts G, French P. Periarthritis of the shoulder. A study of the disease and its treatment. *Br Med J* 1959;1:1569–1574.
3. Neviaser R, Neviaser T. The frozen shoulder: Diagnosis and management. *Clin Orthop* 1987;223:59–64.
4. Bridgman J. Periarthritis of the shoulder and diabetes mellitus. *Ann Rheum Dis* 1972;31: 69–71.
5. Bowman C, Jeffcoate W, Patrick M, Doharty M. Bilateral adhesive capsulitis, oligoarthritis and proximal myopathy as a presentation of hypothyroidism. *Br J Rheumatol* 1988;27: 62–64.
6. Duplay E. De la periarthrite scapulo-humerale et des raideurs de l'epaule qui en son la consequence. *Arch Gen Med* 1872;20:513–542.
7. Codman E. *The Shoulder*. Todd, Boston, MA 1934.
8. Matsen F, Lippitt S, Sidles J, Harryman D. *Practical Evaluation of Management of the Shoulder*. WB Saunders, Philadelphia, PA, 1994.
9. Bunker T. Frozen shoulder: unravelling the enigma. *Ann R Coll Surg Engl* 1997;79:210–213.
10. Harryman D, Lazarus M. The stiff shoulder. In Rockwood C, Matsen F, eds. *The Shoulder*. 2nd Ed. W. B. Saunders, Philadelphia, PA, 1997, pp. 1064–1112.
11. Lundberg B. The frozen shoulder: Clinical and radiographical observations. The effect of manipulation under general anaesthesia. Structure and glycosaminoglycan content of the joint capsule. Local bone metabolism. *Acta Orthop Scand* 1969;119 (Suppl):1–59.
12. Cuomo F. Diagnosis, classification, and management of the stiff shoulder. In Iannotti J, Williams G, eds. *Disorders of the Shoulder; Diagnosis and Management.* Lippincott Williams & Wilkins, Philadelphia, PA, 1999, pp. 397–417.

13. Murnaghan J. Frozen shoulder. In Rockwood C, Matsen F, eds. *The Shoulder*. WB Saunders, Philadelphia, PA, 1990, pp. 837–862.
14. Kozin F. Two unique shoulder disorders: Adhesive capsulitis and reflex sympathetic dystrophy syndrome. *Postgrad Med* 1983;73:207–216.
15. Wiley A. Arthroscopic appearance of frozen shoulder. *Arthroscopy* 1991;7:138–43.
16. Bunker T, Anthony P. The pathology of frozen shoulder. A Dupuytren-like disease. *J Bone Joint Surg Br* 1995;77:677–683.
17. Grubbs N. Frozen shoulder syndrome. *J Orthop Sports Physl Ther* 1993;18:479–487.
18. Reeves B. The natural history of the frozen shoulder syndrome. *Scand J Rheumatol* 1975;4: 193–196.
19. DePalma A. Loss of scapulohumeral motion (frozen shoulder). *Ann Surg* 1952;135:194–204.
20. Simmonds F. Shoulder pain: with particular reference to the frozen shoulder. *J Bone Joint Surg* 1949;31B:426–432.
21. Hannafin J, DiCarlo E, Wickiewicz T, Warren R. Adhesive capsulitis: capsular fibroplasia of the glenohumeral joint. *J Shoulder Elbow Surg* 1994;3:5.
22. Neviaser J. Adhesive capsulitis of the shoulder. *J Bone Joint Surg* 1945;27:211–222.
23. Bulgen D, Binder A, Hazelman B, Park J. Immunological studies in frozen shoulder. *J Rheumatol* 1982;9:893–898.
24. Bulgen D, Hazelman B, Ward M, McCallum M. Immunological studies in frozen shoulder. *Ann Rheum Dis* 1978;37:135–138.
25. Young A. Immunological studies in the frozen shoulder. In Bayley J, Kessel L, eds. *Shoulder Surgery*. Springer-Verlag, Berlin and Heidelberg, Germany, 1982, pp. 110–113.
26. Harryman D. Shoulders: Frozen and stiff. *Instr Course Lect* 1993;42:247–257.
27. Bunker T, Esler C. Frozen shoulder and lipids. *J Bone Joint Surg Br* 1995;77:684–686.
28. Sanderson P, Morris M, Stanley J, Fahmy N. Lipids and Dupuytren's disease. *J Bone Joint Surg Br* 1992;74B:923–927.
29. Rodeo SA, Hannafin JA, Tom J, Warren RF, Wickiewics TL. Immunolocalization of cytokines and their receptors in adhesive capsulitis of the shoulder. *J Orthop Res* 1997;15: 427–436.
30 Grasland A, Ziza J, Raguin G, Pouchot J, Vinceneux P. Adhesive capsulitis of shoulder and treatment with protease inhibitors in patients with HIV infection. *J Rheumatol* 2000;27:2642–2646.
31. Freedman L, Munro R. Abduction of the arm in the scapular plane: scapular and glenohumeral movements. A roentgenographic study. *J Bone Joint Surg Am* 1966;48:1503–1510.
32. Harryman D, Sidles J, Clark J. Translation of the humeral head on the glenoid with passive glenohumeral motion. *J Bone Joint Surg Am* 1990;72:1334–1343.
33. Ticker J, Beim G, Warner JJ. Recognition and Treatment of Refractory Posterior Capsule Contracture of the Shoulder. *Arthroscopy* 2000;16:27–34.
34. Patten C, Hillel A. The 11th nerve syndrome. Accessory nerve palsy or adhesive capsulitis? *Arch Otolaryngol Head Neck Surg* 1993;119:215–220.
35. Simon L, Pujol H, Blotman F, Pelissier J. Aspects of the pathology of the arm after irradiation of breast cancer. *Rev Rhum Mal Osteoartic* 1976;43:133–140.
36. Pineda C, Arana B, Martinez-Lavin M, Dabague J. Frozen shoulder triggered by cardiac catheterization via the brachial artery. *Am J Med* 1994;96:90–91.
37. Shaw D, Deutsch D, Bowling R. Efficacy of shoulder range of motion exercise in hospitalised patients after coronary artery bypass graft surgery. *Heart Lung* 1989;18: 364–369.
38. Tuten H, Young D, Douoguih W, Lenhardt K, Wilkerson J, Adelaar R. Adhesive capsulitis of the shoulder in male cardiac surgery patients. *Orthopaedics* 2000;23:693–6.
39. Lequesene M, Dang N, Bensasson M, Mery C. Increased association of diabetes mellitus with capsulitis of the shoulder and shoulder-hand syndrome. *Scand J Rheumatol* 1977;6: 53–56.

40. Binder A, Bulgen D, Hazelman B, Roberts S. Frozen shoulder: an arthrographic and radionuclear scan assessment. *Ann Rheum Dis* 1984;43:365–369.
41. Ryu K, Lee S, Rhee Y, Lim J. Adhesive capsulitis of the shoulder joint: usefulness of dynamic sonography. *J Ultrasound Med* 1993;12:445–449.
42. Emig E, Schweitzer M, Karasick D, Lubowitz J. Adhesive capsulitis of the shoulder: MR diagnosis. *Am J Roentgenol* 1995;164:1457–1459.
43. Neviaser R. Painful conditions affecting the shoulder. *Clin Orthop* 1983;173:63.
44. Hannafin J, Chiaia T. Adhesive capsulitis: a treatment approach. *Clin Orthop* 2000;372: 95–109.
45. Neviaser J. Adhesive capsulitis and the stiff and painful shoulder. *Orthop Clin North Am* 1980;11:327.
46. Hazleman B. The painful stiff shoulder. *Rheumatol Phys Med* 1972;11:413–421.
47. Kennedy J, Willis R. The effects of local steroid injections on tendons: a biochemical and microscopic correlative study. *Am J Sports Med* 1976;4:11–21.
48. Bulgen D, Binder A, Hazleman B, Dutton J, Roberts S. Frozen shoulder: prospective clinical study with an evaluation of three treatment regimes. *Ann Rheum Dis* 1984;43: 353–360.
49. Dacre J, Beeney N, Scott D. Injections and physiotherapy for the painful stiff shoulder. *Ann Rheum Dis* 1989;48:322–325.
50. Richardson A. The painful shoulder. *Proc R Soc Med* 1975;68:731–736.
51. Miller M, Wirth M, Rockwood CJ. Thawing the frozen shoulder: the "patient" patient. *Orthopedics* 1996;19:849–853.
52. Watson-Jones R. Simple treatment of stiff shoulders. *J Bone Joint Surg Br* 1963;45:207.
53. Griggs S, Ahn A, Green A. Idiopathic adhesive capsulitis. a prospective functional outcome study of nonoperative treatment. *J Bone Joint Surg Am* 2000;82A:1398–1407.
54. Sharma R, Bajekal R, Bhan S. Frozen shoulder syndrome: a comparison of hydraulic distention and manipulation. *Int Orthop* 1993;17:275–278.
55. Haines J, Hargadon E. Manipulation as the primary treatment of the frozen shoulder. *J R Coll Surg Edin* 1982;27:271–275.
56. Thomas D, Williams R, Smith D. The frozen shoulder: a review of manipulative treatments. *Rheumatol Rehabil* 1980;19:173–179.
57. Pollock R, Duralde XA, Flatow E, Bigliani L. The use of arthroscopy in the treatment of resistant frozen shoulder. *Clin Orthop* 1994;304:30–36.
58. Ogilvie-Harris D, Wiley A. Arthroscopic surgery of the shoulder. *J Bone Joint Surg Br* 1986;68:201–207.
59. Warner J, Allen A, Marks P, Wong P. Arthroscopic release for chronic refractory adhesive capsulitis of the shoulder. *J Bone Joint Surg Am* 1996;78:1808–1816.
60. Kieras D, Matsen FI. Open release in the management of refractory frozen shoulder. *Orthop Trans* 1991;15:801.
61. Shaffer B, Tibone JE, Kerlan RK. Frozen shoulder. A long-term follow up. *J Bone Joint Surg Am* 1992;74:738–746.

9

Capsular Shrinkage of the Shoulder

Current Clinical Status

Andrew L. Wallace

INTRODUCTION

Although arthroscopic treatment of the unstable shoulder remains a challenging area of clinical development, in recent years, a better understanding of joint pathomechanics, coupled with significant technological advances, have increased the multitude of techniques at the surgeon's disposal. Successive clinical results have generally improved, but controversy still exists as to whether an arthroscopic approach can be effective for all indications and patients.

The introduction of thermal capsular shrinkage was perceived by many as the ideal solution—using an old idea with a new twist to deal quickly and simply with the complex problem of excess capsular laxity. Unfortunately, the expansion rate of clinical applications has, to some extent, exceeded the rate of discovery of the biological and mechanical effects of capsular tissues derived from basic science. As more experimental studies have emerged, short-term clinical reports have also appeared, and it is now an appropriate time to consider the practical role of this innovation in the treatment of shoulder instability.

Similarly to the evaluation of any new treatment modality, two fundamental factors must be considered: whether it works and whether it is safe.

SCIENTIFIC BASIS

The theoretical basis for thermal shrinkage is well established, and the details of numerous basic science experiments are covered in a series of review articles *(1–3)*. Shrinkage is a property of the major structural component of connective tissues—type I collagen, which is arranged in a fibrillar network. Essentially, the crystalline triple helix undergoes a phase change at a critical temperature, as the heat-labile intramolecular hydrogen bonds dissolve. Analagous to melting, this phenomenon is associated with a significant shortening as the ordered quarter-stagger array of the collagen molecules collapses, leaving a tangled coil of individual α chains still linked together by heat-stable covalent intermolecular bonds. Ultrastructurally, the collagen fibrils enlarge and their margins become less distinct, coalescing with adjacent fibrils in a denatured mass of protein in which the resident fibroblasts also undergo necrosis.

From: *Orthopedic Biology and Medicine: Repair and Regeneration of Ligaments, Tendons, and Joint Capsule*
Edited by: W. R. Walsh © Humana Press Inc., Totowa, NJ

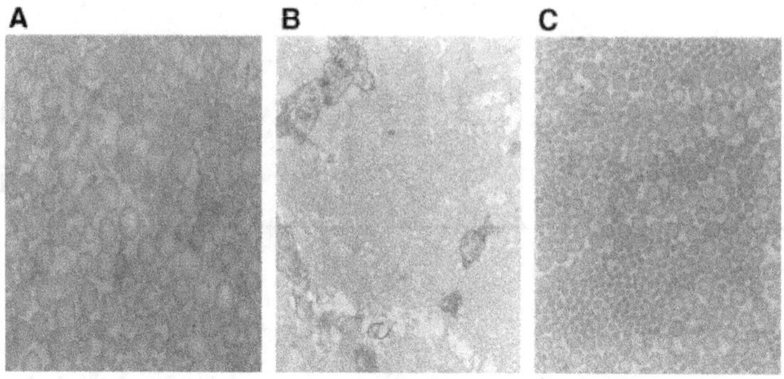

Fig. 1. These transmission electron micrographs represent the medial collateral ligament (MCL) of the adult rabbit **(A)** before treatment, **(B)** at 12 wk after treatment with thermal shrinkage, and **(C)** at 12 wk after surgical division and plication of the ligament.

In vitro, capsular tissues and ligaments can shorten up to 50% of their original unconstrained length, but this may take several minutes. In vivo, most studies have demonstrated shortening in the range of 15–20% during short-term application of thermal energy. This limit may restrict the extent of reduction in capsular volume that can be achieved using the shrinkage technique. Nonetheless, decreased joint laxity and translation have been shown experimentally after shrinkage, but this effect has a consequence in mechanical terms. An inverse relationship exists between the extent of shrinkage and the tissue stiffness; as the tissue shortens, it becomes more elastic and liable to creep and stretch *(4–6)*. Strength is also reduced, but the recovery rate is still somewhat controversial. Some studies have suggested that mechanical properties are back to normal within 30 d, but others have indicated that it may be up to 90 d before strength and stiffness are sufficiently recovered *(7,8)*.

The mechanism of remodeling of the thermally treated tissue is not well understood. The major issue is whether the denatured matrix provides a useful scaffold for rapid repopulation by fibroblasts and new collagen synthesis or instead must first be removed and replaced completely, e.g., when a soft tissue defect heals in classic scar formation. Some in vitro evidence shows that heat-treated tissue can enhance fibroblast migration, and focal areas of new collagen production have been observed. In one study, biopsies from the operated shoulder capsule were taken from 53 patients between 3 and 38 mo after treatment at the time of stabilization of the symptomatic contralateral shoulder. Even at 6 mo, there was increased cellularity when compared with normal capsule, but by 12 mo, the histology appeared normal *(9)*.

Recent work from our laboratory has shown that the ultrastructure of thermally treated rabbit ligament tissue is similar to the scar tissue after gap healing in ligaments, with a shift seen from the normal bimodal distribution of large and small collagen fibrils toward a unimodal population of smaller fibrils *(10)*. The ultrastructure of ligaments that have been surgically plicated to achieve shortening is distinctly different; the large fibrils are still present, but there are bundles of smaller fibrils interspersed between them, suggesting another mechanism of matrix production (Fig. 1). Although the pattern of remodeling is different, viscoelastic properties in both groups are similar at 90 d, but still far from those of the intact control ligaments (Fig. 2).

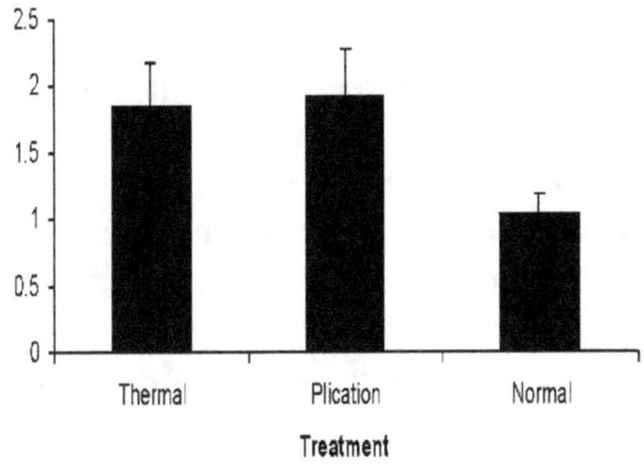

Fig. 2. The chart demonstrates that the creep strains in both thermal and plication groups were almost identical at 12 wk but about twice as liable to creep as the intact control ligaments.

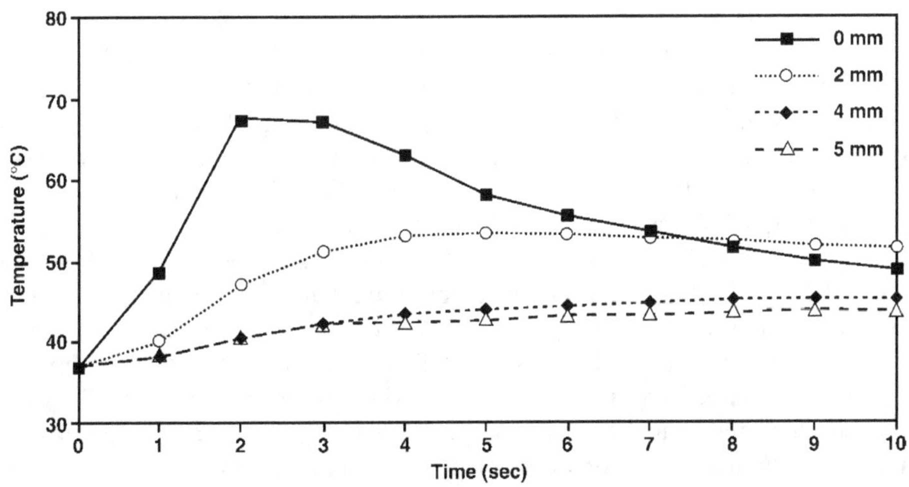

Fig. 3. Temperature profiles for a bipolar end-effect thermal electrode using bovine capsular tissue in vitro. Using fluoroptic thermometry, temperatures were measured between 0 and 5 mm deep to the tissue surface. Temperatures exceeded 45°C within 2 mm of the electrode tip. Reproduced with permission from ref. *12*.

MODALITIES OF THERMAL ENERGY DELIVERY

Initial studies of thermal shrinkage used the Holmium-YAG laser—the first laser system designed for use with fiberoptic cables and in a saline environment. However, the laser relies on absorption of light by water molecules in the tissue; therefore, the probe tip must be held away from the tissue surface. Because of the relative expense of laser generation and associated safety issues, many clinicians have preferred electrothermal energy generation using either monopolar or bipolar probes.

In theory, bipolar probes should have a more "local" effect than monopolar probes, where the circuit is completed by transmission of current through the remote electrode. But recent studies have shown that the temperature profile in the tissues below the surface is remarkably similar in both types *(11,12)*. The temperature is highest at the surface, decreasing with depth of penetration (Fig. 3).

TECHNIQUES

In our practice (as in many centers) arthroscopic shoulder surgery is performed under interscalene regional anesthesia, where the patients are sedated and placed in the beach-chair position on the operating table. The beach-chair position facilitates examination under anesthesia (EUA) and functional assessment during arthroscopy. However, these evaluations can also be undertaken using the lateral decubitus position, but the traction apparatus must be temporarily disengaged.

The EUA is an important component of the procedure, because it provides a link between the patient's subjective history and clinical signs and the arthroscopic findings. Passive anterior, posterior, and inferior translation are estimated using the load and shift test specified by Hawkins *(13)*. Elevation and rotation are added and translation is reassessed and graded 1–4 as described by Cofield *(14)*, as many patients with multidirectional laxity may not necessarily have multidirectional instability (MDI).

Following insertion of the arthroscope through the standard posterior-viewing portal, a diagnostic routine is followed. Starting at the biceps anchor, the anterior glenoid margin and labrum is inspected. The arthroscope is then pushed forward between the humeral head and glenoid so that the tip of the instrument lies in the anterior compartment. By elevating the hand, the arthroscope is allowed to slide inferiorly; if it passes into the axillary recess without resistance, the "drive-through" sign is positive. The axillary recess is often enlarged. The arthroscope is then withdrawn posteriorly, allowing inspection of the inferior and posterior labrum, returning to the biceps anchor. The inspection is then completed by tracing the biceps tendon to its exit hiatus, then laterally along the insertion of the supraspinatus tendon on the humerus, noting the presence of any osteochondral (Hill-Sachs) defect. This defect is distinguished from the bare area by the presence of an intervening intact ridge of normal cartilage. To fully inspect the anterior labrum and exclude the presence of the anterior labral periosteal sleeve avulsion or humeral avulsion of the glenohumeral ligaments lesion, an anterior-viewing portal is recommended.

In the absence of any validated quantitative measurement technique for intraoperative assessment of humeral translation, the drive-through sign is useful. But it should be emphasized that although the drive-through sign is correlated with increased shoulder laxity, it does not always infer a diagnosis of instability, because it may be positive in shoulders with other diagnoses *(15)*. Nonetheless, elimination of the drive-through sign and volume reduction of the axillary recess can be utilized as an indicator of the effectiveness of shrinkage at the time of application.

For application of thermal energy, we use an additional anterosuperior portal, through which the probe can be inserted parallel to the arthroscope in the anterior portal for shrinkage of the posterior capsule. The posteroinferior capsule can be reached with the probe in the posterior portal. The arthroscope is then reinserted in the posterior portal, and shrinkage is applied to the axillary recess and anterior capsule. Although a supplementary posteroinferior portal has been described, its use may be hazardous because of its association with injury to the axillary nerve *(16)*.

The pattern of thermal energy application has been addressed in a recent study using monopolar radiofrequency (RF) probes *(8)*. Using the ovine joint capsule, a comparison was made between a "paint" technique, where contiguous areas are treated, with a "grid" technique in which corridors of normal tissue were left untreated. Surprisingly, there was no difference in the degree of shrinkage (paint 29% vs grid 27%). However, whereas the grid pattern was regarded as "healed" by 6 wk, there were still areas of nonviable tissue in the paint group, and the tissue was weaker and less stiff. This evidence suggests that the grid approach is just as effective and may facilitate more rapid remodeling during the postoperative phase.

Because axillary nerve injury can have devastating consequences in terms of duration of rehabilitation and return to functional activity, caution should be taken when using the probe in the axillary recess. In experimental studies using monopolar RF probes, temperatures in the axillary nerve can frequently exceed 45°C using a conventional paint technique and may even exceed the maximum "set point" (for example 67°C) established for the generator *(17)*. This is probably owing to delay in the feedback loop from the thermocouple to the probe tip but may also be a result of flow effects of the irrigant solution, where the probe tip temperature may be falsely suppressed. To reduce this risk, the probe tip should be kept in constant motion while in contact with the tissue, and retreating areas already thermally treated should be avoided, especially in the 5–7 o'clock zone *(16)*. Reducing the energy settings on the generator and lowering the in-flow irrigation pressure may also be useful precautions *(18)*.

CLINICAL RESULTS

The first clinical reports published in the peer-reviewed literature on thermal shrinkage were centered on its use as adjunctive treatment in the arthroscopic management of posttraumatic anterior instability. In 1996, Hardy et al. *(19)* researched 18 patients who had labral repairs using an absorbable tack and then had laser-assisted capsular shrinkage. At 1 yr postsurgery, there were no recurrences. In a similar review of patients treated with monopolar RF shrinkage after labral repair with longer follow-up (2–4 yr), Mishra *(20)* had a recurrence rate of 7%, and 38 of 42 patients were able to return to the same level of sports activity. The Rowe score improved from a preoperative mean of 38–89 postoperatively. Range of motion was normal in 74% of cases, and the remainder had a loss of less than 10° of rotation in the abducted externally rotated position.

In 53 patients with anteroinferior instability managed arthroscopically, reviewed at a minimum of 2 yr, Gartsman *(21)* described the use of laser thermal shrinkage in 48 patients in addition to labral repair using suture anchors. Using this combined technique, failure occurred in only four cases between 9 and 18 mo after surgery. The maximum reduction in motion was 5° strength improved by 60% after surgery, and 91% of patients achieved a good or excellent rating using the Rowe score. More than 80% returned to sports activity; although the authors regarded the technique as "developmental," they felt that the results were comparable with those of open stabilization.

Monopolar RF shrinkage has also been used to treat the internal impingement syndrome seen in baseball pitchers when there is overuse and gradual stretching of the anteroinferior capsule, presumed to be owing to "repetitive microtrauma." As this injury can be career-threatening, and the risk of restriction of motion from open-stabilization surgery is considerable, shinkage is an appealing concept. Players undergoing arthroscopy and debridement of lesions of the rotator cuff and labrum were compared with those additionally having thermal shrinkage. Those players treated with shrinkage had a higher rate of return to competition (97% at a mean of 8 mo vs 80% at a mean of 7 mo) and appeared to avoid reinjury, because at 30-mo follow-up,

Table 1
Outcome of Arthroscopic Treatment for Multidirectional Instability

Technique	Number in group	Average follow-up	Return to sports	Recurrence	Revision surgery
Suture	26	52 mo	82%	3 (10%)	1 (3%)
Laser	32	27 mo	88%	1 (3%)	2 (6%)
Monopolar RF	30	28 mo	93%	2 (6%)	1 (3%)

87% were still competent at the preoperative level in comparison to 61% in the control group *(22)*.

Lyons et al. *(23)* reported on 26 patients with MDI who had been treated using laser-assisted thermal capsulorrhaphy. Data was collected prospectively for a minimum 2 yr follow-up after surgery. There was one recurrence in the group (4%), and 12 of 14 athletes (86%) were able to return to their previous level of sports activity.

Electrothermal shrinkage has also been compared with laser-assisted shrinkage and arthroscopic suture plication in recent reports. Savoie and Field *(24)* reviewed three consecutive series of patients with symptomatic MDI managed with suture plication, laser or monopolar electrothermal shrinkage. Postoperatively, active movements were restricted for 3–4 wk. Although not randomized, the results (*see* Table 1) were broadly similar and highly satisfactory according to standardized outcome scales (UCLA, Rowe and Neer-Foster measures).

However, these results were not replicated by Levy et al. *(25)*, who also compared laser and electrothermal shrinkage in patients with capsular or MDI-type instability. In 56 patients treated with laser-assisted shrinkage, recurrent symptoms occurred in 36% at an average follow-up of 40 mo; in 34 patients treated using monopolar electrothermal shrinkage, the failure rate was 24% at an average follow-up of 23 mo. Of course, it is possible that the failure rate in the electrothermal group may have increased with longer review, but it should also be noted that in most of these patients, active motion was allowed between 4 and 7 d after surgery. This early active mobilization may explain the discrepancy in comparison with the series reported by Savoie *(24)*. Nonetheless, the authors concluded that the minimal morbidity associated with arthroscopic thermal shrinkage justified its role as an alternative to the open capsular shift procedure for patients with MDI. Similar recurrence rates for the open capsular shift procedure have been reported by Hamada *(26)*, but follow-up was much longer.

The most up-to-date reports continue to support a favorable outcome for this procedure. In a study of naval recruits, Fitzgerald et al. *(27)* reviewed 30 patients with MDI at a minimum of 24 mo after electrothermal shrinkage with a bipolar device. The majority (70%) were able to return to full active military duties, including strenuous physical exercise. There were no recurrent dislocations, but three patients (10%) reported symptomatic episodic subluxations, and two subsequently had open-revision procedures. Although these findings were encouraging, the authors regarded them as too premature to ascertain the "specific beneficial role" of shrinkage in the treatment of MDI; yet, they did recognize a tendency for the rating scale scores to improve even beyond 12 mo postsurgery.

A similar-sized cohort of patients with MDI was followed prospectively by Frostick et al. *(28)*, who found a significant improvement in the Constant score from 59 to 81 when assessed 2 yr following capsular shrinkage. Even with a fairly conservative rehabilitation program (avoiding combined external rotation and abduction for at least 6 wk after surgery), the authors found a complication rate of 16%, including recurrence (three cases) and adhesive capsulitis (one case). They concluded that the early results were positive but warned that the failure rate would probably increase in the longer term.

REHABILITATION

Based on evidence from basic scientific studies and general concern about the risk of recurrent stretching during the remodeling phase *(6)*, there has been a return to more conservative rehabilitation programs in many centers *(16)*. During the first 3–4 wk, external rotation in adduction is generally limited to the neutral position, with elevation in the scapular plane permitted to 90°. After the first month, the passive range of motion is usually tight at these extremes, and a gentle active stretching program is initiated for the next 4–8 wk *(24,27)*. Proprioceptive retraining is also important at this stage to restore a functional range *(25)*. By 8–10 wk, isometric strengthening may commence, progressing to isokinetic- and dynamic-resisted strengthening from 12 to 16 wk. During this latter phase, specific sports-related conditioning is begun, but contact and collision sports should likely be avoided until 6 months after surgery. Using this format, it has been shown that after 12 wk, 50% of patients regain full shoulder motion, whereas in the remainder, deficits were less than 10–15° in abduction and rotation. In this same group of 20 patients, external rotation strength was back to normal in 60% at this stage. Isokinetic testing can be a useful objective quantitative method of defining fitness to return to sports activity *(29)*.

COMPLICATIONS

Set against the encouraging early clinical results, particularly in athletes for whom open surgery poses major risks of stiffness and lengthy rehabilitation, concern exists about the specific risks of the thermal procedure. Case reports of necrosis of the capsule *(30)*, leading to recurrence, and axillary nerve palsy *(18)* have demanded a cautious approach both to patient selection and technical application.

In a retrospective review, Anderson *(31)* attempted to define risk factors for early failure in 106 patients following monopolar RF shrinkage. Failure was defined as recurrent dislocation, the requirement for a revision operation, or a score of less than 70 on the L'Insalata scale. They found a failure rate of 14% using these criteria at an average 13 mo follow-up. Failure occurred at an average of 6 mo after surgery but ranged up to 16 mo. Definitive risk factors included a history of previous surgery for the same condition and a history of multiple dislocations. Evidence of involvement in contact sports or evidence of MDI were probable risk factors. Surprisingly, neither age nor the presence of other pathologic lesions were implicated as risk factors.

The most comprehensive attempt to define the incidence of problems was undertaken by Wong and Williams *(16)* when they surveyed 379 arthroscopic shoulder surgeons in North America and performed 14,277 arthroscopic procedures involving thermal shrinkage for shoulder instability in the 5 yr preceding the survey. Recurrence rates were 8.4% for the laser technique, 8.3% for monopolar probe, and 8.4% for the bipolar probes. Of these failures, about one third went on to undergo revision surgery. Axillary nerve injury was reported in 1.4% and was notably more common after electrothermal procedures, but nearly all were purely sensory and recovered in 2–4 mo. There was no association with either the lateral decubitus or beach-chair position for the procedure. Protracted shoulder stiffness—described as adhesive capsulitis—was a rare complication and occurred in less than 0.1% of cases.

FUTURE ROLE

The current available evidence suggests that thermal capsular shrinkage can be effective in the arthroscopic management of shoulder instability, either as an adjunctive agent for capsular redundancy following labral repair or as a first-line option in unidirectional or MDI that is possibly related to repetitive microtrauma, where there is no caposulolabral avulsion. Furthermore, the risks or morbidity associated with the technique appear to be acceptably low and certainly favorably comparable with those related to open surgery. Following shrinkage, there is a definite compromise of the material properties of the capsular tissue, but whether this is a temporary or permanent effect is not yet fully known. In fact, it may not ultimately matter. Although the scar-like lesion produced by thermal energy application may have a poor mechanical performance, if there is sufficient volume produced by the remodeling process, then the structural requirements of the tissue may still be met.

Shoulder instability is a clinical spectrum of conditions with a range of pathologies, both at the structural level of the joint and at the neuromuscular control level. It may be that shrinkage facilitates a recovery at both levels, effectively bringing the patient back to stability without compromising mobility. Further work quantifying the respective contribution of these components is required for its efficacy to be more fully understood.

At a more fundamental level, the introduction of this technology heralds a new era in biological intervention in musculoskeletal injury and disease. Arnocsky has argued that shrinkage is simply the stimulant for a new biological process, i.e., a "second chance" to heal the soft-tissue defect and restore the anatomy of the joint to its original condition. It should be also remembered that the initial effect seen at the time of surgery may bear little relation to the final result, but a poor response to shrinkage generally predicts a poor outcome for the patient *(25)*. In some individuals, thermal alteration of capsular tissue may be sufficient to offer a new foundation or platform for a coordinated dynamic rehabilitation program. However, in others, the extent of redundancy of the capsule and overall joint volume may preclude the shrinkage effect and may not provide any additional benefit.

REFERENCES

1. Arnocsky SP, Aksan A. Thermal modification of connective tissue: basic science considerations and clinical implications. *Instr Course Lect* 2001;50:3–11.
2. Medvecky MJ, Ong BC, Rokito AS, Sherman OH. Thermal capsular shrinkage: basic science and clinical applications. *Arthroscopy* 2001;17:624–635.
3. Wallace AL, Hollinshead RM, Frank CB. The scientific basis of thermal capsular shrinkage. *J Shoulder Elbow Surg* 2000;9:354–360.
4. Lopez ML, Hayashi K, Vanderby R, Thabit G, Fanton GS, Markel MD. Effects of monopolar radiofrequency energy on ovine joint capsular mechanical properties. *Clin Orth* 2000;374:286–297.

5. Wallace AL, Hollinshead RM, Frank CB. Electrothermal shrinkage reduces laxity but alters creep behavior in a lapine ligament model. *J Shoulder Elbow Surg* 2001;10:1–6.
6. Wallace AL, Hollinshead RM, Frank CB. Creep behavior of a rabbit model of ligament laxity after electrothermal shrinkage in vivo. *Am J Sports Med* 2002;30:98–102.
7. Hayashi K, Hecht P, Thabit G, Peters DM, Vanderby R, Cooley AJ, Fanton GS, Orwin JF, Markel MD. The biologic response to laser thermal modification in an in vivo sheep model. *Clin Orthop* 2000;373:265–276.
8. Lu Y, Hayashi K, Edwards RB, Fanton GS, Thabit G, Markel MD. The effect of monopolar radiofrequency treatment pattern on joint capsular healing. *Am J Sports Med* 2000;28:711–719.
9. Hayashi K, Massa KL, Thabit G, Fanton GS, Dillingham MF, Gilchrist KW, Markel MD. Histologic evaluation of the glenohumeral joint capsule after the laser-assisted capsular shift procedure for glenohumeral instability. *Am J Sports Med* 1999;27:162–167.
10. Jones IT, Hansen U, Sandison A, Moss J, Wallace AL. A comparison of thermal shrinkage with suture plication in a lapine ligament model. *Trans Orthop Res Soc* 2002.
11. Obrzut SL, Hecht P, Hayashi K, Fanton GS, Thabit III G, Markel MD. The effect of radiofrequency energy on the length and temperature properties of the glenohumeral joint capsule. *Arthroscopy* 1998;14:395–400.
12. Shellock FG, Shields CL. Temperature changes associated with radiofrequency energy-induced heating of bovine capsular tissue: evaluation of bipolar RF electrodes. *Arthroscopy* 2000;16:348–358.
13. Hawkins RJ, Schutte JP, Janda DH, Huckell GH. Translation of the glenohumeral joint with the patient under anesthesia. *J Shoulder Elbow Surg* 1996;5:286–292.
14. Cofield RH, Nessler JP, Weinstabl R. Diagnosis of shoulder instability by examination under anesthesia. *Clin Orthop* 1993;291:45–53.
15. McFarland EG, Neira CA, Gutierrez MI, Cosgarea AJ, Magee M. Clinical significance of the arthroscopic drive-through sign in shoulder surgery. *Arthroscopy* 2001;17:38–43.
16. Wong KL, Williams GR. Complications of thermal capsulorrhaphy of the shoulder. *J Bone Joint Surg* 2001;83A(Suppl):151–155.
17. Gryler EC, Greis PE, Burks RT, West J.Axillary nerve temperatures during radiofrequency capsulorrhaphy of the shoulder. *Arthroscopy* 2001;17:567–572.
18. Greis PE, Burks RT, Schickendantz MS, Sandmeier R. Axillary nerve injury after themal capsular shrinkage of the shoulder. *J Shoulder Elbow Surg* 2001;10:231–235.
19. Hardy P, Thabit G, Fanton GS, Blin JL, Lortat-Jacob A, Benoit J. Arthroscopic treatment of recurrent anterior glenohumeral luxations by combining a labrum suture with holmium:YAG laser-assisted capsular shrinkage. *Orthopade* 1996;25:91–93.
20. Mishra DK, Fanton GS. Two-year outcome of arthroscopic Bankart repair and electrothermal-assisted capsulorrhaphy for recurrent traumatic anterior shoulder instability. *Arthroscopy* 2001;17:844–849.
21. Gartsman GM, Roddey TS, Hammermann SM. Arthroscopic treatment of anterior-inferior glenohumeral instability. *J Bone Joint Surg* 2000;82A:991–1003.
22. Levitz CL, Dugas J, Andrews JR. The use of arthroscopic therml capsulorrhaphy to treat internal impingement in baseball players. *Arthroscopy* 2001;17:573–577.
23. Lyons TR, Griffith PL, Savoie FH, Field LD. Laser-assisted capsulorrhaphy for multidirectional instability of the shoulder. *Arthroscopy* 2001;17:25–30.
24. Savoie FH, Field LD. Thermal versus suture treatment of symptomatic capsular laxity. *Clin Sports Med* 2000;19:63–75.
25. Levy O, Wilson M, Williams H, Bruguera JA, Dodenhoff R, Sforza G, Copeland S. Thermal capsular shrinkage for shoulder instability. *J Bone Joint Surg* 2001;83B:640–645.
26. Hamada K, Fukuda H, Nakajima T, Yamada N. The inferior capsular shift operation for instability of the shoulder. *J Bone Joint Surg* 1999;81B:218–225.

27. Fitzgerald BT, Watson T, Lapoint JM. The use of thermal capsulorrhaphy in the treatment of multidirectional instability. *J Shoulder Elbow Surg* 2002;11:108–113.
28. Frostick SP, Sinopidis C, Al-Muskari S, Gibson J, Kemp GJ, Richmond JC. Arthroscopic capsular shrinkage of the shoulder for the treatment of patients with multidirectional instability: Minimum 2-year follow-up. *Arthroscopy* 2003;19:227–233.
29. Ellenbecker TS, Mattalino AJ. Glenohumeral joint range of motion and rotator cuff strength following arthroscopic anterior stabilization with thermal capsulorrhaphy. *J Orthop Sports Phys Ther* 1999;29:160–167.
30. Rath E, Richmond JC. Capsular disruption as a complication of thermal alteration of the glenohumeral capsule. *Arthroscopy* 2001;17:E10.
31. Anderson K, Warren RF, Altchek DW, Craig EV, O'Brien SJ. Risk factors for early failure after thermal capsulorrhaphy. *Am J Sports Med* 2002;30:103–107.

Part IV

Research and Advances

10

Biomechanical and Clinical Evaluation of Tendons and Ligaments

David Hartright, Adam M. Butler, R. Mark Gillies, Warwick J. Bruce, and William R. Walsh

INTRODUCTION

Ligaments and tendons are important connective tissues throughout the body. Ligaments are the soft-tissue connections between bones, whereas tendons are the attachments between muscle and bone. Allowing movement at a joint, ligaments provide physical restraints to unwanted ranges of motion. Tendons, through their origins and insertions, enable a muscle to act upon a particular joint while also giving some structural support. Both share similar structures and properties, which allows them to be discussed simultaneously, but there are differences between the two. This chapter explores current clinical and biomechanical test methods used to evaluate the normal, diseased, and healing properties of these collagenous structures.

Both are composed of water (60–80% wet weight), elastin, glycolipids, proteoglycans, fibroblasts, and collagens. Type I collagen comprises 60–86% of the dry weight arranged in tightly packed, parallel bundles often longitudinally along the axis of the tendon or ligament. Each tendon/ligament is a complex bundle of fibers *(1)* arranged in a hierarchal organization of ever-smaller fibrils down to collagen strands. Silver and coworkers recently reviewed aspects of collagen self-assembly and its role in mechanical properties *(2)*. The in vivo formation of collagen fibers, and ultimately the connective tissues, is an area of continued research and interest.

Collagen is one of the strongest fibrous proteins; given its propensity and parallel longitudinal arrangement in tendons and ligaments, these structures have high tensile strengths. As both tissues transmit tensile loading, the axis of the tissue is orientated across a joint, such that it lies in the optimal position for the transmission of force. Given this function, the main goal of testing these tissues is first to assess their integrity, then establish their respective biomechanical properties. These properties are often used as a generic term in the literature and can be further clarified through structural properties that are obtained from load vs displacement data or material properties from stress vs strain. Static and viscoelastic, time-dependent properties of these tissues are not only important from an experimental point of view but clinically as well.

Evaluation of the tendon and ligament properties has important clinical and biomechanical relevance. Clinically, tendons and ligaments have a vital role in the kinemat-

From: *Orthopedic Biology and Medicine: Repair and Regeneration of Ligaments, Tendons, and Joint Capsule*
Edited by: W. R. Walsh © Humana Press Inc., Totowa, NJ

ics of the musculoskeletal system. Evaluating their in vivo function has evolved as our understanding of anatomy and biomechanics has progressed. Biomechanical testing of tendons and ligaments in the laboratory setting has had a similar evolution in sophistication with continued development of new testing methods, techniques, and equipment. This chapter examines the development of clinical- and laboratory-based testing of tendon and ligaments from basic clinical examination, tensile experiments, to current techniques using robotics.

CLINICAL EVALUATION

Clinical evaluation of tendons and ligaments is a complex issue that should consider the region of the body being examined based on the complex nature of joints. All clinical assessments begin with an understanding of the native anatomy of the bone as well as soft-tissue constraints. These are complex problems given the varied kinematic and clinical requirements of each individual joint. Three main classes can be examined with the clinical function of a tendon or ligament in any joint, including a basic clinical examination, imaging techniques, and operative assessment (when appropriate).

Clinical Examination

The clinical assessment of tendons involves detailed anatomical knowledge of the musculoskeletal system, especially regarding the action of a particular muscle upon a joint. When that has been established, assessing the ability of the subject to perform specific movements indicates the integrity of the tendon in question. Confusion may sometimes arise when several muscles act upon a joint in a similar manner, e.g., in the shoulder. Here, accurate assessment is extremely difficult. It should also be noted that if a subject has any abnormality along the neuromuscular pathway, this may also lead to inaccurate results.

Ligaments provide physical restraints to unwanted movements at joints, thus providing stability. Testing relies on moving the particular joint into the position of instability so that maximum tension is placed within the ligament. Clearly, if the ligament is absent or damaged, the joint will become unstable, and the unwanted position will be attainable. Again, these tests depend on a detailed knowledge of anatomy and joint biomechanics. As with tendon testing, problems arise in joints where a complex arrangement of ligaments generate multidirectional stability, and assessment of an individual ligament is impossible.

Because of the large number of ligaments in the body, many tests exist to review their integrity. Grading systems have been proposed that relate to whether the ligament is intact, partially torn, or completely ruptured as determined by clinical findings. Overall, these are inaccurate and difficult to reproduce. Examples of specific ligament tests include the anterior draw test, the Lachman test, and the pivot-shift test, which are all associated with just the anterior cruciate ligament. Specific testing machines are available that are not necessarily more accurate than manual testing. However, they do provide a more objective measure of ligament integrity, which is particularly important following surgical repair of a ligament.

The use of equipment to monitor the specific range of knee laxity has become clinically appropriate following cruciate ligament injuries. Instrumented devices, such as the KT 1000, provide a reliable measure of anterior *(3–14)* and posterior knee laxity

(3,10). Roentgen stereophotogrammetric analysis (RSA) has also been recently applied to assess anteroposterior knee laxity *(14–17)*. The RSA technique is well known in the arthroplasty field and utilizes Ta markers to determine the three-dimensional positional changes. This technique provides greater insight into the knee motion after injury or reconstruction but does require the implantation of permanent markers into the knee and radiographs at low energy to document marker position in space.

Imaging

Imaging techniques help to determine the ligament or tendon integrity, but they do not provide much information about the mechanical properties. Several useful imaging techniques are available that allow assessment of both ligaments and tendons and include arthrography, ultrasound, and magnetic resonance imaging (MRI). Arthrography is an indirect method of evaluating ligament and tendon continuity. It relies on ligaments and tendons to be arranged in such a way to create an enclosed space. A radio-opaque dye is injected into this space, and a standard roentgenographic assessment is made. If there is a breach in this envelope, the radio-opaque dye extravasates from the space, giving characteristic appearances. This method can be used for assessing the integrity of the rotator cuff in the shoulder and the triangular fibrocartilage (TFCC) in the wrist.

Ultrasound imaging also provides an effective modality to examine ligament and tendon integrity. It is a safe, quick, and inexpensive method relying on the transmission of sound waves through tissue and reflections back to the transducer. The ultrasound images provide a real-time assessment of the area of interest, but there are many limitations based on transducer frequency, imaging site, and resolution. The results of ultrasound diagnosis of rotator cuff tears have been reported to be highly user-dependent, especially in the case of the rotator cuff *(18)*, but these results are controversial *(19,20)*.

Ultrasound has been used to assess the mechanical properties of the tendon in vivo *(21,22)*. Its measurements of tendon-aponeurosis elongation were taken during tensile loading applied by contraction of the in-series muscle. Manganaris reports values similar to in vitro testing results, as well as differential strain along the tendon and evidence of creep in vivo *(21,22)*. The in vivo monitoring of strain with ultrasound overcomes many classic biomechanical concerns about the testing environment, clamping or holding issues, and loading conditions. Further consideration of these in vivo techniques will be very important in the future evaluation of the biomechanical properties of tendons and ligaments in vivo.

MRI is an extremely powerful tool for tendon and ligament evaluation because it enables direct visualization of tissue composition owing to the high contrast. Not only does it give information about the continuity of the tissues, but it also offers information about any inflammation or healing in or around them. It is an extremely accurate diagnostic modality, but the image quality is dependent on the strength of the magnet. MRI has become the gold standard for the assessment of cruciate ligament injury *(23–35)*. It is also used extensively in the investigation of shoulder injuries, such as the rotator cuff *(36–40)*, and has become the preferred technique for these injuries.

Operative Assessment

With the advent of arthroscopy, minimally invasive surgery has become the method of choice for the direct visualization of ligaments and tendons. This is particularly true in the knee and shoulder; yet, arthroscopic examination of the wrist, elbow, ankle, and hip are possible and have gained popularity. It allows for instrumentation and, consequently, therapeutic measures may be undertaken at the same time. To date, this has been limited to the evaluation of cartilage stiffness.

EXPERIMENTAL BIOMECHANICAL TESTING

The mechanical properties of intact and injured tendons and ligaments in animals and humans have been a topic of intense scrutiny for decades. Excellent review chapters have been published over the years detailing the static and viscoelastic properties of tendons and ligaments. Work published by Woo and his group *(41–54)*, Professor Butler and his research group, along with Amis can provide the interested reader with endless information related to tendon and ligament biomechanics. This chapter does not seek to replicate or reproduce this vast amount of previously published works in detail but rather to provide an overview and reference list of this early work and focus on new testing methods and recent advancements in this field.

By their ultrastructure organization and composition, tendons and ligaments are primarily considered as tensile-bearing structures. However, other forces (e.g., compression and shear) may be very important in a larger scheme. Although not completely understood, connective tissue cells do respond to various mechanical forces in the production and regulation of the extracellular matrix *(55,56)*. Mechanical testing of tendon and ligaments is an all-encompassing field with studies that involve surgeons, pathologists, anatomists, biologists, and engineers. Newcomers continue to enter the field as new research pathways open, such as tissue engineering and gene therapy. However, the foundation of mechanical testing is based on classic engineering with techniques used to monitor load and displacement that establishes the basis for all measurements.

Tensile properties of tendon and ligaments have been reported as isolated subunits from a variety of anatomic sites in human and animal species as well as bone–ligament–bone *(42,50)* or bone–tendon–muscle preparations *(21,22)*. Although tensile testing forms the core of most biomechanical investigations of tendons and ligaments, there are many other parameters that may be measured and reported. Structural properties can be obtained from load-vs-displacement data and often includes the ultimate load (in N), displacement (in mm), energy (Nmm), and stiffness (N/mm). The material properties are obtained by considering the cross-sectional area and gauge length to reduce the load-vs-displacement data to stress vs strain and report the tensile stress (in Pa), strain (without dimension), and elastic modulus (in Pa).

The classic sigmoid-shaped curve of tendons and ligaments have been emphasized over the years to demonstrate the unique arrangements of these tissues. The initial nonlinear or toe region, followed by the linear region, where stiffness is usually reported, and the failure region have been the foundation of many studies. Beyond a static or quasistatic tensile test of tendons and ligaments, other testing methods have been reported. These include: low-load properties *(57)* biaxial tensile testing, viscoelastic properties [creep *(21)* and stress relaxation *(85)*, hysteresis *(64)*, free vibration, forced oscillation]; and thermoelastic tests. Professor Woo and his group introduced the technique of a universal force sensor and robotics *(44–46,48–50,53,58)* to evaluate the mechanical properties of ligaments under more realistic physiological loading. Clearly, the evolution in biomechanical testing protocols will continue in collaboration with clinical-based measures to provide information to diagnose and treat injuries to this region.

General Principles of Mechanical Testing of Tendon and Ligaments

As with any experimental technique, consideration must be made prior to testing about the factors that may influence your results. The literature on mechanical testing of tendons and ligaments often varies greatly from study to study. Although tensile testing is fundamentally an easy test to perform, there are numerous obstacles to maneuver and variables to consider before accurate biomechanical results can be obtained. Tissue-specific factors, e.g., age of the sample and treatment (if any), along with experimental factors, e.g., testing equipment (strain measurements and cross sectional area), tissue storage and handling, and test methods (testing environment, gripping or clamping, rate, and orientation) all have an important impact. These factors must be considered regardless of the testing modality chosen (sample storage, gripping, loading orientation, testing rate, method of cross-sectional area measurements, and method of strain measurements). Sample storage in phosphate-buffered saline is traditionally employed and has been reported not to significantly affect the properties of these tissues.

Gripping of the Sample

To determine the load and displacement characteristic for any material, it has to be held firmly in the testing apparatus. Mechanical testing of tendons and ligaments can be performed on the tissue itself or the bone–tendon–muscle or bone–ligament bone complexes, respectively. The method of gripping the sample is an important influence on the overall data. Fixation can be achieved either directly or indirectly. In direct fixation, the sample is simply held using the clamps of the tensile testing equipment. With indirect fixation, the bone attached to the test material is used for clamp fixation, which is particularly useful for testing ligaments. However, with the latter mode of fixation, it is essential to differentiate between the biomechanical properties of the bone–tissue unit and the tissue itself.

Given that the (tendon and ligament) tissue has the surface of a hydrated soft biomaterial, is relatively smooth, and has a partially independent arrangement of the fascicles, fixation may not be easily achieved. The ideal goal of fixation is to uniformly hold each fiber, but this rarely (if ever) achieved. Often, the sample will fail at the points of fixation rather than midsubstance owing to the high stress concentration. Tissues may be altered at their ends so that "hold" of the sample is easier without changing the biomechanical properties, e.g., air-drying of the tendon ends. Haut described a method where the tendon ends are allowed to dry and consequently become rigid while keeping the central portion of the tendon hydrated.

Fixation of isolated ligaments, tendons, or muscle–tendon junctions is often required for experimentation. Riemersma and Schambadt developed a system in which the tendon is frozen into the jaws of the clamp *(59)*. Once frozen, the clamp is then tightened to securely grip the frozen portion of tissue. It has been named "cryojaw" and has produced good results because of the decreased stress concentrations at the tendon–clamp interface. We have used this technique to provide fixation of isolated tendon-braided constructs *(60–63)*, and muscle–tendon subunits *(64)*. Care should be taken with this technique to not freeze the sample too long in the grips to prevent potentially freezing the testing length of the sample.

Cross-Sectional Area

In the calculation of the stress–strain relationship, it is essential to accurately determine the cross-sectional area. This calculation allows comparisons to be made between the biomechanical properties of materials of different dimensions. Given the complex shape and geometry of the tissues, measurement of their dimensions is difficult and, if inaccurate, ultimately produces errors in the stress-strain calculations. Methods for measuring the tissue dimensions can be divided into contact and non-contact approaches.

The gravimetric method was popular in the 1960s and was employed extensively by VanBrocklin and Ellis *(65)*. Volumetric displacement (Archimedes' principle) was measured, and the cross-sectional area was calculated through division of the volume by length. Direct conventional measurements traditionally use calibrated vernier calipers. Geometric approximations must be assumed to exploit this method of measurement; thus, it is only an approximation of the area. Unfortunately, because of the tissue deformability, the area measured is dependent on the pressure applied and consequently may lead to inaccuracies in area determination.

Noncontact approaches have been developed as a result of the difficulties faced with the above methods of cross-sectional measurement. These rely on image reconstruction techniques and employ various visual media to measure dimensions, e.g., the laser micrometer system as reported by Lee and Woo *(66)*. Accurate determination of area is clearly vital in the determination of the stresses. Considerable differences in area method measurements in various studies make direct comparison of stress data difficult.

Strain

Monitoring deformation of the test sample is vital in any mechanical testing experiment. The technique used to monitor deformation of the test sample has a major role in the overall meaning of the strain data reported. Strain is defined as the change in length of a substance normalized by the original length. This deformation system is often used to determine the strain but is limited by the gripping factors and test specimen (i.e., bone–ligament–bone), as all may impact the overall deformation. The use of linear variable differential transformers (LVDTs) accurately define deformation in a prescribed gauge length *(67)*. A video-based noncontact method has been reported by Woo *(68,69)*. Two or more reference lines (gauge lengths) are made on the sample perpendicular to the direction of the loading axis, while a video dimension analyzer records a video image of the sample and deformation of the markers during an applied load. This method is particularly effective because of its lack of contact, it allows strain measurements to be made at any point along the tissue, and enables the measurement of midsubstance strains independent from bony insertions.

Other Factors

Numerous other factors that can influence the results of biomechanical testing of tendons and ligaments have been well described *(70)*. For example, the biomechanical properties of tendons and ligaments vary depending on the sample orientation. As a rule, the maximal tensile strength is found longitudinally along the tissue axis. Consequently, if the sample is not tested in that orientation, discrepancies arise with the results. Other factors are tissue hydration, age, and source of the tissue. Regarding the properties of healing tendons, ligaments, or tendon–bone interfaces, surgical procedure, fixation techniques, and postoperative recovering programs can all affect the results.

VISCOELASTIC PROPERTIES

Considering the complex hierarchical organization of tendons and ligaments, surrounding proteins, and ground substance, it is not surprising that they demonstrate nonlinear viscoelastic properties that are both time- and history-dependent. This essentially means that the elongation of the tissue is based not only on the amount of force but on the time and history of force application. A Medline search reveals published literature as early as 1969 on the viscoelastic properties of collagenous tissues *(71,72)*. Time-dependent behavior of connective tissues has classically been examined using creep *(21,71,73–84)*, stress relaxation, or hysteresis experimental methods.

Creep is fundamentally simple to measure, where a constant load is applied to a tissue and the progressive time-dependent elongation is measured. The elongation amount should be measured with reference to markers on the sample rather than the separation of the grips to ensure no slippage occurs. Stress relaxation is measured when the sample is held at a fixed displacement and the corresponding load is measured vs time. Lynch and coworkers *(85)* recently reported the stress relaxation behavior of ovine tendons relating to fiber orientation and strain rate. These authors examined samples aligned with the transverse to the tendon fiber direction to determine the anisotropic properties of toe-region modulus (E_0), linear-region modulus (E), and Poisson's ratio (ν). Interestingly, they reported the fiber-aligned linear-region modulus (E_1) to be strain-rate–dependent. Poisson's ratio values were not found to be rate-dependent in either the fiber-aligned or transverse direction. They concluded that the lack of strain-rate dependence of transverse properties demonstrates that slow constant strain-rate tests represent elastic properties in the transverse direction. In contrast, when tested along the long axis of the samples, the strain-rate dependence of the modulus in the linear region suggests that incremental stress-relaxation tests are required to determine the tendon's equilibrium elastic properties *(85)*. This study indicates continued advances in our understanding of tendons and ligaments.

Hysteresis is another viscoelastic property that has been considered in the literature. A single cyclic loading and unloading of a tendon or ligament produces two separate curves corresponding to whether a load is applied or withdrawn. These curves form a hysteresis loop on the load-elongation graph. With repeated/cyclical loading of a sample, its properties alter, and the amount of elongation increases with each given load. Increasing cycles cause the loops to become more constant. When a tendon or ligament is exposed to repeated loading, the area of hysteresis for the first few loading cycles is comparatively greater than with later load cycles (Fig. 1). Hence, with repeated loading, the load-elongation curve becomes more constant and is referred to as preconditioning. This effect is important when testing tendons and ligaments and should be calculated into experimental design to prevent inaccurate results.

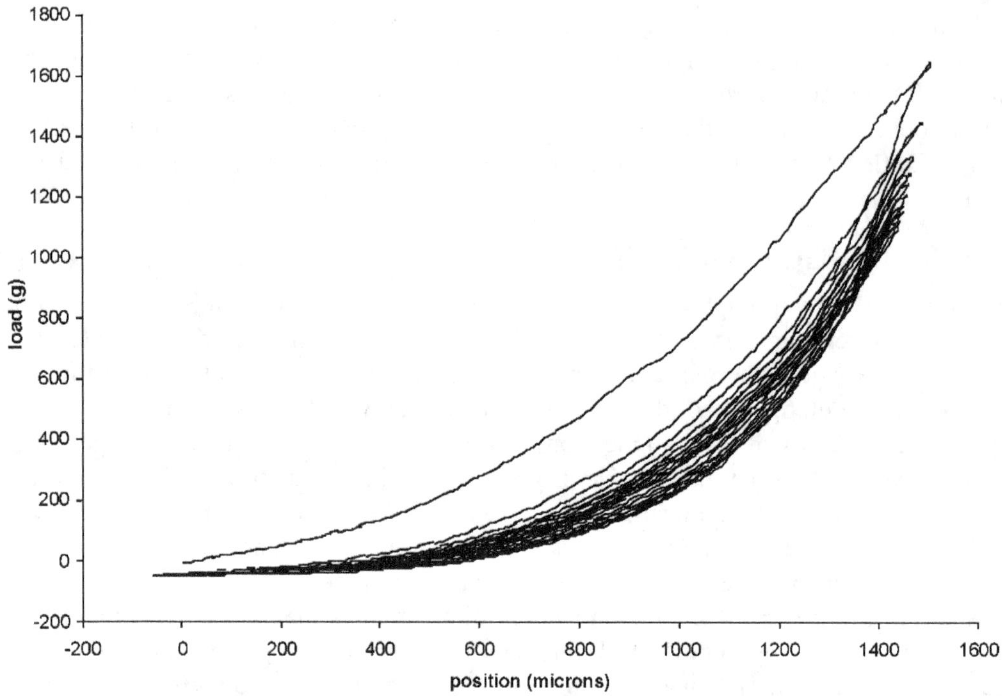

Fig.1 Example of preconditioning a human ankle ligament.

Quasilinear Viscoelasticity

The quasilinear viscoelasticity (QLV) theory developed by Fung *(86)* has been used successfully to describe these time- and history-dependent viscoelastic properties for many soft tissues. This theory has also been used for ligaments and tendons *(87)*. Recently, the QLV theory has been further refined to account for a constant strain rate (rather than an infinite strain rate or true step load, which is physically impossible to achieve experimentally) and the subsequent stress relaxation. The QLV theory assumes that the stress-relaxation function of the tissue can be expressed in the form:

$$\sigma(t) = G(t)\sigma^e(\varepsilon) \tag{1}$$

where $\sigma^e(\varepsilon)$ is the elastic response, i.e., the maximum stress in response to an instantaneous step input of strain ε. $G(t)$ is the reduced relaxation function that represents the time-dependent stress response of the tissue, which is normalized by the stress at the time of step input of strain. If the strain history is considered as a series of infinitesimal step strains ($\Delta\varepsilon$), then the overall stress-relaxation function will be the sum of all individual relaxations. Thus, for a general strain history, the stress at time t, $\sigma(t)$, is given by the strain history and convolution integral over time of $G(t)$:

$$\sigma(t) = \int_{-\infty}^{t} G(t-\tau)\frac{\partial\sigma^e(\varepsilon)}{\partial\varepsilon}\frac{\partial\varepsilon}{\partial\tau}d\tau \tag{2}$$

The lower limit of integration is taken as negative infinity to imply inclusion of all past strain history. In the experimental setting, one assumes that the history begins at $t = 0$. Once $G(t)$, $\sigma^e(\varepsilon)$, and the strain history are known, the time- and history-dependent stress can be completely described by Eq. 2. For soft tissues whose stress–strain relationship and hysteresis are not over sensitive to strain rates, Fung has proposed the following expression for $G(t)$:

$$G(t) = \frac{1 = C\left[E_1\frac{t}{\tau_2} - E_1\frac{t}{\tau_1}\right]}{1 + C\ln\frac{\tau_2}{\tau_1}} \tag{3}$$

where

$$E_1(y) = \int_y^\infty \frac{e^{-z}}{z}dz \tag{3a}$$

is the exponential integral, and C, τ_1, and τ_2 are material coefficients.

An exponential approximation has been chosen to describe the elastic stress–strain relationship during a constant strain rate test:

$$\sigma^e(\varepsilon) = A\left(e^{B\varepsilon} - 1\right) \tag{4}$$

where A and B are material coefficients. It is impossible to experimentally apply an instantaneous strain to the test material and therefore impossible to directly measure $\sigma^e(\varepsilon)$. To better approximate actual experimental conditions, it is necessary to replace the instantaneous step load with a ramp load of constant finite strain rate γ to a strain level ε at time t_0. The corresponding stress rise during $0 < t < t_0$ can then be written by combining Equations 3 and 4 as:

$$\sigma(t) = \frac{AB\gamma}{1 + C\ln\frac{\tau_2}{\tau_1}} \int_0^t \left\{1 + C\left[E_1\frac{(t-\tau)}{\tau_2} - E_1\frac{(t-\tau)}{\tau_1}\right]\right\} e^{B\gamma\tau}d\tau \tag{5}$$

Similarly, the subsequent stress relaxation $\sigma(t)$ from t_0 to t can be described as:

$$\sigma(t) = \frac{AB\gamma}{1 + C\ln\frac{\tau_2}{\tau_1}} \int_0^{t_0} \left\{1 + C\left[E_1\frac{(t-\tau)}{\tau_2} - E_1\frac{(t-\tau)}{\tau_1}\right]\right\} e^{B\gamma\tau}d\tau \tag{6}$$

Equations 5 and 6 are then normalized by dividing by the peak stress $\sigma(t_0)$ to eliminate constant A.

$$\frac{\sigma(t)}{\sigma(t_0)} = \frac{\int_0^{\min(t,t_0)} \left\{1 + C\left[E_1\frac{(t-\tau)}{\tau_2} - E_1\frac{(t-\tau)}{\tau_1}\right]\right\} e^{B\gamma\tau}d\tau}{\int_0^{t_0} \left\{1 + C\left[E_1\frac{(t-\tau)}{\tau_2} - E_1\frac{(t-\tau)}{\tau_1}\right]\right\} e^{B\gamma\tau}d\tau} \tag{7}$$

With data from a stress-relaxation experiment, the material coefficients B, C, τ_1, and τ_2 can be determined by a nonlinear, least-square, curve-fitting procedure *(88)*. Constant A can be then computed by using either Eqs. 5 or 6. For a known strain history, these five constants, together with $G(t)$ and $\sigma^e(\varepsilon)$, can be then used to determine the stress at any time t, $\sigma(t)$, by using Eq. 3.

COMBINED ROBOTIC/UNIVERSAL FORCE SENSOR ASSESSMENT OF TENDONS AND LIGAMENTS

A recent advance in biomechanical testing techniques and understanding of the properties of tendons, ligaments, and their reconstruction comes once again from the work of Professor Savio Woo and colleagues *(44,50,89)*. The use of robotic technology and a universal force sensor that combines a six-degree freedom robotic manipulator and a six-degree freedom force-moment sensor and control system represents a new era in biomechanical testing of tendons and ligaments *(44–46,48–51,53,58,89–102)*. Along with providing information about the passive knee flexion path (for controlling the knee flexion positions) and straining specific knee structures, it can be used to measure the *in situ* forces in tendons and ligaments. These forces are measured by recording differences in forces and moments when repeating a prerecorded movement before and after the removal of the ligament or tendon to be tested.

The testing of ligaments and tendons is relatively easy in principle. Yet, with the unique biological properties of the tissues, the inaccuracies of clinical assessment, the difficulties with experimental apparatus and sample maintenance (in vitro), testing of these tissues is far from straightforward. Indeed, there is uncovered ground in this area with exciting work still to be done.

REFERENCES

1. Kastelic J, Galeski A, Baer E. The multicomposite structure of tendon. *Connect Tissue Res* 1978;6:11–23.
2. Silver FH, Freeman JW, Seehra GP. Collagen self-assembly and the development of tendon mechanical properties. *J Biomech* 2003;36:1529–1553.
3. Anderson AF, Lipscomb AB. Preoperative instrumented testing of anterior and posterior knee laxity. *Am J Sports Med* 1989;17:387–392.
4. Harter RA, Osternig LR, Singer KM. Instrumented Lachman tests for the evaluation of anterior laxity after reconstruction of the anterior cruciate ligament. *J Bone Joint Surg Am* 1989;71:975–983.
5. Highgenboten CL, Jackson A, Meske NB. Genucom, KT-1000, and Stryker knee laxity measuring device comparisons. Device reproducibility and interdevice comparison in asymptomatic subjects. *Am J Sports Med* 1989;17:743–746.
6. Steiner ME, Brown C, Zarins B, Brownstein B, Koval PS, Stone P. Measurement of anterior-posterior displacement of the knee. A comparison of the results with instrumented devices and with clinical examination. *J Bone Joint Surg Am* 1990;72:1307–1315.
7. Anderson AF, Snyder RB, Federspiel CF, Lipscomb AB. Instrumented evaluation of knee laxity: a comparison of five arthrometers. *Am J Sports Med* 1992;20:135–140.
8. Kowalk DL, Wojtys EM, Disher J, Loubert P. Quantitative analysis of the measuring capabilities of the KT-1000 knee ligament arthrometer. *Am J Sports Med* 1993;21:744–747.
9. Queale WS, Snyder-Mackler L, Handling KA, Richards JG. Instrumented examination of knee laxity in patients with anterior cruciate deficiency: a comparison of the KT-2000, Knee Signature System, and Genucom. *J Orthop Sports Phys Ther* 1994;19:345–351.

10. Hewett TE, Noyes FR, Lee MD. Diagnosis of complete and partial posterior cruciate ligament ruptures. Stress radiography compared with KT-1000 arthrometer and posterior drawer testing. *Am J Sports Med* 1997;25:648–655.
11. Huber FE, Irrgang JJ, Harner C, Lephart S. Intratester and intertester reliability of the KT-1000 arthrometer in the assessment of posterior laxity of the knee. *Am J Sports Med* 1997; 25:479–485.
12. Balasch H, Schiller M, Friebel H, Hoffmann F. Evaluation of anterior knee joint instability with the Rolimeter. A test in comparison with manual assessment and measuring with the KT-1000 arthrometer. *Knee Surg Sports Traumatol Arthrosc* 1999;7:204–208.
13. Uh BS, Beynnon BD, Churchill DL, et al. A new device to measure knee laxity during weightbearing and non-weightbearing conditions. *J Orthop Res* 2001;19:1185–1191.
14. Fleming BC, Brattbakk B, Peura GD, Badger GJ, Beynnon BD. Measurement of anterior-posterior knee laxity: a comparison of three techniques. *J Orthop Res* 2002;20:421–426.
15. Karrholm J, Selvik G, Elmqvist LG, Hansson LI, Jonsson H. Three-dimensional instability of the anterior cruciate deficient knee. *J Bone Joint Surg Br* 1988;70:777–783.
16. Karrholm J, Elmqvist LG, Selvik G, Hansson LI. Chronic anterolateral instability of the knee. A roentgen stereophotogrammetric evaluation. *Am J Sports Med* 1989;17:555–563.
17. Fleming BC, Peura GD, Abate JA, Beynnon BD. Accuracy and repeatability of Roentgen stereophotogrammetric analysis (RSA) for measuring knee laxity in longitudinal studies. *J Biomech* 2001;34:1355–1359.
18. Goldberg JA, Bruce WJ, Walsh W, Sonnabend DH. Role of community diagnostic ultrasound examination in the diagnosis of full-thickness rotator cuff tears. *ANZ J Surg* 2003; 73:797–799.
19. Olive Jr RJ, Marsh HO. Ultrasonography of rotator cuff tears. *Clin Orthop* 1992;282: 110–113.
20. Paavolainen P, Ahovuo J. Ultrasonography and arthrography in the diagnosis of tears of the rotator cuff. *J Bone Joint Surg Am* 1994;76:335–340.
21. Maganaris CN. Tensile properties of in vivo human tendinous tissue. *J Biomech* 2002;35: 1019–1027.
22. Maganaris CN, Paul JP. Tensile properties of the in vivo human gastrocnemius tendon. *J Biomech* 2002;35:1639–1646.
23. Turner DA, Prodromos CC, Petasnick JP, Clark JW. Acute injury of the ligaments of the knee: magnetic resonance evaluation. *Radiology* 1985;154:717–722.
24. Lee JK, Yao L, Phelps CT, Wirth CR, Czajka J, Lozman J. Anterior cruciate ligament tears: MR imaging compared with arthroscopy and clinical tests. *Radiology* 1988;166: 861–864.
25. Tung GA, Davis LM, Wiggins ME, Fadale PD. Tears of the anterior cruciate ligament: primary and secondary signs at MR imaging. *Radiology* 1993;188:661–667.
26. Robertson PL, Schweitzer ME, Bartolozzi AR, Ugoni A. Anterior cruciate ligament tears: evaluation of multiple signs with MR imaging. *Radiology* 1994;193:829–834.
27. Lerman JE, Gray DS, Schweitzer ME, Bartolozzi A. MR evaluation of the anterior cruciate ligament: value of axial images. *J Comput Assist Tomogr* 1995;19:604–607.
28. Yao L, Gentili A, Petrus L, Lee JK. Partial ACL rupture: an MR diagnosis? *Skeletal Radiol* 1995;24:247–251.
29. Brandser EA, Riley MA, Berbaum KS, el-Khoury GY, Bennett DL. MR imaging of anterior cruciate ligament injury: independent value of primary and secondary signs. *AJR Am J Roentgenol* 1996;167:121–126.
30. Friedman RL, Jackson DW. Magnetic resonance imaging of the anterior cruciate ligament: current concepts. *Orthopedics* 1996;19:525–532.
31. Roychowdhury S, Fitzgerald SW, Sonin AH, Peduto AJ, Miller FH, Hoff FL. Using MR imaging to diagnose partial tears of the anterior cruciate ligament: value of axial images. *AJR Am J Roentgenol* 1997;168:1487–1491.

32. Chen WT, Shih TT, Tu HY, Chen RC, Shau WY. Partial and complete tear of the anterior cruciate ligament. *Acta Radiol* 2002;43:511–516.
33. Ho CP, Marks PH, Steadman JR. MR imaging of knee anterior cruciate ligament and associated injuries in skiers. *Magn Reson Imaging Clin N Am* 1999;7:117–130.
34. Moore SL. Imaging the anterior cruciate ligament. *Orthop Clin North Am* 2002;33:663–674.
35. Vande Berg BC, Lecouvet FE, Poilvache P, Maldague B, Malghem J. Spiral CT arthrography of the knee: technique and value in the assessment of internal derangement of the knee. *Eur Radiol* 2002;12:1800–1810.
36. Vahlensieck M. MRI of the shoulder. *Eur Radiol* 2000;10:242–249.
37. Recht MP, Resnick D. Magnetic resonance-imaging studies of the shoulder. Diagnosis of lesions of the rotator cuff. *J Bone Joint Surg Am* 1993;75:1244–1253.
38. Zlatkin MB, Falchook FS. Magnetic resonance pathology of the rotator cuff. *Top Magn Reson Imaging* 1994;6:94–120.
39. Fritz RC, Stoller DW. MR imaging of the rotator cuff. *Magn Reson Imaging Clin N Am* 1997;5:735–754.
40. Miniaci A, Salonen D. Rotator cuff evaluation: imaging and diagnosis. *Orthop Clin North Am* 1997;28:43–58.
41. Woo SL, Orlando CA, Camp JF, Akeson WH. Effects of postmortem storage by freezing on ligament tensile behavior. *J Biomech* 1986;19:399–404.
42. Boardman ND, Debski RE, Warner JJ, et al. Tensile properties of the superior glenohumeral and coracohumeral ligaments. *J Shoulder Elbow Surg* 1996;5:249–254.
43. Pfaeffle HJ, Tomaino MM, Grewal R, Xu J, Boardman ND, Woo SL, Herndon JH. Tensile properties of the interosseous membrane of the human forearm. *J Orthop Res* 1996;14: 842–845.
44. Rudy TW, Livesay GA, Woo SL, Fu FH. A combined robotic/universal force sensor approach to determine in situ forces of knee ligaments. *J Biomech* 1996;29:1357–1360.
45. Woo SL, Chan SS, Yamaji T. Biomechanics of knee ligament healing, repair and reconstruction. *J Biomech* 1997;30:431–439.
46. Fox RJ, Harner CD, Sakane M, Carlin GJ, Woo SL. Determination of the in situ forces in the human posterior cruciate ligament using robotic technology. A cadaveric study. *Am J Sports Med* 1998;26:395–401.
47. Hildebrand KA, Woo SL, Smith DW, et al. The effects of platelet-derived growth factor-BB on healing of the rabbit medial collateral ligament. An in vivo study. *Am J Sports Med* 1998;26:549–554.
48. Debski RE, Wong EK, Woo SL, Sakane M, Fu FH, Warner JJ. In situ force distribution in the glenohumeral joint capsule during anterior-posterior loading. *J Orthop Res* 1999;17: 769–776.
49. Hoher J, Vogrin TM, Woo SL, Carlin GJ, Aroen A, Harner CD. In situ forces in the human posterior cruciate ligament in response to muscle loads: a cadaveric study. *J Orthop Res* 1999;17:763–768.
50. Woo SL, Debski RE, Wong EK, Yagi M, Tarinelli D. Use of robotic technology for diathrodial joint research. *J Sci Med Sport* 1999;2:283–297.
51. Woo SL, Debski RE, Withrow JD, Janaushek MA. Biomechanics of knee ligaments. *Am J Sports Med* 1999;27:533–543.
52. Woo SL, Debski, RE, Zeminski, J, Abramowitch, SD, Saw, SS, Fenwick, JA. Injury and repair of ligaments and tendons. *Annu Rev Biomed Eng* 2000;2:83–118.
53. Abramowitch SD, Yagi M, Tsuda E, Woo SL. The healing medial collateral ligament following a combined anterior cruciate and medial collateral ligament injury—a biomechanical study in a goat model. *J Orthop Res* 2003;21:1124–1130.
54. Abramowitch SD, Woo SL, Clineff TD, Debski RE. An evaluation of the quasi-linear viscoelastic properties of the healing medial collateral ligament in a goat model. *Ann Biomed Eng* 2004;32:329–335.

55. Chiquet M. Regulation of extracellular matrix gene expression by mechanical stress. *Matrix Biol* 1999;18:417–426.
56. Chiquet M, Renedo AS, Huber F, Fluck M. How do fibroblasts translate mechanical signals into changes in extracellular matrix production? *Matrix Biol* 2003;22:73–80.
57. Butler AM, Walsh WR. Mechanical response of ankle ligaments at low loads. *Foot Ankle Int* 2004;25:8–12.
58. Livesay GA, Fujie H, Kashiwaguchi S, Morrow DA, Fu FH, Woo SL. Determination of the in situ forces and force distribution within the human anterior cruciate ligament. *Ann Biomed Eng* 1995;23:467–474.
59. Riemersa DJ, Schamhardt HC. The cryo-jaw, a clamp designed for in vitro rheology studies of horse digital flexor tendons. *J Biomech* 1982;15:619–620.
60. Nicklin S, Waller C, Walker P, Chung WK, Walsh WR. In vitro structural properties of braided tendon grafts. *Am J Sports Med* 2000;28:790–793.
61. Millett PJ, Miller BS, Close M, Sterett WI, Walsh W, Hawkins RJ. Effects of braiding on tensile properties of four-strand human hamstring tendon grafts. *Am J Sports Med* 2003;31: 714–717.
62. Dowling BA, Dart AJ, Hodgson DR, Rose RJ, Walsh WR. The effect of recombinant equine growth hormone on the biomechanical properties of healing superficial digital flexor tendons in horses. *Vet Surg* 2002;31:320–324.
63. Dowling BA, Dart AJ, Hodgson DR, Rose RJ, Walsh WR. Recombinant equine growth hormone does not affect the in vitro biomechanical properties of equine superficial digital flexor tendon. *Vet Surg* 2002;31:325–330.
64. Nightingale EJ, Allen CP, Sonnabend DH, Goldberg J, Walsh WR. Mechanical properties of the rotator cuff: response to cyclic loading at varying abduction angles. *Knee Surg Sports Traumatol Arthrosc* 2003;11:389–392.
65. Vanbrocklin JD, Ellis DG. A study of the mechanical behavior of toe extensor tendons under applied stress. *Arch Phys Med Rehabil* 1965;46:369–373.
66. Lee TQ, Woo, SL. A new method for determining cross-sectional shape and area of soft tissues. *J Biomech* Eng 1988;110:110–114.
67. Kristal P, Tencer AF, Trumble TE, North E, Parvin D. A method for measuring tension in small ligaments: an application to the ligaments of the wrist carpus. *J Biomech* Eng 1993; 115:218–224.
68. To SY, Kwan MK, Woo SL. Simultaneous measurements of strains on two surfaces of tendons and ligaments. *J Biomech* 1988;21:511–514.
69. Woo SL, Gomez MA, Seguchi Y, Endo CM, Akeson WH. Measurement of mechanical properties of ligament substance from a bone-ligament-bone preparation. *J Orthop Res* 1983;1:22–9.
70. Woo SL, Livesay G, Runco T, Yung E. Structure and function of tendon and ligaments. In: Mow V, WC Hayes, eds. *Basic Orthopaedic Biomechanics*. Lippincott-Raven, Philadelphia, PA, 1997, pp. 209–252.
71. Morchio R, Ciferri A. The role of calcium and of in vitro aging on the creep behavior of collagen tendons. *Biophysik* 1969;5:327–330.
72. Stromberg DD, Wiederhielm CA. Viscoelastic description of a collagenous tissue in simple elongation. *J Appl Physiol* 1969;26:857–862.
73. Cohen RE, Hooley CJ, McCrum NG. Viscoelastic creep of collagenous tissue. *J Biomech* 1976;9:175–184.
74. Monleon Pradas M, Diaz Calleja R. Nonlinear viscoelastic behaviour of the flexor tendon of the human hand. *J Biomech* 1990;23:773–781.
75. Wang XT, Ker RF. Creep rupture of wallaby tail tendons. *J Exp Biol* 1995;198:831–845.
76. van Driel WD, van Leeuwen EJ, Von den Hoff JW, Maltha JC, Kuijpers-Jagtman AM. Time-dependent mechanical behaviour of the periodontal ligament. *Proc Inst Mech Eng [H]* 2000;214:497–504.

77. Boorman RS, Thornton GM, Shrive NG, Frank CB. Ligament grafts become more susceptible to creep within days after surgery: evidence for early enzymatic degradation of a ligament graft in a rabbit model. *Acta Orthop Scand* 2002;73:568–574.
78. Ozenci AM, Panjabi MM. Creep behavior of a rabbit model of ligament laxity after electrothermal shrinkage in vivo. *Am J Sports Med* 2002;30:630.
79. Thornton GM, Shrive NG, Frank CB. Ligament creep recruits fibres at low stresses and can lead to modulus-reducing fibre damage at higher creep stresses: a study in rabbit medial collateral ligament model. *J Orthop Res* 2002;20:967–974.
80. Wallace AL, Hollinshead RM, Frank CB. Creep behavior of a rabbit model of ligament laxity after electrothermal shrinkage in vivo. *Am J Sports Med* 2002;30:98–102.
81. Thornton GM, Boorman RS, Shrive NG, Frank CB. Medial collateral ligament autografts have increased creep response for at least two years and early immobilization makes this worse. *J Orthop Res* 2002;20:346–352.
82. Wood ML, Luthin WN, Lester GE, Dahners LE. Tendon creep is potentiated by NKISK and relaxin which produce collagen fiber sliding. *Iowa Orthop J* 2003;23:75–79.
83. Wren TA, Lindsey DP, Beaupre GS, Carter DR. Effects of creep and cyclic loading on the mechanical properties and failure of human Achilles tendons. *Ann Biomed Eng* 2003;31: 710–717.
84. Hingorani RV, Provenzano PP, Lakes RS, Escarcega A, Vanderby R, Jr. Nonlinear viscoelasticity in rabbit medial collateral ligament. *Ann Biomed Eng* 2004;32:306–312.
85. Lynch HA, Johannessen W, Wu JP, Jawa A, Elliott DM. Effect of fiber orientation and strain rate on the nonlinear uniaxial tensile material properties of tendon. *J Biomech Eng* 2003;125:726–731.
86. Fung YC. Biorheology of soft tissues. *Biorheology* 1973;2:139–155.
87. Woo SL. Mechanical properties of tendons and ligaments-quasistatic and nonlinear viscoelastic properties. *Biorheology* 1982;3:385–296.
88. Kwan MK, Lin TH, Woo SL. On the viscoelastic properties of the anteromedial bundle of the anterior cruciate ligament. *J Biomech* 1993;26:447–452.
89. Fujie H, Livesay GA, Woo SL, Kashiwaguchi S, Blomstrom G. The use of a universal force-moment sensor to determine in-situ forces in ligaments: a new methodology. *J Biomech Eng* 1995;117:1–7.
90. Sakane M, Fox RJ, Woo SL, Livesay GA, Li G, Fu FH. In situ forces in the anterior cruciate ligament and its bundles in response to anterior tibial loads. *J Orthop Res* 1997;15: 285–293.
91. Debski RE, Sakone M, Woo SL, Wong EK, Fu FH, Warner JJ. Contribution of the passive properties of the rotator cuff to glenohumeral stability during anterior-posterior loading. *J Shoulder Elbow Surg* 1999;8:324–329.
92. Li G, Rudy TW, Sakane M, Kanamori A, Ma CB, Woo SL. The importance of quadriceps and hamstring muscle loading on knee kinematics and in-situ forces in the ACL. *J Biomech* 1999;32:395–400.
93. Pfaeffle HJ, Fischer KJ, Manson TT, Tomaino MM, Herndon JH, Woo SL. A new methodology to measure load transfer through the forearm using multiple universal force sensors. *J Biomech* 1999;32:1331–1335.
94. Kanamori A, Sakane M, Zeminski J, Rudy TW, Woo SL. In-situ force in the medial and lateral structures of intact and ACL-deficient knees. *J Orthop Sci* 2000;5:567–571.
95. Kanamori A, Woo SL, Ma CB, et al. The forces in the anterior cruciate ligament and knee kinematics during a simulated pivot shift test: A human cadaveric study using robotic technology. *Arthroscopy* 2000;16:633–639.
96. Parsons IM, Apreleva M, Fu FH, Woo SL. The effect of rotator cuff tears on reaction forces at the glenohumeral joint. *J Orthop Res* 2002;20:439–446.

97. Tsuda E, Fukuda Y, Loh JC, Debski RE, Fu FH, Woo SL. The effect of soft-tissue graft fixation in anterior cruciate ligament reconstruction on graft-tunnel motion under anterior tibial loading. *Arthroscopy* 2002;18:960–967.
98. Woo SL, Kanamori A, Zeminski J, Yagi M, Papageorgiou C, Fu FH. The effectiveness of reconstruction of the anterior cruciate ligament with hamstrings and patellar tendon. A cadaveric study comparing anterior tibial and rotational loads. *J Bone Joint Surg Am* 2002; 84:907–914.
99. Fukuda Y, Woo SL, Loh JC, et al. A quantitative analysis of valgus torque on the ACL: a human cadaveric study. *J Orthop Res* 2003;21:1107–1112.
100. Kanamori A, Lee JM, Haemmerle MJ, Vogrin TM, Harner CD. A biomechanical analysis of two reconstructive approaches to the posterolateral corner of the knee. *Knee Surg Sports Traumatol Arthrosc* 2003;11:312–317.
101. Ma CB, Kanamori A, Vogrin TM, Woo SL, Harner CD. Measurement of posterior tibial translation in the posterior cruciate ligament-reconstructed knee: significance of the shift in the reference position. *Am J Sports Med* 2003;31:843–848.
102. Gabriel MT, Wong EK, Woo SL, Yagi M, Debski RE. Distribution of in situ forces in the anterior cruciate ligament in response to rotatory loads. *J Orthop Res* 2004;22:85–89.

11

Healing of Ligament and Tendon to Bone

Andreas Weiler, Sven Scheffler, and Maria Apreleva

INTRODUCTION

Proper healing of tendon or ligament tissue to bone after injury or surgical repair is a basic premise for the full restoration of the involved functional locomotor unit. While during injury most ligament structures fail in midsubstance or by bony avulsion, tissue failure directly at the ligament insertion site is relatively rare. Even in situations where the ligament or tendon tissue shows degenerative changes prior to failure, e.g., in tears of the rotator cuff, failure occurs close to the tendon insertion site but does not directly involve the tissue insertion to bone itself in most cases. In contrast, direct tendon or ligament healing to bone is a mechanism that occurs after surgical repair of tendon and ligaments, such as in rotator cuff repair, reconstruction of the cruciate ligaments with soft-tissue grafts, or with other surgical procedures of tendon grafting and tendon repair to bone, as in hand or foot and ankle surgery.

Particularly in cruciate ligament reconstruction, solid osseous tendon incorporation is essential for the long-term survival of the grafted tissue. In earlier years the bone-patellar tendon–bone (BPTB) graft was the predominant graft source, but soft-tissue grafts (e.g., hamstring tendons and the proximal part of the distal quadriceps tendon) have recently become more popular. If a bone–tendon–bone graft is used, its osseous incorporation inside the bone tunnel progresses via bone-to-bone healing. This mechanism has been studied in the past, and a certain shear stability of the construct could be expected around the fourth to sixth week *(1–3)*. Alternatively, when a soft-tissue graft is used in cruciate ligament reconstruction, its osseous integration in the bone tunnel must progress by tendon-to-bone healing. This process has been previously investigated in several animal models, and different timeframes of a solid tendon-to-bone healing have been reported *(4–14)*. Because biological and mechanical boundary conditions may have a strong influence on tendon-to-bone healing, including its resulting clinical relevance, controversy still remains on the mechanisms that could be found during early and late tendon-to-bone healing *(15,16)*.

LIGAMENT AND TENDON INSERTIONS

The firm attachment of tendons and ligaments to the underlying bone is essential for the force transmission between soft and hard tissue. These insertion sites present a highly differentiated tissue structure that serves as a stress absorber during mechanical

From: *Orthopedic Biology and Medicine: Repair and Regeneration of Ligaments, Tendons, and Joint Capsule*
Edited by: W. R. Walsh © Humana Press Inc., Totowa, NJ

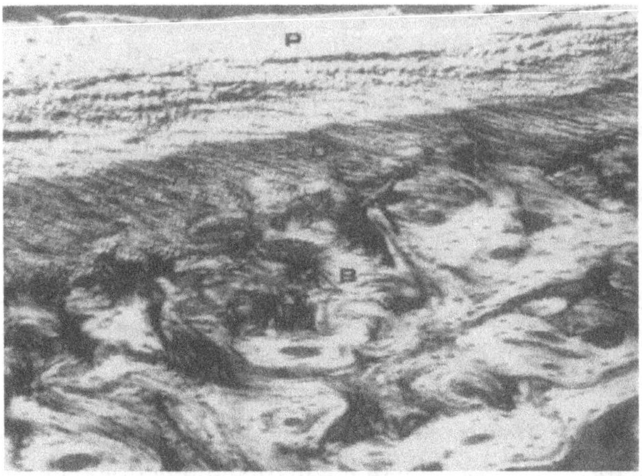

Fig. 1. An indirect type of ligament insertion. There is a broad zone of fibrous tissue (O) connecting the periosteum (P) with the underlying bone (B) by a high density of Sharpey fibers (From ref. *67*.)

loading. In 1691, Havers described two principally different types of ligament or tendon insertion into bone *(17)*. He wrote:

> "The tendons of many muscles do propagate their fibers to make some part of the periosteum; yet, I have observed that some of them, which have often great stress or dependence upon them, when they act, have not been so kind, but penetrated this membrane and were immediately inserted into the bone, so that I could distinguish the periosteum, which lay like a circle round them" *(17)*.

In this report, Havers first described the presence of a direct and indirect type of tendon insertion to bone, which can be distinguished by its distinct histological structure. In 1957 and 1958, Biermann and Knese, two anatomists from Kiel, Germany, reported on bone growth at tendon and ligament insertion sites and differentiated between periosteal-diaphyseal (indirect) insertions *(18)* and chondral-apophyseal (direct) insertions *(19)*.

An indirect type of insertion or so-called "periosteal insertion" is characterized by a high number of collagen fibers that continue from the tendon into the underlying periosteum and then into bone (Fig. 1). These fibers are named "Sharpey's fibers," in recognition of their first description by William Sharpey in 1856 *(20)*. He described perforating collagen fibers extending across bone lamellae "like nails driven perpendicularly or slantingly through a board" and "as it were, bolt them together. The periosteum also contributes to give firmer hold to the tendons and ligaments where they are fixed to bone; indeed, these fibrous structures become continuous and incorporated with it at their attachment" (Fig. 2; *20,21*). (A typical example for an indirect type of ligament insertion is the tibial insertion of the medial collateral ligament of the knee. In general, indirect insertion sites are mainly present with short ligaments or tendons, which have a relatively large and broad insertion area to bone. The typical characteristic of an indirect insertion type is the continuity of the periosteum distal and proximal to the insertion site; thus, this type of insertion is also called a periosteal insertion.

In contrast, with a direct type of ligament insertion, the periosteum is noncontinuous, and the tendon or ligament tissue is in direct contact with the underlying bone *(22)*.

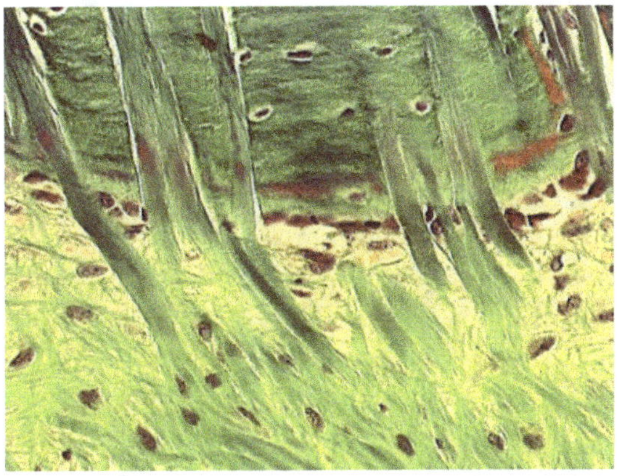

Fig. 2. Sharpey fibers extending from the soft tissue deep into bone (Masson Goldner's trichrome stain, ×400 original magnification)

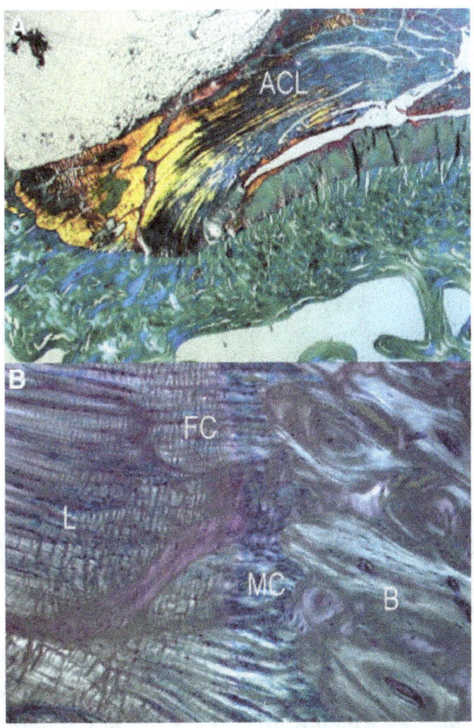

Fig. 3 **(A)** Femoral insertion site of the ACL in a sheep, presenting a typical direct type of ligament insertion (Masson Goldner's trichrome stain, polarized light, ×16 original magnification). **(B)** Higher magnification of the direct ligament insertion. There are four distinct zones: Lamellar bone (B), mineralized cartilage (MC), fibrocartilage (FC), and ligament tissue (L) (Alcian Blue stain, polarized light, ×100 original magnification).

The typical histological appearance of a direct insertion was initially described by Dolgo-Saburoff in 1929 *(23)*. At such attachment sites, there are four zones, consisting of tendon, fibrocartilage, mineralized fibrocartilage, and bone (Fig. 3). Later studies have confirmed this specific insertion anatomy using light and electron microscopy

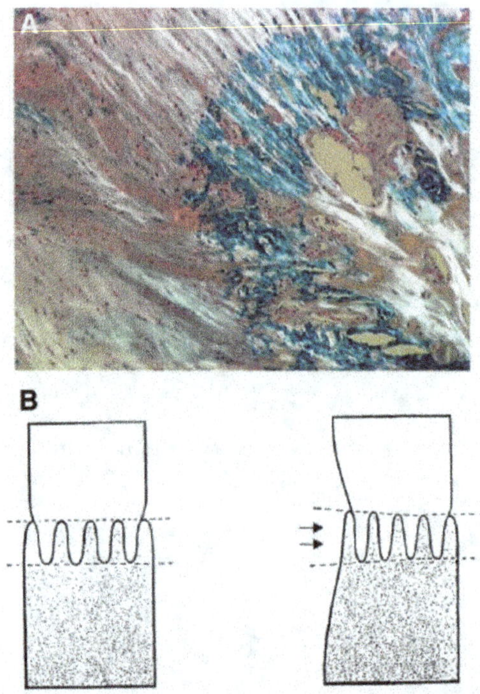

Fig. 4. (**A**) Mineralized cartilage tidemark (blue) between bone and fibrocartilage 24 wk after ACL reconstruction in a sheep. Note the deep interdigitations extending into the lamellar bone, thereby increasing the surface area (Alcian Blue stain, polarized light, ×200 original magnification). (**B**) Schematic drawing to demonstrate the resistance against shear forces by building deep interdigitations between two materials of different stiffness. A separation of the two materials is impossible. The shear stress results in a compression of both elastic materials, which is proportional to its magnitude. (Reprinted from ref. *22*.)

(*18,19,21,22,24–31*) and found it to be present with the cruciate ligaments, supraspinatus tendon, patellar tendon, Achilles tendon, deltoid muscle insertion, and many other ligament and tendon insertions around the body. Dolgo-Saburoff further described the presence of a "blue line", the mineralized cartilage tidemark or cement line between the fibrocartilage and the bone *(23)*. The mineralized cartilage tidemark forms deep interdigitations (Fig. 4), thus increasing the contact area between these mechanically different tissues and the strength of this unit to resist shear and tensile forces, as described in 1956 by Schneider *(22)*. This tidemark has similarities to the mineralized cartilage tidemark between the hyaline articular cartilage and subchondral bone, which also acts as a shock absorber by reducing the stiffness gradient between the articular cartilage and underlying bone, thus decreasing the likelihood of chondral shear injuries.

Schneider then found that the amount of fibrocartilage at the insertion site is not only associated with the strength of the insertion, but also with the amount of soft-tissue bending that occurs during motion *(22,32)*. By embedding the collagen fibers into a zone of fibrocartilage, their resistance (especially against shear) is increased (Fig. 5). Messner investigated the development of the cruciate ligament insertions during growth and found fibrocartilaginous tissue at the insertion where the epiphyseal cartilage was

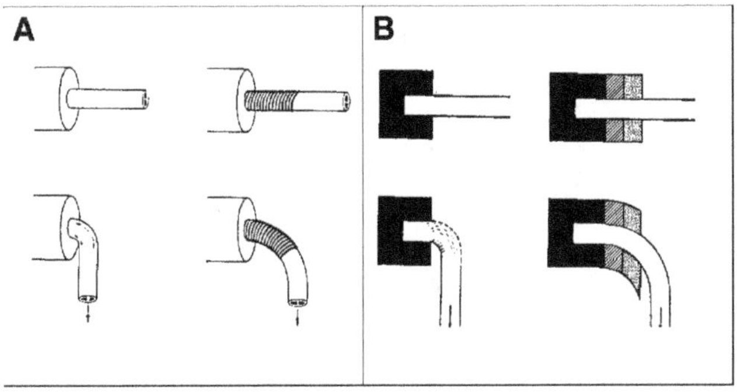

Fig. 5. **(A)** Schematic drawing of the resistance to shear stress by a metal spring in an electronic cable. **(B)** Schematic drawing of the damping of shear stress in direct tendon insertion zones. Black area, bone; stripe area, mineralized fibrocartilage; dotted area, nonmineralized fibrocartilage. (Left) Incorporation of a tendon into bone without a fibrocartilage zone. When the load is not aligned with the direction of the interdigitating channels of the tendon fibers, an angulation of the tendon in front of its entrance into bone occurs during movement. This causes tension stress at the convex site of the tendon angulation and results in rupture of the respective tendon fibers. The compressive force at the concave site causes compressive damages at the respective tendon fibers. (Right) Direct tendon insertion. By adding a zone of mineralized and non-mineralized fibrocartilage in front of the bone, a reduction of the tendon angulation (with a load direction as seen on the left side of the figure) can be achieved to an extent that no further shear stress occurs. Special attention should be paid to the deformation of the cartilaginous zones! The appearance of the mineralized fibrocartilage is only minimally altered, whereas the nonmineralized fibrocartilage undergoes significant deformation. (Reprinted from ref. *22*.)

replaced by bone. Thus, she concluded that the interposition of a fibrocartilagous zone in the insertion may diminish the sudden change in stiffness between ligament soft-tissue and bone *(28)*. All these findings clearly indicate that the transition zone, composed of mineralized cartilage and fibrocartilage, acts as a stress absorber by reducing the stiffness gradient between the hard bone and the ligament or tendon.

It might be reasonable to conclude that in a direct ligament insertion, the mineralized cartilage tidemark acts as a stress absorber between the insertion site itself and the underlying bone, whereas the fibrocartilage layer also reduces the stiffness gradient but, more importantly, protects the tendon or ligament tissue against shear (Fig. 5). In 1960, Pauwels, described the morphological cell transformation into chondroid cells when the soft-tissue is exposed to compressive loads *(33)*. Compressive loads are generated when fibers are bent or become under tension. Electron microscopy studies have shown that chondral cells, which lie between the collagen fibers, get compressed because the fibers create a figure-of-eight course around the cells. (Fig. 6; *24,30*).

In summary, the insertion site morphology reflects the local mechanical boundary conditions. However, it remains unclear whether the mechanical environment also influences the development of a direct chondroid or an indirect periosteal insertion. Evidence suggests that the development of an indirect type of tendon insertion may be related to growth. Hurov studied different ligament and tendon insertion sites around the knee during growth in a rabbit model *(29)*. He concluded that evidence exists that

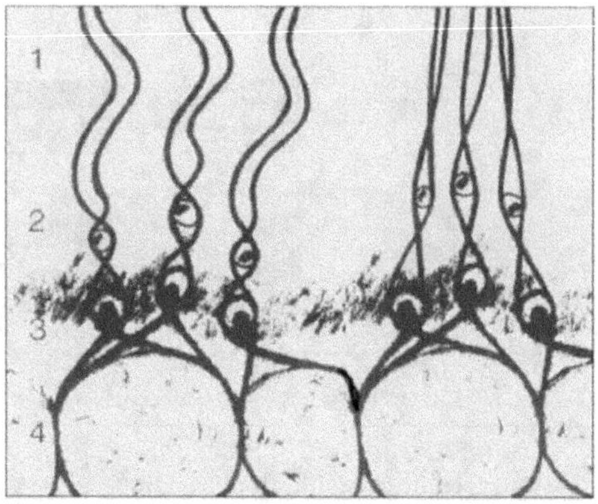

Fig. 6. Schematic drawing of the four histological zones of a direct ligament insertion: (1) tendon, (2) fibrocartilage, (3) mineralized cartilage tidemark, (4) lamellar bone. The relationship between the chondroid cells and collagen fibers is shown (left, relaxed status; right, status under tension). By tensing the collagen fibers, the cells get compressed, thus acting as an additional stress absorbent. (From ref. *24.*)

periosteal attachments (indirect insertion) are a necessary structural prerequisite for compensatory movements and invariance of the relative positions of muscles, tendons, and ligaments during long bone growth.

TENDON HEALING IN A BONE TUNNEL

The major indication for tendon tissue to be implanted into a bone tunnel is the reconstructive surgery of the cruciate ligaments. Especially with soft-tissue grafts, (hamstring tendons or the proximal part of a quadriceps tendon graft) and special allograft tissues, two major problems are encountered. The first is to regain a neoligament with normal tissue morphology and mechanical properties after graft remodeling; the second is to reestablish the normal insertion to bone, thus reconstructing these highly specialized transition zones between soft-tissue and bone, which is necessary for normal ligament function.

Animal Models

To study tendon-to-bone healing, an adequate animal model needs to be considered. Furthermore, when interpreting results of other studies, the animal model needs to be fully understood, as different models may display vastly different results, and their clinical relevance may be variable. Most studies investigating tendon-to-bone healing in a bone tunnel used extra-articular tendon transfer procedures *(4,7,10,12,13,34–40).* There are several advantages of extra-articular models. The implanted tendon tissue does not undergo an extensive remodeling; therefore, the mechanical interface–strength relationship is easier to study *(4).* In contrast, with an intra-articular model, as in anterior cruciate ligament (ACL) reconstructions, the tendon tissue undergoes intensive remodeling, which results in decreased mechanical properties of the tendon tissue during the early remodeling phase, causing midsubstance failure of the graft. This precludes any conclusions about the strength of the tendon–bone interface *(16).* Another advantage of an extra-articular model is that it can be easily performed in small animals, such as in rats and rabbits. Yet, an ACL reconstruction model in rats or rabbits is generally questionable, because the dimensions of these knee joints hardly allow a precise tunnel placement, which ultimately influences the outcome of reconstruction. Even with larger animals (sheep, goats, or dogs), reconstructive surgery of the ACL or posterior cruciate ligament are sometimes difficult to perform, as the dimensions of these knees are still far from the human equivalent. Therefore, even studies on cruciate ligament reconstruction in larger animals are somewhat limited regarding their clinical relevance *(41)*. When studying specific variables, such as biologic intervention procedures or details of the mechanical boundary conditions, extra-articular models are advantageous, because they present fewer variables (ligament remodeling, synovial contact, and so on; *4,35)*.

When studying tendon-to-bone healing in the context of ACL reconstruction procedures, an intra-articular model should be considered because of its closer resemblance of the clinical situation. Recently, more literature shows the investigation of tendon-to-bone healing of soft-tissue grafts in an intra-articular setting *(5,6,9,11,14,16,42–49)*. The clear advantage of these models is that graft-tunnel motion and a possible synovial in-flow into the tunnel could be assessed, which are believed to be responsible for tunnel enlargement, thereby improving the clinical relevance of these models. However, only a few studies used larger animals, such as dogs, sheep, or goats *(11,14,16,43,44,48)*. Knowledge of tendon-to-bone healing pertaining to ACL reconstruction is therefore still limited. However, intra-articular models in small animals are generally questionable, and rats and rabbits should only be considered for extra-articular tendon-to-bone healing studies.

With extra-articular models, tendon transfer procedures around the calcaneus in rabbits *(7,12,13)*, or implantation of the digital extensor tendon into the proximal metaphyseal tibia in dogs, sheep, and rabbits *(4,35–39)*, have been shown to be effective. But what is the most appropriate graft source to investigate tendon-to-bone healing of soft-tissue grafts? Numerous studies utilize a BPTB graft in sheep, goats, monkeys, or dogs. This graft can be easily harvested and requires only one incision: the arthrotomy. However, with soft-tissue grafts, controversy concerns the appropriate equivalent to the human hamstring tendon in the animal model. Shino et al. used a single-stranded patellar tendon graft without bone plugs *(44)*. Goradia et al. described the possibility of harvesting a semitendinosus tendon in sheep to reconstruct the ACL.

> "A 20-cm medial parapatellar incision was made. The subcutaneous tissue and superficial fascia were sharply incised along the same line as the skin incision to reveal the insertion of the semitendinosus tendon on the tibia" *(14)*.

Yet during anatomical dissection studies, we found that the semitendinosus tendon presents a more fascia-like structure in sheep rather than a solid tendon strand (Fig. 7), making it unsuitable for this type of reconstruction. Therefore, we utilized a split Achilles tendon graft or a long-flexor tendon graft that can be easily harvested. This procedure was well tolerated by the animals *(16,43)*. Yamazaki et al. made a similar observation in dogs and determined that the semitendinosus tendon was inappropriate as an ACL graft. Consequently, they used a flexor digitorum superficialis tendon to reconstruct the ACL in dogs *(11)*.

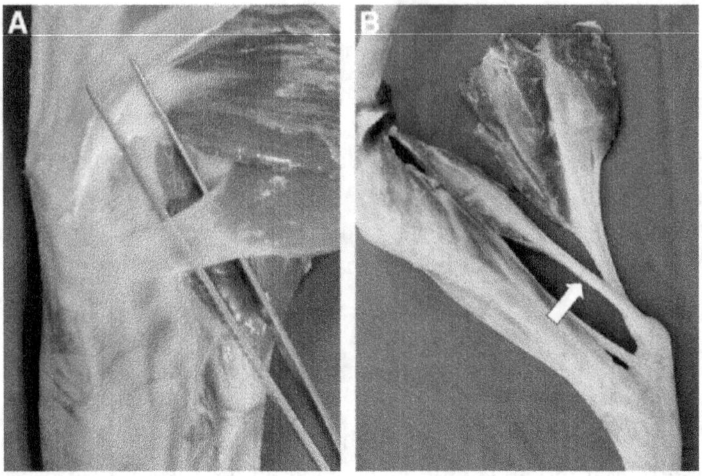

Fig. 7. **(A)** Insertion site of the semitendinosus tendon in sheep (forceps placed below). This tissue presents more a fascia-like structure than a solid tendon. **(B)** An alternative graft to study soft-tissue graft-to-bone healing is the long flexor digitorum tendon (arrow), which is embedded into a tendon sheet (removed) of the Achilles tendon.

Principals of Tendon-to-Bone Healing

The initial motivation to study tendon-to-bone healing in a bone tunnel is derived from a group of hand surgeons. In 1942, Kernwein transplanted extensor carpi radialis longus tendons in a dog model and found that the tensile strength of the tendon at its insertion site decreased after initial fixation *(34)*. Whiston and Walmsley conducted similar experiments in 1960, and found that the tendon tissue undergoes progressive degeneration combined with intensive bone tunnel remodeling *(12)*. Three years later, Forward and Cowan used different techniques of tendon-to-bone sutures in an Achilles tendon model in rabbits. The authors concluded:

> "Anchorage of tendon to bone is effected first by a temporary attachment formed by a connective tissue sleeve, which surrounds and adheres to the inserted portion of the tendon and weaves in between the intact bone trabeculae of the marrow cavity... Permanent mooring of the tendon to the bone is effected by actual ingrowth of bone tissue into the implanted tendon and the formation of a rough-walled bone tube about the implanted tendon. The collagen fibers of the implanted tendon attach directly to and become buried in the osseous tissue. These collagen fibers resemble the Sharpey fibers seen in normal tendon-to-bone insertions" *(13)*.

In this paper, Forward and Cowan described the basic principles of tendon-to-bone healing, as it has been later specified by Rodeo et al. *(4)*. Forward and Cowan further examined the chondroid cell transformation close to bone tissue, where the collagen fibers were inserted *(13)*. However, they discussed this chondroblastic reaction as part of the healing callus. In 1986, Jones et al. compared tendon transfer and tendon grafting into bone tunnels in a rabbit model. They were the first to draw attention to the development of a direct tendon insertion anatomy. However, they found that the normal four-zone tendon junction was not reproduced histologically in either group *(10)*.

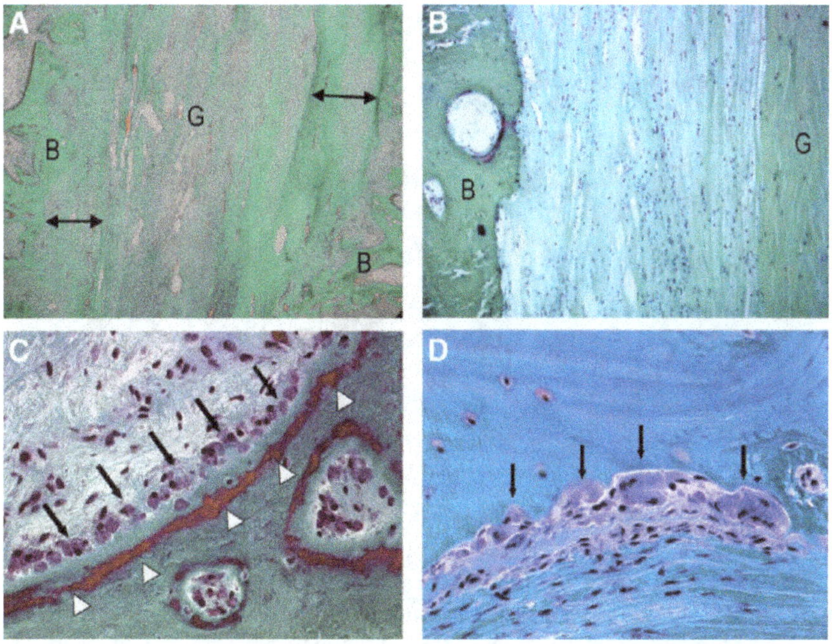

Fig. 8. **(A)** Longitudinal section through a tibial tunnel 6 wk after ACL reconstruction in sheep. There is a broad FIZ (in between arrows) between the graft tissue (G) and the surrounding bone (B). The graft itself is less organized and hypercellular owing to the early remodeling (Masson Goldner's trichrome stain, ×15 original magnification). **(B)** Higher magnification of the FIZ 9 wk after ACL reconstruction. The tissue is hypercellular and hypervascular. Note the fiber alignment parallel to the graft tissue (G) and the bone (B) surface (Masson Goldner's Trichrom stain, ×100 original magnification). **(C)** Bone–FIZ interface 9 wk postsurgery. There is an intensive appositional bone growth with a high amount of osteoblasts (arrows) and a continuous seam of uncalcified osteoid (arrow heads) (Masson Goldner's trichrome stain, original magnification ×400). **(D)** Bone–FIZ interface 6 wk postsurgery. There is a high amount of osteoclasts (arrows) removing bone tissue, signifying bone tunnel remodeling (Masson Goldner's trichrome stain, ×400 original magnification).

Pertaining to the question of tendon integration in a bone tunnel after cruciate ligament reconstruction, the first report was written by Shino et al. in 1984 *(44)*. They studied the remodeling of allograft vs autograft tissue for ACL replacement in a dog model. Regarding the controversies of tendon-to-bone healing that exist today, Shino et al. studied the columnation of fibrocartilage, which is seen in a normal ligament–bone junction *(44)*, but their initial goal was to study the remodeling process of the allograft tissue alone. Then in 1993, Rodeo et al. studied the tendon-to-bone healing in an extra-articular tendon transfer model in dogs with the aim to define the histological mechanisms and biomechanical characteristics of the healing of soft-tissue to bone *(4)*.

In an extra-articular model in dogs, Rodeo et al. described the development of an interface between the implanted tendon and the surrounding bone *(4)*. This interface, which we defined as the fibrous interzone (FIZ) because it may broaden if a tunnel enlargement occurs *(16,43)*, consists of disorganized, highly cellular, and highly vascular connective granulation tissue (Fig. 8).

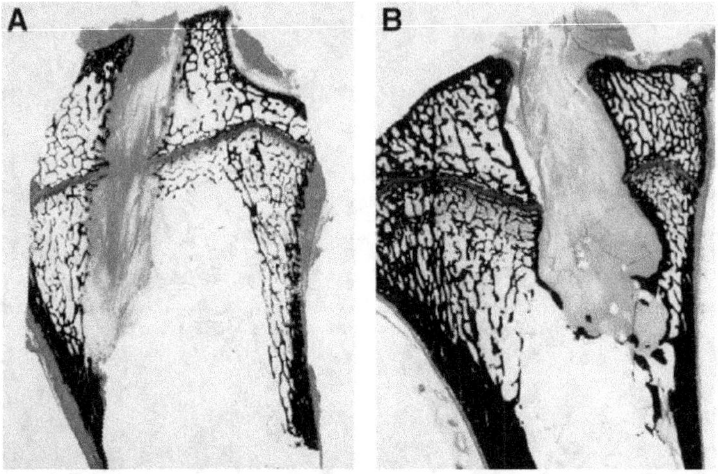

Fig. 9. (**A**) Sagital cut through a proximal tibia 6 wk post-ACL reconstruction with a soft-tissue graft in sheep. The initially drilled tunnel of 4.5 mm increased to a diameter of 5 mm; thus, the FIZ must have grown 0.25 mm on each side (Safranin O–van Kossa stain). (**B**) Sagital cut through a tibia 24 wk after ACL reconstruction in sheep, showing an intensive tunnel enlargement. The tunnel diameter increased from 4.5 mm to a maximum of 11 mm. Therefore, the FIZ must have increased by 3.25 mm on each side (Safranin O–van Kossa stain). (Reprinted from ref. *54*.)

During early healing, there is an intensive bone tissue remodeling with appositional growth of woven bone and simultaneous bone resorption (Fig. 8). The FIZ thickness may vary significantly and may depend on the fit between the tendon and bone tunnel at the time of implantation, the occurrence of a subsequent tunnel enlargement, or the intensity of the appositional bone growth during early healing (Figs. 9 and 10; *11,36, 43*). With further healing, the FIZ–tendon and FIZ–bone interfaces show the following developments:

- The FIZ tissue gets less cellular and vascular. The extracellular matrix becomes oriented until its fibers are longitudinally aligned and the FIZ–tendon interface becomes indistinct.
- There is an early development of Sharpey-like collagen fibers bridging the FIZ–bone interface, sometimes spanning from the tendon tissue directly into the bone. The amount of fibers increases over time.
- The bone at the FIZ–bone interface grows until all open intertrabecular spaces are closed for the bone to form a continuous line along the entire tunnel length. Later, a slight osseous narrowing occurs with no further tunnel enlargement, and the bone at the FIZ–bone interface becomes sclerotic (Fig. 10).

The development of Sharpey-like fibers has been perceived as the earliest sign of osseous soft-tissue graft incorporation *(4–7)*. In an immunohistochemical study, Liu et al. demonstrated that these fibers are immunoreactive for type III collagen. The authors further described an expression of type II collagen at the insertion site, but a chondroid cell transformation was not found *(7)*. However, it is unclear how high the density of Sharpey fibers must be to be seen as a sign for a solid-graft incorporation,

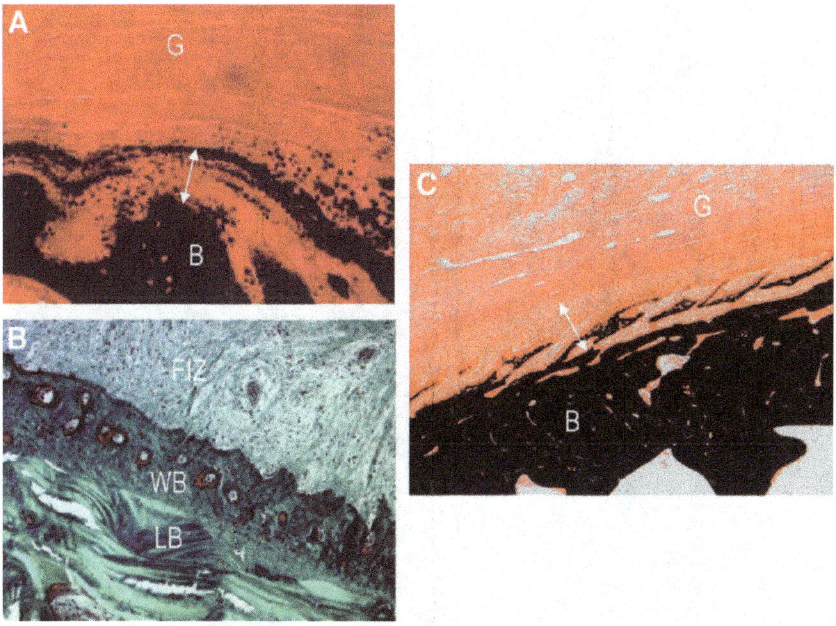

Fig. 10. **(A)** Sagital cut through a proximal tibia 6 wk after ACL reconstruction with a soft-tissue graft and extracortical fixation in sheep. There is an intensive granulation-like calcification of the FIZ (double-headed arrow) between the bone (B) and the graft (G) (Safranin O–van Kossa stain, ×200 original magnification).**(B)** Sagital cut through a proximal tibia 6 wk after ACL reconstruction with a soft-tissue graft and extracortical fixation in sheep. There is appositional bone growth (woven bone, WB) narrowing the FIZ (LB, lamellar bone; Safranin O–van Kossa stain, ×200 original magnification). **(C)** Sagital cut through a proximal tibia 24 wk following ACL reconstruction with a soft-tissue graft and extracortical fixation in sheep. There is an intensive in-growth of bone trabeculae into the FIZ (double-headed arrow) between the dense sclerotic bone surface (B) and the graft (G) (Safranin O–van Kossa stain, ×100 original magnification).

because several authors described a sparse occurrence in their animal models, as well as in human tissue harvested during second-look arthroscopies *(6,7,36,38,45–47,50, 51)*. Yet, we believe that a sparse occurrence of these interconnecting fibers could be found all around the body where there is a soft-tissue–bone interface, despite the fact that the tissue has no weight-bearing capacity. We made the observation that the granulation tissue, which forms inside a drill hole in bone, is anchored somehow to the bone by the development of Sharpey-like fibers, but the tissue is not exposed to any load (Fig. 11). Therefore, we consider it essential that a high density of Sharpey-like fibers (as described by Rodeo et al. *[4]*, Goradia et al. *[14]*, and Grana et al. *[5]*) is necessary, which might then be viewed as a solid indirect tendon insertion (Fig. 11). Although we consider an indirect type of ligament insertion to be mechanically inferior when compared to a direct type of insertion *(16,46,52)*, most studies investigating the tendon-to-bone healing within the tunnel showed only the development of an indirect insertion *(4–7,9,47, 49)*; thus, a direct type of insertion, as it is found with the native ACL, could not be identified within the tunnel.

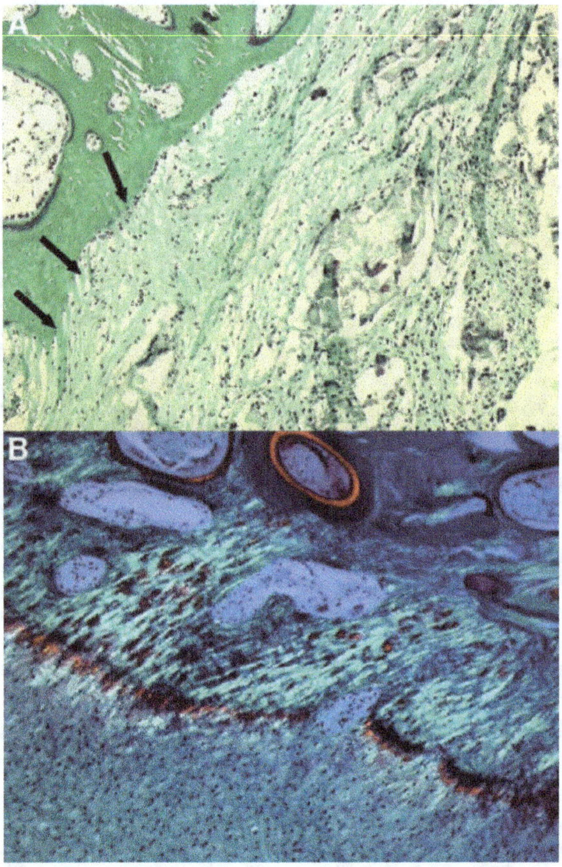

Fig. 11. **(A)** Microphotograph made 24 wk after tunneling bone tissue without an insertion of a tendon graft. The newly developed fibrous granulation is connected to the surrounding bone (B) by Sharpey-like fibers (arrows), but there is no load transmission via the soft-tissue (Masson Goldner's trichrome stain, ×100 original magnification). **(B)** FIZ-bone interface 12 wk after ACL reconstruction in sheep. Note the tight alignment and high density of Sharpey fibers. There is still appositional bone growth with active osteoblasts and a dense stripe of uncalcified osteoid (orange stain) (Masson Goldner's trichrome stain, ×200 original magnification).

Because most authors viewed the intratunnel part of the grafted tissue in a histological perspective, only a few saw the development of a chondroid transition zone *(13,35, 44)*, which might indicate that a direct type of ligament insertion develops. During our own investigations *(16,43)*, we studied the tendon-to-bone healing process at the intratunnel part of the grafted tissue, as well as at the articular tunnel aperture site, and found that different healing mechanisms may apply. The early intratunnel healing may be linked with the development of an indirect insertion, and in the later surface healing, a direct ligament insertion might develop with certain mechanical boundary conditions *(16,35,43)*. Therefore, it is our belief that most controversies regarding the development of an indirect vs a direct ligament insertion resulted from methodological inconsistencies from the different sites of the healing tissue being studied.

As the histological appearance is only one essential parameter to judge the progress and quality of the tendon-to-bone healing process, knowledge about the strength of the newly developed tendon–bone junction is important to better tailor rehabilitation protocols. In their extra-articular model, Rodeo et al. described that between 2 and 8 wk, the graft tissue failed by pullout, whereas at 12 and 26 wk, the tissue failed in midsubstance or at the clamp *(4)*. This suggests that there was a change of failure mode between wk 8 and 12, indicating that the tendon–bone interface was the weak link only in the early healing period.

Rodeo et al. further calculated the interface strength and the strength-to-length ratio and found the most obvious improvement in strength between the second and fourth week *(4)*. Goradia et al., who used an intra-articular model of soft-tissue graft ACL reconstruction in sheep, found that all reconstruction after 4 and 8 wk and two/thirds after 12 wk failed by pullout from the tunnel *(14)*. Their specimens at 24 and 52 wk failed in midsubstance; thus, the data of Goradia et al. are somewhat comparable to data by Rodeo et al., although an intra-articular model was used. Goradia et al. found the most prominent improvement in strength between wk 12 and 24, contrasting to the work by Rodeo et al. *(4,14)*. In our own series using extracortical graft fixation in an intra-articular ACL reconstruction model in sheep, we found the most significant increase in strength between the sixth and the twelfth week *(53)*. Furthermore, we found that some of the specimens failed by a so-called "degloving mechanism" even 24 wk after surgery (Fig. 12). Failing by degloving signifies that the central part of the graft is pulled out of the tunnel, whereas the peripheral part is still attached to the bony tunnel wall. Our histological investigation of these specimens indicates that the failure occurs at the FIZ–tendon interface. Although there might be a solid anchorage of the FIZ–bone interface, the FIZ–tendon interface is still the weak link, even 24 wk after reconstruction.

Relating to a BPTB graft, which is preferred for an accelerated rehabilitation program, it is important to consider the data on tendon-to-bone healing in comparison to healing of a bone plug in a bone tunnel. Tomita et al. studied the intraosseous graft healing in an intra-articular model in rabbits and compared a BPTB graft and flexor tendon graft for ACL reconstruction *(9)*. They found a significantly lower maximum load to failure for the flexor tendon graft group after only 3 wk. After 6 and 9 wk, there was no difference between the BPTB and flexor tendon graft *(9)*. Park et al. studied the osseous integration of a bone–tendon and bone tendon–bone graft in rabbits. They found a significantly lower failure load of the bone–tendon specimens at 4 and 6 wk, but there was no difference at 2 and 12 wk *(49)*. Yamazaki et al. studied the intraosseous healing of two different kinds of tunnel preparation with flexor tendon grafts for ACL reconstruction in dogs and compared them to a BPTB graft *(11)*. Similarly to Tomita et al., only a notable difference was found between both grafts at 3 wk. Although we consider intra-articular models in rabbits to be less clinically relevant, the study by Yamazaki et al. clearly indicates that at the time when more strenuous activities are allowed during rehabilitation, no variation in strength exists between both graft sources.

Influence of Local Boundary Conditions

The exposure of healing hard and soft-tissue to the mechanical load is an essential factor that influences biochemical and biomechanical characteristics of the healing tissue. Therefore, the influence of mechanical boundary conditions on tendon-to-bone

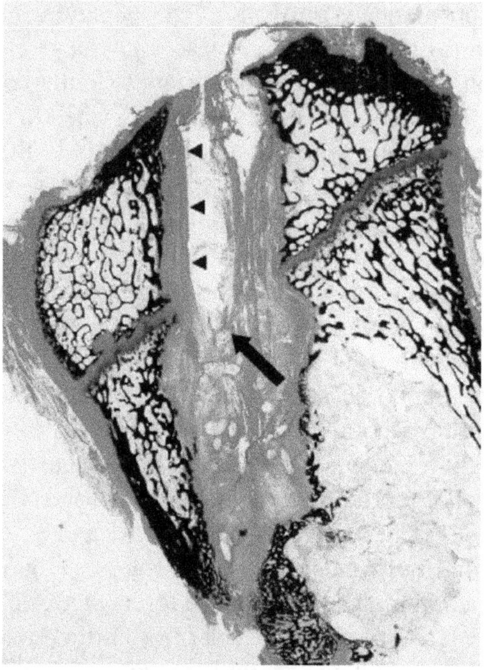

Fig. 12. Sagital section through a proximal tibia 24 wk after ACL reconstruction in sheep. During mechanical testing, the graft failed by a "degloving mechanism," which indicates that the FIZ–bone interface is stronger than the FIZ–tendon interface (arrowheads). Note that the graft failed at its suture attachment site (arrow), and the FIZ tissue (small arrows) remained attached to the tunnel wall. In this specimen, there was a tunnel enlargement of 4.5 to 8 mm (Safranin O–van Kossa stain). (Reprinted from ref. *114*.)

healing should not be neglected. Recently, Yamakado et al. published a significant study, investigating the quality of tendon-to-bone healing under different load conditions *(35)*. In an extra-articular model in rabbits, they implanted the extensor digitorum tendon almost perpendicular to the bone axis into the metaphyseal tibia, thus creating a tensile and a compressive site at the tunnel entrance. They found that tensile stress enhances the healing process of the tendon–bone junction and that compressive stress promotes a chondroid cell transformation. However, after 6 mo, a direct type of ligament insertion was developed in two out of nine specimens on the tensile site and none of the specimens on the compressive site, which might contrast the authors' claim that compressive forces lead to a chondroid tissue transformation *(35)*. However, according to the findings of Schneider and Küsswetter, the tensile forces transmitted by the collagen fibers create compressive forces to which the cells are exposed that lay in between the fibers. Thus, a zone of fibrocartilage develops *(22,24)*.

In our own series, two different techniques of ACL soft-tissue graft fixation were compared: one with biodegradable interference screw fixation and the other with extracortical Endobutton and tibial postfixation (Fig. 13). We found substantially different healing mechanisms *(43)*. With the Endobutton specimens, essentially comparable to the setup of Goradia et al. and principally comparable to all other studies, in which the

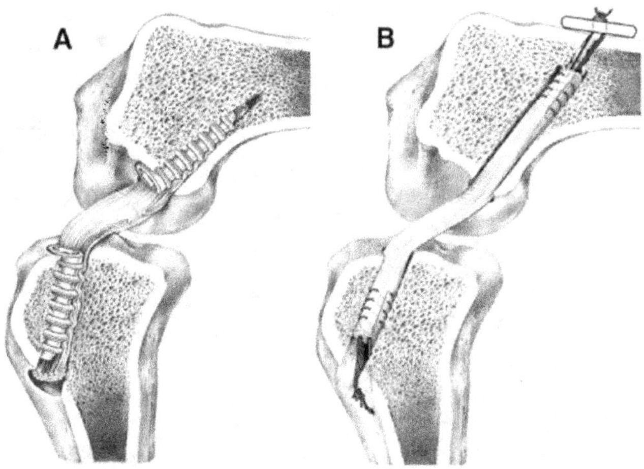

Fig. 13. Models used to study tendon-to-bone healing with two different fixation techniques. (**A**) The flexor tendon graft was directly fixed with biodegradable interference screws in an inside-out direction. (From ref. *42*.) (**B**) Graft fixation with Endobutton and sutures, as a typical example for an extracortical and indirect type of soft-tissue graft fixation. Note the posterior aspect of the tibial tunnel aperture site presents the compressive side, whereas the anterior aspect presents the tensile side.

graft was fixed outside the tunnel, a direct type of ligament insertion was partially present in four out of six tibial specimens after 24 wk. On the femur, none of the specimens developed such a direct type of ligament insertion *(43)*. Interestingly, the partially developed direct type of insertion in the Endobutton specimen was found at the anterior aspect of the tibial tunnel, which we considered to be the tensile site according to Yamakado's description (Fig. 14; *35,43*).

With the interference fit fixation specimens, all specimens developed a direct type of ligament insertion at the tibia and at the femur at 24 weeks (Fig. 15; *16,43*). During tendon-to-bone healing at the aperture site (surface healing), there was an initial blending between graft tissue and mineralized cartilage after 9 wk and a further maturation with interdigitating fibers after 12 wk (Fig. 16; *16*). With the intratunnel part of the graft tissue, a FIZ was only partially developed or was already replaced by bone; thus, the graft was in direct contact with the surrounding bone (Fig. 17; *16*). Using fluorescence microscopy, a continuous shift of bone growth and remodeling is shown from the intra-tunnel region toward the articular surface site, underlining the hypothesis that there is an early intratunnel and a later surface healing (Fig. 18; *16*).

When suggesting this hypothesis, the phenomenon of stress shielding or stress protection of the graft within the tunnel after surface healing has occurred needs to be further discussed. In our series of ACL reconstruction in sheep with soft-tissue graft interference fit fixation, around 1 yr postsurgery, a thinning of the graft tissue was found inside the tunnel with narrowing of the adjacent bone and resorption of the grafted tissue (Fig. 19; *16*). After 2 yr of implantation, the graft inside the tunnel was completely resorbed and replaced by bone in some specimens (Fig. 19). Because of

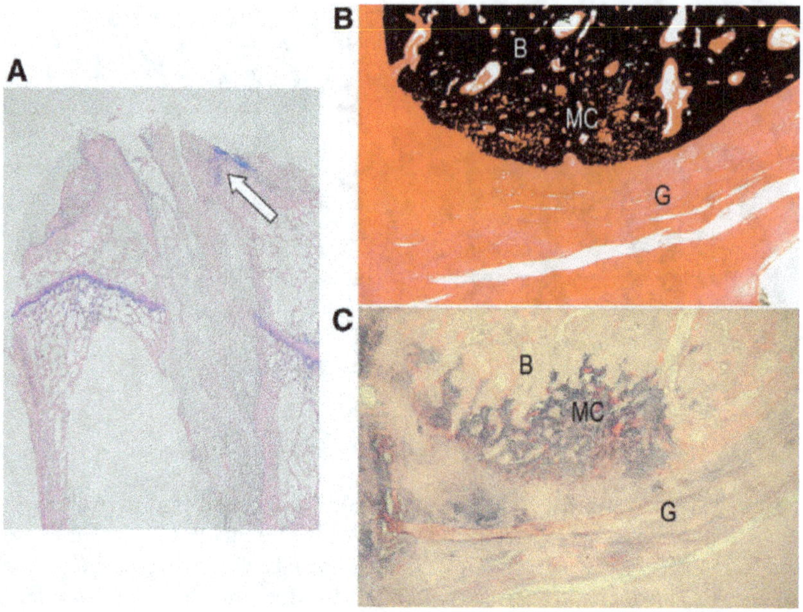

Fig. 14. **(A)** Sagital section through a tibial specimen with extracortical graft fixation 24 wk after surgery. Note the blue-stained tissue (arrow) at the anterior aspect of the tibial tunnel aperture site, indicating the development of a direct type of ligament insertion (Alcian Blue stain). **(B)** Higher magnification photomicrograph of the anterior aspect of the tunnel aperture site. Note the calcified tissue (black) with its chondroid cells embedded between the calcified matrix, indicating the development of a mineralized cartilage (MC) tidemark (G, graft; B, Bone; Safranin O–van Kossa stain, ×15 original magnification). **(C)** Serial section of the same specimen showing the broad area of the mineralized cartilage (MC) tissue (G, graft; B, bone; Alcian Blue stain, ×15 original magnification).

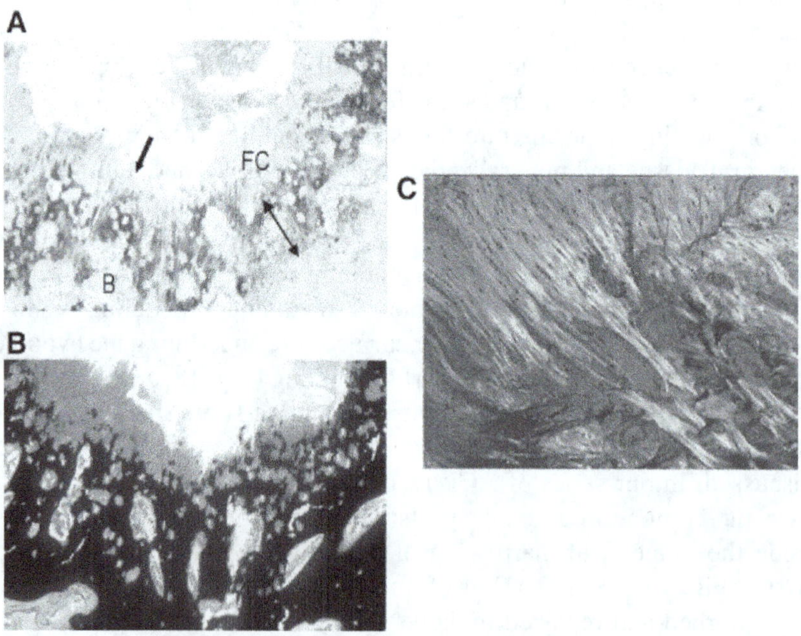

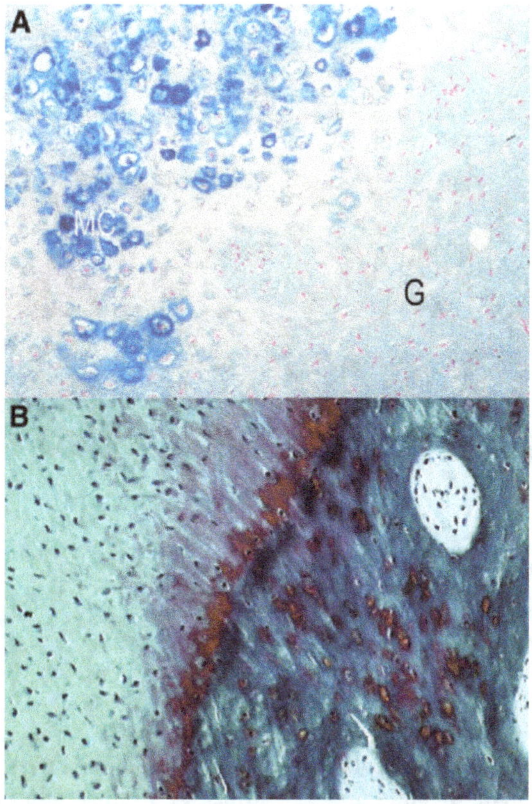

Fig. 16. **(A)** Tibial specimen 9 wk following ACL reconstruction with interference screw fixation. A blending already occurs between the mineralized cartilage tissue (MC) and the graft (G) (Alcian Blue stain, ×200 original magnification). (Reprinted from ref. *16*.) **(B)** Tibial specimen 12 wk after ACL reconstruction. A further maturation of the interface is present with a large amount of fibers extending into the zone of mineralized cartilage and woven bone. Note the appositional bone growth, similar to an apophyseal bone growth, with a broad seam of uncalcified osteoid (orange color) (polarized light, Masson Goldner's trichrome stain, ×100 original magnification).

Fig. 15. *(opposite page)* **(A)** Tibial graft insertion site 24 wk after ACL reconstruction with a soft-tissue graft and biodegradable interference screw fixation. A broad seam of mineralized cartilage (blue, in between arrows) has been formed, which lays between the lamellar bone (B) and the layer of fibrocartilage (FC). Note the site of tissue rupture after mechanical testing (arrow), which is located where the ligament tissue blends with the fibrocartilage (Alcian Blue stain, ×63 original magnification). **(B)** Same as Part **(A)**, confirming that a zone of mineralized cartilage has been formed using the Safranin O–van Kossa method. Note the chondrocyte islets in between the calcified tissue (Safranin O–van Kossa stain, ×63 original magnification). (Reprinted from ref. *16*.) **(C)** Tibial graft insertion site 24 wk after ACL reconstruction in another specimen with interference screw fixation. Note how deep the collagen fibers extend into the zone of mineralized cartilage and underlying lamellar bone (polarized light, Masson Goldner's trichrome stain, ×200 original magnification).

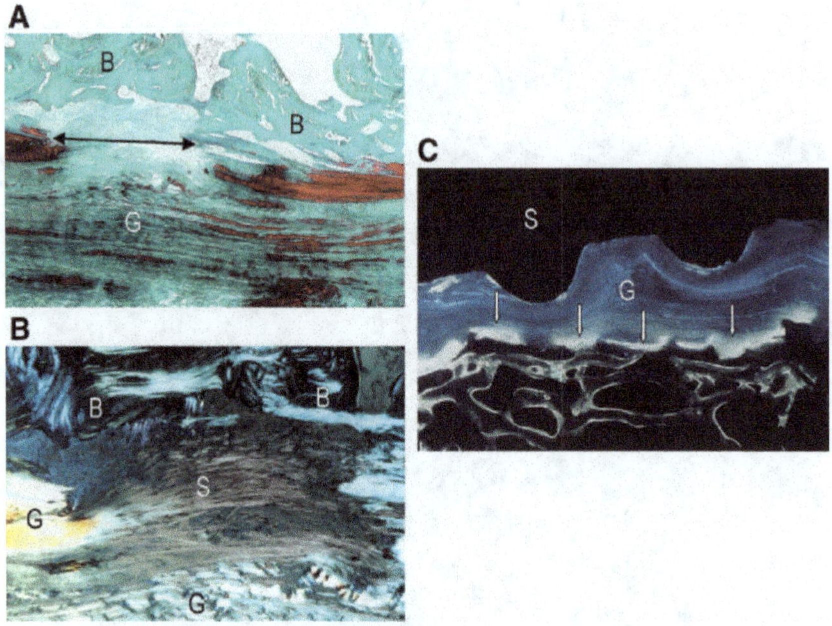

Fig. 17. **(A)** Tibial specimen 6 wk post-ACL reconstruction with interference screw fixation, demonstrating the interface between the graft (G) and the bone (B). The graft is immediately adjacent to the bone, and a FIZ is only developed in parts (between arrows) (Masson Goldner's trichrome stain, ×15 original magnification). (Reprinted from ref. *54*.) **(B)** Same as part **(A)** with a higher magnification under polarized light, illustrating the development of a FIZ (arrows) in an area where the graft (G) is not in direct contact with the adjacent bone tissue (B). In the area where a FIZ has been developed, a high number of Sharpey-like fibers (S) extend into the bone (polarized light, Masson Goldner's trichrome stain, ×63 original magnification). **(C)** Fluorescence microscopy of a longitudinal tibial section at 9 wk, presenting tetracycline fluorescence. The intense islet-like fluorescence (arrows) at the tendon–bone interface indicates an osseous bridging of the partially developed FIZ between 4 and 8 wk (S, screw site; G, graft tissue).

this finding, we concluded that owing to the development of a direct ligament insertion at the joint surface, the forces acting on the insertion site are mainly transmitted via this newly developed insertion, whereas the intratunnel part of the graft is stressshielded and is resorbed over time *(54)*.

In summary, the compressive forces acting on the tendon–bone interface are beneficial for the development of a direct type of ligament insertion. However, whether this is a result of the chondroid cell transformation being induced by compressive forces or the simple neutralization of graft-tunnel motions (e.g., by a press-fit mechanism with screw fixation and the sealing effect against the synovial in-flow into the tunnel) remains unclear.

Another local factor that might influence the strength of the healing tendon–bone unit is the length of the implanted tendon and the matching between graft and tunnel diameter. Greis et al. studied the strength of the healing tendon when implanted over a length of 1 or 2 cm into a bone tunnel. They used an extra-articular model in dogs based

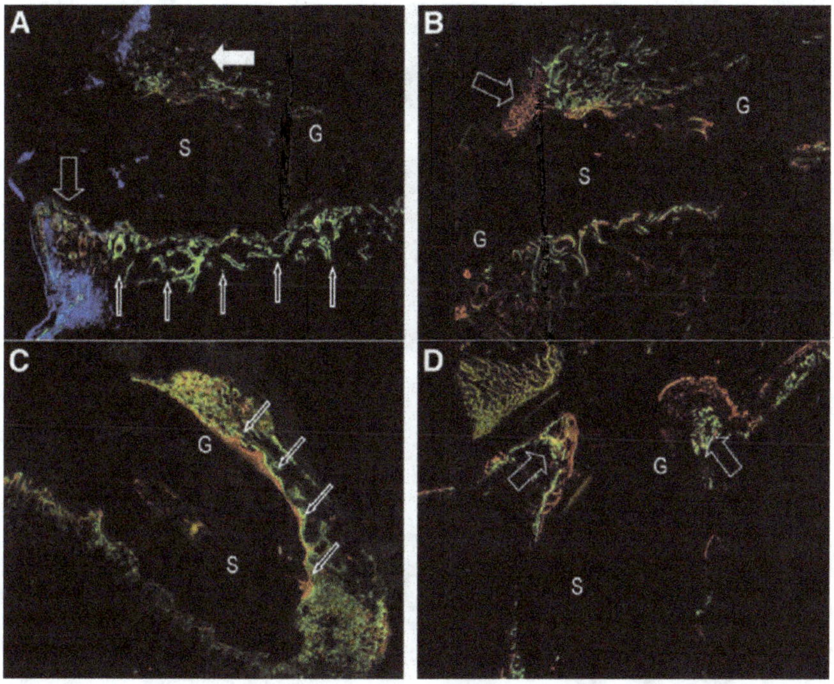

Fig. 18. **(A)** Fluorescence microscopy of a longitudinal tibial section at 6 wk. There is an intense bone growth after 1 wk close to the graft fixation site as indicated by the calcein green fluorescence (small arrows). At 3 wk, intense bone growth is seen closer to the articular tunnel aperture (transparent arrow) and more peripheral to the graft fixation site (white arrow). (S, screw site; G, graft tissue). **(B)** Fluorescence microscopy of a longitudinal tibial section at 9 wk. There is still intense bone growth close to the graft fixation site as indicated by all three given fluorochromes (4–8 wk). Note the intense xylenol orange fluorescence at the articular site (arrow) indicating a narrowing of the tunnel aperture at 6 wk. (S, screw site; G, graft tissue). **(C)** Fluorescence microscopy of a longitudinal femoral section at 12 wk. There is almost no osseous activity at the implant–bone interface, whereas there is markedly still remodeling activity at the tendon–bone interface (small arrows). Note the intense fluorescence of all three fluorochromes at the articular tunnel aperture site (arrow), indicating a continuous bone growth and remodeling at the surface over the whole labeling period (7–11 wk). (S, screw site; G, graft tissue). **(D)** Fluorescence microscopy of a longitudinal tibial section at 24 wk presenting all three given fluorochromes. Note that there is almost no osseous activity neither at the implant–bone interface nor the tendon–bone interface between 13 and 23 wk, whereas there is still intense bone growth and remodeling at the articular tunnel aperture site (arrows). The xylenol orange labeling (small arrows) indicates that the calcified cartilage tidemark develops around wk 18. (S, screw site; G, graft tissue). (Reprinted from ref. *16*.)

on the model initiated by Rodeo et al. *(4,36)*. Greis et al. found that a longer tendon length inside the tunnel revealed significantly higher load to failure data 6 wk after implantation *(36)*.

Greis et al. further studied the difference between a tightly and a loosely implanted tendon graft in a bone tunnel and compared 4.2- vs 6-mm tunnel diameters. With a tight tendon-tunnel fit, they found a significantly higher failure load 6 wk following

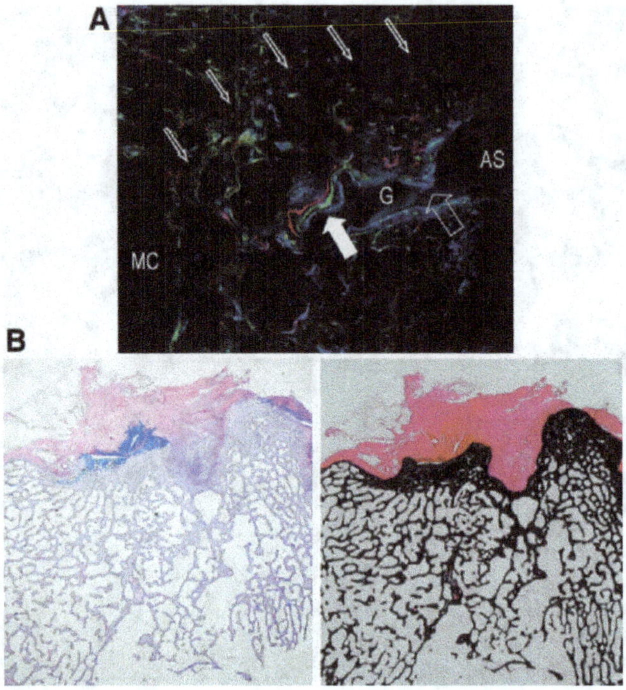

Fig. 19. **(A)** Fluorescence microscopy of a longitudinal tibial section at 52 wk presenting all three given fluorochromes. The former screw site (approximately outlined by the small arrow) is partially replaced by dense lamellar bone. A narrowing of the graft tunnel (transparent arrow) by a continuous bone in-growth is indicated by the homogenous and broad fluorochrome bands (white arrow). (G, graft tissue; MC, medullary cavity; AS, articular tunnel aperture site). (Reprinted from ref. *16*.) **(B)** Tibial specimen 2 yr after ACL reconstruction. Note the broad zone of mineralized fibrocartilage at the articular aperture site (left, Alcian blue staining,) and the replacement of the former screw site, as well as of the graft within the tunnel by lamellar bone (right, SafraninO–van Kossa stain). (Reprinted from ref. *54*.)

surgery *(36)*. Thus, they concluded that both factors—tendon length and tendon fit—are essential parameters to influence the strength of the healing tendon–bone interface. However, Yamazaki et al. studied the effect of tendon fit on tendon-bone healing in an intra-articular model in dogs and found no significant difference for the failure load between a tightly and a loosely implanted tendon graft *(11)*.

The main difference between the studies is that Greis et al. used an extra-articular model and Yamazaki et al. used an intra-articular model. Regarding the standardization of the experimental setup, the extra-articular model might be superior. Yet, the intra-articular model may have a higher clinical relevance. Because of this, we should follow the recommendations of Yamazaki et al., which might imply that a loosely implanted tendon graft during cruciate ligament reconstruction has no direct influence on the outcome. But it should be noted that the critical diameter difference between tendon and bone tunnel is unknown. Furthermore, it is obvious that a loosely implanted tendon graft is more likely to induce a tunnel enlargement, and this has been demonstrated to influence outcome after ACL reconstruction *(55)*.

In our own series, we have found that a tunnel enlargement is likely to occur with extracortical graft fixation in an intra-articular animal model and that it disturbs tendon-to-bone healing *(43)*. However, Yamazaki et al. have not reported the occurrence of a tunnel enlargement in their animal series *(11)*. We believe a tight graft insertion into the bone tunnel, especially an extracortical fixation should be considered.

Relating to an intra-articular tendon transfer for ACL reconstruction, it has been described that the healing capabilities may vary between the femoral and tibial fixation site. Our series found that it is more likely to have a direct ligament insertion develop at the tibial site than on the femur *(43)*. As mentioned above, the different mechanical boundary conditions are likely responsible for this finding. Alternatively, Grassman et al. used a rabbit model and discovered that the tendon-to-bone healing is accelerated with the cancellous-filled femoral site when compared to the more marrow-dominated tibial site *(40)*. The authors suggested that graft healing may also depend on the cancellous bone architecture at the graft insertion site. This finding is important, particularly when discussing results from previous investigations, because the animal model may be not only responsible for different results but also the site of tendon implantation that has been studied.

TENDON HEALING TO A BONE SURFACE

Tendon healing to a bone surface can be observed in numerous structures, including the rotator cuff tendons in the shoulder, flexor tendons in the hand, tibial insertion site of the medial collateral ligament in the knee, and the Achilles tendon in the foot. This section focuses on the rotator cuff and the supraspinatus tendons, particularly, as representatives. It is interesting to note that the number of studies investigating tendon-to-bone healing in the knee joint far exceed those performed for the shoulder. This could be somewhat explained by the lack of an appropriate animal model of the rotator cuff tendons.

Injuries of the rotator cuff tendons in the shoulder are among the most common problems that cause shoulder pain and dysfunction in adults. Cuff tear can be partial- or full thickness, acute or chronic, and traumatic or degenerative *(56,57)*. Rotator cuff surgery is considered when nonoperative treatment fails to reduce pain and does not improve shoulder function. The most common types of surgical treatment for rotator cuff tears include open or arthroscopic repair that involves reapproximating the tendon edge to a bony surface of the humeral head. In cases of complex or irreparable tears, tendon transfers are often performed *(58–60)*. The major goal of a rotator cuff repair is to provide a sufficient initial strength of fixation to allow appropriate rehabilitation during early stages of the healing process when the tendon–bone interface is still weak and complete functional recovery has yet to take place. However, high failure rates of the rotator cuff repairs remains a significant postoperative complication that often requires revision surgeries *(61–64)*. Several factors contribute to these failures: poor quality and elasticity of the involved muscle-tendon unit, neurovascular damage, tendon degeneration, osteoporosis of the humeral head, inadequate fixation of tendon to the bone, and lack of tendon-to-bone healing at the tendon–bone interface *(63,65,66)*.

The supraspinatus tendon is the most frequently injured rotator cuff tendon and is often used for clinical and basic science studies of various repair techniques. The supraspinatus insertion to the superior aspect of the humeral head greater tuberosity is considered to be a direct insertion and can be categorized into four distinct zones. Zone 1 consists of the tendon proper and contains only fibroblastic cells. Zone 2 consists of fibrocartilage, where the cells become larger and change from thin flat fibroblasts to more rounded chondrocyte-like cells. Zone 3 is characterized by a sudden transition from nonmineralized to mineralized fibrocartilage, separated by a tidemark. Zone 4 is represented by bone *(21,67)*. The changes in the tendon tissue properties as it transitions from zone to zone are gradual and continuous, and there are no clearly defined boundaries between the zones.

Several authors have investigated the collagen content of the supraspinatus insertion site in human cadaveric tissue, as well as in several animal models *(68–71)*. Fallon et al. have pointed out that fibrocartilagenous region of the supraspinatus tendon extends well beyond the normal 500–700 μm to approx 2 cm *(21,27,68)*. The histological characteristics of this collagen structure were similar to those described in compressional fibrocartilage *(71)*. Neer has suggested that this region of the supraspinatus tendon is being compressed between the acromion and humeral head *(72,73)*. Therefore, the morphology and composition of the attachment fibrocartilage region may function to resist not just tension but also compression. Fan et al. and Kumagai et al. found that type I was the predominant collagen, but significant amounts of type III and possibly some types II and V were also present at the attachment zone of the supraspinatus tendon *(70)*. The predominant labeling in the fibrocartilage was for collagen type II, and the tidemark showed inconsistent labeling for all of the collagen types. Interestingly, there appeared to be more type III collagen in the insertion zone than in the tendon substance. The authors concluded that this differential collagen composition may contribute to the high incidence of tear associated with this rotator cuff tendon *(69,70,74)*.

Restoration of the natural insertion site is critical for the proper functioning of the tendon–bone structure. Although numerous investigations have focused on finding the strongest repair technique for the rotator cuff tears, much remains unknown about the healing and repair of the torn rotator cuff insertion *(65,76–82)*. This is partly because of the lack of a suitable animal model of the healing rotator cuff tendons. In one of the first animal models, St. Pierre et al. used goats to compare the healing process of the infraspinatus tendon after two repair techniques at 6 and 12 wk postoperatively *(75)*. In the first technique, the supraspinatus tendon was reattached to a trough in cancellous bone, while the second repair used direct fixation of a tendon to cortical bone. The authors reported a progressive maturation and reorganization of the bone–tendon interface with reestablishment of collagen-fiber continuity between the tendon and bone in both groups. The parallel array of collagen fibers extending perpendicular to the tendon was found to be histomorphologically identical to the Sharpey fibers of normal tendon-to-bone attachment. This evidence suggests that the tendon healing process was equivalent whether the tendon was attached to cortical or cancellous bone, provided that close apposition was maintained during healing. The authors concluded that there was no variation between the two repair groups; therefore, there is no benefit from a creation of a bone trough to expose tendon to cancellous bone.

Soslowsky and coworkers proposed the rat's supraspinatus tendon as a suitable model to study human rotator cuff disorders *(83)*. This group studied the healing response of a controlled defect in the supraspinatus tendon and evaluated the role of intrinsic injury (modeled as an acute insult to the tendon) and extrinsic injury (modeled as external subacromial impingement), as well as overuse factors on rotator cuff tendinosis *(84,85)*. Carpenter et al. concluded that there was an active, but inadequate, repair response to a defect in the supraspinatus tendon of rats *(84)*.

From the same group, Thomopoulos et al. described the localized expression of extra-cellular matrix components at the tendon insertion side using histology and *in situ* hybridization methods *(86)*. Their histologic results indicated a poor healing response to the injury, with only partial recreation of the insertion site by 8 wk. *In situ* hybridization results indicated a specific pattern of genes expressed in each zone of the insertion site (i.e., tendon, fibrocartilage, mineralized cartilage, and bone). Expression of collagen types I and XII, aggrecan, and biglycan was increased, whereas expression of collagen type X and decorin was decreased. Over time, expression of collagen type I, type XII, and biglycan decreased, but remained above normal at 8 weeks. Their research found that the rat supraspinatus tendon is ineffective in recreating the original insertion site, even at 8-wk postinjury, in the absence of biological or biomechanical enhancements.

Bjorkenheim et al. monitored supraspinatus tendon healing by measuring intra-articular hydrodynamic pressure and observed healing or closure of the defect in a rabbit model after 9 wk *(87)*. Kumagai et al. demonstrated a repair response with type III collagen that was initially formed and was gradually replaced with type I collagen in a transected supraspinatus tendon model in rabbits *(88)*.

In another model, Choi and coauthors investigated the spontaneous healing process of a surgically created supraspinatus tendon tear in rabbits with particular reference to the expression of matrix metalloproteinase-2 (MMP-2) and its time-course change in enzymatic activity, along with the expression of tissue inhibitors of metalloproteinases (TIMPs; *89*). The authors found that MMP-2–positive cells were mainly localized at both cutting ends of the tendon, and reparative tissue encroached into the gap from the bursal side. The expression of TIMP-1 was induced in the cells at not only the tendon edges, but also at the reparative tissue during the healing process. TIMP-2 was constitutively expressed in both the tendon and reparative tissue. Latent and active forms of MMP-2 and characteristic time-linked changes of the enzymatic activity were also shown. These results may suggest that MMP-2 is expressed and activated during the healing process of acute supraspinatus tendon tear and can have an important role in the remodeling process.

The importance of the subacromial bursa for the supraspinatus healing process was emphasized by Uhthoff and coauthors *(90,91)*. They determined the origin of the cells affecting healing of the supraspinatus tendon inserted into a bony trough in a rabbit model. After 2 wk, both the cellularity of the underlying bone and the thickness of the subacromial bursa were significantly increased in the operated when compared with the control shoulders, thus contributing to the process of repair. In an earlier examination of the biopsy specimens obtained during surgery on patients with complete rotator cuff rupture, the authors found vascularized connective tissue covering the area of rupture and proliferating cells in the fragmented tendons. The main source of this fibrovascular tissue was the wall of the subacromial bursa, which might significantly influence tendon reconstitution and remodeling *(90)*.

These results are consistent with the work of Kobayashi et al., who studied *in situ* hybridization of α1(I) and α1(III) procollagen mRNA during healing of full-thickness tears of avian supracoracoid tendons *(92)*. The authors found high-level expression of procollagen mRNA in the proliferating peritendon cells on the bursal side, contributing to the repair process that progressed to the joint side.

Recently, attempts have been made to improve and enhance healing of the rotator cuff tendons to the bone surface *(76,93–95)*. Gerber et al. and Koh et al. independently used a polylactide plate and polylactide scaffold, respectively, to improve the initial strength of the rotator cuff repair in a sheep model and compared these augmented repair techniques to traditional fixation methods *(76,93)*. Both groups concluded that the augmentation increased the functional surface area, over which the stresses of the repair are distributed, therefore decreasing the peak load on any one area and resulting in a superior strength of the repair vs the traditional fixation techniques.

BIOLOGICAL INTERVENTION

Several approaches to the improvement of tendon-to-bone healing exist. The application of growth-enhancing factors and different delivery tools, such as gene therapy and direct or carrier-mediated indirect transfer, have been investigated in numerous studies *(38,45,46,96–98)*. From studies in the early 1970s, the potential of periosteum to induce new bone formation has been known *(99–101)*. However, recent studies applied this knowledge to the concept of tendon-to-bone healing and showed the advantage of graft augmentation with periostal flaps to improve bony in-growth and take advantage of their potential osteoinductivity *(102–104)*. Youn et al. found that an augmentation of a free-tendon graft with a periosteum patch, whose cambium layer was facing the surrounding bone, was able to significantly improve the biomechanical properties of the newly formed tendon-to-bone insertion at 6 wk after implantation in comparison to a periosteum free-tendon graft *(102)*. They used an extra-articular model of implanting a free-tendon graft into a bone tunnel in the calcaneus process of rabbits. They observed an increased bone formation around the tendon graft and found a direct relationship between the periosteal osteogenesis and the application of mechanical stress at the tendon-to-bone interface *(102)*. In another study by Kyung et al., the long digital extensor tendon of rabbits was detached from its femoral insertion, wrapped either into a periosteal patch with its cambium layer facing the tendon or left as a free-tendon graft and rerouted into a tibial bone tunnel *(104)*. Histological and biomechanical analysis at 3 and 6 wk showed more extensive bone formation and closer apposition of bone around the tendon graft in the periosteal group, also with notably improved biomechanical properties at both time points. Ohtera et al. used an identical model, comparing freshly harvested and frozen periosteum flaps as an augmentation of a free-tendon autograft to improve tendon-to-bone healing *(105)*. They found the development of an early stage of a direct insertion type with fibrocartilage formation as early as 4 wk postimplantation in the group with fresh periosteal patches in comparison to the development of a fibrous interzone in the frozen periosteal group.

In summary, the augmentation of a free-tendon graft with periosteal tissue is a promising technique to accelerate tendon-to-bone healing without the application of growth factors. Therefore, it can be easily applied to humans without the possible side effects of biologically active substances *(103)*.

Numerous studies researched the effect of different growth factors, such as platelet-derived growth factor, basic fibroblast growth factor (FGF), insulin-like growth factor, and transforming growth factor-β (TGF-β) on tendon and ligament healing *(53,106–111)*. However, only a few studies looked at the enhancement of the tendon-to-bone incorporation with the application of biological agents. In 1991, Itoh used bone morphogenic protein (BMP) combined with fibrin sealant to study the influence on tendon-to-bone healing in an extra-articular model in rabbits *(112)*. Itoh reported that BMP increases the failure strength but did not contribute to the early formation of an enthesis. In 1999, Rodeo et al. used BMP-2 to study its effect on tendon-to-bone healing *(38)*. They used a collagen carrier in an extra-articular model in dogs and found that the effect of BMP on the mechanical strength was only significant after 2 wk, whereas no major difference to the control after 4 and 8 wk *(38)*. Nicklin et al. used BMP-7 to study the histological changes during tendon-to-bone healing after ACL reconstruction in sheep *(48)*. They found an increased bone formation around the grafted tendons but did not report on results of mechanical testing. Anderson et al. reported on the use of a bone growth factor in 2001 that presents a bone-derived extract (different BMPs, TGF-β and FGF) to augment tendon-to-bone healing after soft-tissue graft ACL reconstruction in rabbits. Bone growth factor was shown to increase load to failure at 2, 4, and 6 wk.

Recently, attempts have been made to enhance the tendon-to-bone healing process from a biological standpoint using tissue engineering methods via gene transfer *(46,96–98)*. The concept is based on the manipulation of cellular and biochemical mediators to affect protein synthesis and improve tissue remodeling. Cell therapy involves the introduction of mesenchymal progenitor cells as a pluripotent cell source into the healing environment. The combination of cell therapy with growth factor application by gene transfer offers new avenues to improve ligament and tendon healing. Recent studies have shown the feasibility of transferring marker genes to synovium, chondrocytes, meniscal fibrochondrocytes, tenocytes, and ligamental fibroblasts, prompting optimism for the eventual success of this approach *(98)*. Despite this optimism, a number of technical issues remain and need to be addressed before gene transfer might be considered as an approach to improve the structural and functional properties of healing ligaments and tendons. However, just recently Martinek and coworkers reported on the adenovirus-based gene transfer of BMP-2 to the tendon-bone healing site after ACL reconstruction in rabbits *(46)*. The authors found an increased load to failure 8 wk after surgery of the gene transfer-treated specimens (45 N control vs 108.8 N study).

However, although the aforementioned reports have proven that the local increase in growth factor concentration is beneficial for tendon-to-bone healing, we still believe that the first step in improving this healing should include an optimization of local mechanical boundary condition *(43)*. Furthermore, we need a more basic knowledge about the differentiation of cell types involved in normal tendon-to-bone healing *(113)*. More information should also be obtained on growth factor expression prior to the use of growth factors shown to be effective in bone healing, in which completely different healing patterns could be found.

REFERENCES

1. Kasperczyk W, Bosch U, Oestern H, Tscherne H. Staging of patellar tendon autograft healing after posterior cruciate ligament reconstruction. A biomechanical and histological study in a sheep model. *Clin Orthop* 1993;286:271–282.

2. Jackson D, Corsetti J, Simon T. Biologic incorporation of allograft anterior cruciate ligament replacements. *Clin Orthop* 1996;324:126–133.
3. Nagano M, Yoshiya S, Kuroda F, Kurosaka M, Mizuno K. Remodeling and healing process of bone-patellar tendon-bone graft in a bone tunnel: a histological study in dogs. *Trans Orthop Res Soc* 1997;43:78.
4. Rodeo S, Arnoczky S, Torzilli P, Hidaka C, Warren R. Tendon-healing in a bone tunnel. A biomechanical and histological study in the dog. *J Bone Joint Surg* 1993;75A:1795–1803.
5. Grana WA, Egle DM, Mahnken R, Goodhart CW. An analysis of autograft fixation after anterior cruciate ligament reconstruction in a rabbit model. *Am J Sports Med* 1994;22: 344–351.
6. Blickenstaff K, Grana W, Egle D. Analysis of a semitendinosus autograft in a rabbit model. *Am J Sports Med* 1997;25:554–559.
7. Liu S, Panossian V, Al-Shaikh R, et al. Morphology and matrix composition during early tendon to bone healing. *Clin Orthop* 1997;339:253–260.
8. Shino K, Kawasaki T, Hirose H, Gotoh I, Inoue M, Ono K. Replacement of the anterior cruciate ligament by an allogenic tendon graft. *J Bone Joint Surg* 1984;66B:672–681.
9. Tomita F, Yasuda K, Mikami S, Sakai T, Yamazaki S, Tohyama H. Comparison of intraosseous graft healing between the doubled flexor tendon graft and the bone-patellar tendon-bone graft in anterior cruciate ligament reconstruction. *Arthroscopy* 2001;17: 461–476.
10. Jones JR, Simbert JG, Mccullough CJ, Price AB, Hutton WC. Tendon implantation into bone: an experimental study. *J Hand Surg* 1987;12:306–312.
11. Yamazaki S, Yasuda K, Tomita F, Minami A, Tohyama H. The effect of graft-tunnel diameter disparity on intraosseous healing of the flexor tendon graft in anterior cruciate ligament reconstruction. *Am J Sports Med* 2002;30:498–505.
12. Whiston T, Walmsley R. Some observations on the reaction of bone and tendon after tunneling of bone and insertion of tendon. *J Bone Joint Surg* 1960;42B:377–386.
13. Forward A, Cowan R. Tendon suture to bone: An experimental investigation in rabbits. *J Bone Joint Surg* 1963; 45A:807–823.
14. Goradia V, Rochat M, Grana W, Rohrer M, Prasad H. Tendon-to-bone healing of a semitendinosus tendon autograft used for ACL reconstruction in a sheep model. *Am J Knee Surg* 2000;13:143–151.
15. Brand J, Weiler A, Caborn D, Brown C, Johnson D. Current concepts: Graft fixation in cruciate ligament surgery. *Am J Sports Med* 2000;28:761–774.
16. Weiler A, Hoffmann R, Bail H, Rehm O, Südkamp NP. Tendon healing in a bone tunnel—Part II: Histological analysis after biodegradable interference fit fixation in a model of anterior cruciate ligament reconstruction in sheep. *Arthroscopy* 2002;18:124–135.
17. Havers C. *Osteologia Nova*. Smith, London, UK, 1691.
18. Biermann H. Die knochenbildung im bereich periostaler-diaphysärer sehnen- und bandansätze. *Z Zellforsch* 1957;46:635–671.
19. Knese K, Biermann H. Die knochenbildung an Sehnen- und Bandansätzen im Bereich ursprünglich chondraler Apophysen. *Z Zellforsch* 1958;49:142–187.
20. Sharpey W, Ellis G. *Elements of Anatomy*. Walton and Moberly, London, UK, 1856.
21. Cooper R, Misol S. Tendon and ligament insertion: a light and electron microscopic study. *J Bone Joint Surg* 1970;52A:1–20.
22. Schneider H. Zur struktur der sehnenansatzzonen. *Z Anat Entwicklungsgesch* 1956; 119:456.
23. Dolgo-Saburoff B. Über ursprung und insertion der skelettmuskeln. *Anat Anz* 1929;68: 80–87.
24. Küsswetter W, Refior H. Vergleichende licht- und rasterelektronenmikroskopische untersuchungen zum morphologischen aufbau der knöchernen bandinsertionen. *Z Orthop* 1985;123:876–879.

25. Senst W. Beitrag zur feingeweblichen struktur der band-knochenverbindung. *Zbl Chir* 1974;99:275–283.
26. Vis H. Histological investigations into the attachment of tendons and ligaments to the mammalian skeleton. *Proc kon Ned Akad v Went* 1957;60:147–157.
27. Benjamin M, Evans E, Copp D. The histology of tendon attachments to bone in man. *J Anat* 1986;149:89–100.
28. Messner K. Postnatal development of the cruciate ligament insertions in the rat knee - morphological evaluation and immunohistochemical study of collagens type I and II. *Acta Anat* 1997;160:261–268.
29. Hurov J. Soft-tissue bone interface: How do attachments of muscles, tendons, and ligaments change during growth? A light microscopic study. *J Morphol* 1986;189:313–325.
30. Becker W. Elektronenmikroskopische untersuchung der insertion von sehnen am knochen. *Arch Orthop Unfall Chir* 1971;69:315–329.
31. Gao J, Messner K. Quantitative comparison of soft-tissue-bone interface at chondral ligament insertions in the rabbit knee joint. *J Anat* 1996;188:367–373.
32. Vasseur P, Rodrigo J, Stevenson S, Clark G, Sharkley N. Replacement of the anterior cruciate ligament with a bone-ligament-bone anterior cruciate ligament allograft in dogs. *Clin Orthop* 1987;219:268–277.
33. Pauwels F. Eine neue theorie über den Einfluß mechanischer reize auf die differenzierung der stützgewebe. zehnter beitrag zur funktionellen anatomie und kausalen morphologie des stützapparates. *Z Anat Entwicklungs Gesch* 1960;121:478–515.
34. Kernwein G. A study of tendon implantations into bone. *Surg Gynecol Obstet* 1942;75: 794–902.
35. Yamakado K, Kitaoka K, Yamada H, Hashiba K, Nakamura R, Tomita K. The influence of mechanical stress on graft healing in a bone tunnel. *Arthroscopy* 2002;18:82–90.
36. Greis P, Burks R, Bachus K, Luker M. The influence of tendon length and fit on the strength of a tendon-bone tunnel complex: a biomechanical and histologic study in the dog. *Am J Sports Med* 2001;29:493–497.
37. Singhatat W, Lawhorn K, Howell S, Hull M. How four weeks of implantation affect the strength and stiffness of a tendon graft in a bone tunnel: a study of two fixation devices in an extraarticular model in ovine. *Am J Sports Med* 2002;30:506–513.
38. Rodeo S, Suzuki S, Deng X, Wozney J, Warren R. Use of recombinant human bone morphogenetic protein-2 to enhance tendon healing in a bone tunnel. *Am J Sports Med* 1999; 27:476–488.
39. Shoemaker S, Reschl H, Campell P, Kram H, Sanchez M. Effect of fibrin sealant on incorporation of autograft and xenograft tendons within bone tunnels. *Am J Sports Med* 1989; 17:318–324.
40. Grassman S, McDonald D, Thornton G, Shrive N, Frank C. Early healing processes of free tendon grafts within bone tunnels is bone-specific: a morphological study in a rabbit model. *Knee* 2002;9:21–26.
41. Weiler A, Peters G, Mäurer J, Unterhauser F, Südkamp NP. Biomechanical properties and vascularity of an anterior cruciate ligament graft can be predicted by contrast enhanced magnetic resonance imaging. *Am J Sports Med* 2001;29:751–761.
42. Weiler A, Peine R, Pashmineh-Azar R, Abel C, Südkamp NP, Hoffmann RFG. Tendon healing in a bone tunnel—Part I: Biomechanical results after biodegradable interference fit fixation in a model of anterior cruciate ligament reconstruction in sheep. *Arthroscopy* 2002;18:113–123.
43. Weiler A, Unterhauser F, Faensen B, Hunt P, Bail H, Haas N. Comparison of tendon-to-bone healing using extracortical and anatomic interference fit fixation of soft-tissue grafts in a sheep model of ACL reconstruction. Proceedings from the 48th Annual Meeting of the Orthropaedic Research Society, Dallas, TX. *Trans Orthop Res Soc* 2002; 48:0173.

44. Shino K, Kawasaki T, Hirose H, Gotoh I, Inoue M, Ono K. Replacement of the anterior cruciate ligament by an allogeneic tendon graft. *J Bone Joint Surg Br* 1984;66:672–681.
45. Anderson K, Seneviratne A, Izawa K, Atkinson B, Potter H, Rodeo S. Augmentation of tendon healing in an intraarticular bone tunnel with use of a bone growth factor. *Am J Sports Med* 2001;29:689–698.
46. Martinek V, Lattermann C, Usas A, et al. Enhancement of tendon-bone integration of anterior cruciate ligament grafts with bone morphogenic protein-2 gene transfer. *J Bone Joint Surg* 2002;84A:1123–1131.
47. Papachristou G, Tilentzoglou A, Efstathopoulos N, Khaldi L. Reconstruction of the anterior cruciate ligament using the doubled tendon graft technique: An experimental study in rabbits. *Knee Surg Sports Traumatol Arthrosc* 1998;6:246–252.
48. Nicklin S, Morris H, Harrison J, Walsh W. OP-1 augmentation of tendon-to-bone healing in an ovine ACL reconstruction. Proceedings from the 46th Annual Meeting of the Orthropaedic Research Society, Dallas, TX. *Trans Orthop Res Soc* 2000;46:155.
49. Park M, Lee M, Seong S. A comparative study of the healing of tendon autograft and tendon-bone autograft using patellar tendon in rabbits. *Int Orthop* 2001;25:35–39.
50. Scranton P, Lanzer W, Ferguson M, Kirkman T, Pflaster D. Mechanism of anterior cruciate ligament neovascularization and ligamentization. *Arthroscopy* 1998;14:716.
51. Pinczewski L, Clingeleffer A, Otto D, Bonar S, Corry I. Integration of hamstring tendon graft with bone in reconstruction of the anterior cruciate ligament—case report. *Arthroscopy* 1997;13:641–643.
52. Sheh M, Butler D, Stoffer D. Correlation between structure and material properties in human knee ligament and tendons. *Am Soc Mech Eng AMD* 1985;68:17–20.
53. Weiler A, Förster C, Falk R, Schmidmaier G, Südkamp NP. Locally applied platelet-derived growth factor-BB ameliorates structural properties of a free tendon graft after anterior cruciate ligament reconstruction. Proceedings from the 47th Annual Meeting of the Orthropaedic Research Society, Dallas, TX. *Trans Orthop Res Soc* 2001; 47:0327.
54. Weiler A, Scheffler S, Südkamp NP. Aktuelle aspekte in der verankerung von hamstringsehnen-transplantaten in der kreuzbandchirurgie. [Current aspects of anchoring hamstring tendon transplants in cruciate ligament surgery.] *Chirurg* 2000;71:1034–1044.
55. Stange R, Russel V, Salmon L, Pinczewski L. Tibial tunnel widening after ACL reconstruction: a 2 and 5 year comparison of patellar tendon autograft and 4-strand hamstring tendon autograft. *Arthoscopy Association of North America 20th Annual Meeting*, Abstract 67, 2001.
56. Cofield RH. Rotator cuff disease of the shoulder. *J Bone Joint Surg Am* 1985;67:974–979.
57. Matsen FA, Lippitt SB, Sidles JA, Harryman DT2. *Practical Evaluation and Management of the Shoulder*. W.B. Saunders Company, Philadelphia, PA, 1994, pp. 1–242.
58. Warner JJ. Management of massive irreparable rotator cuff tears: the role of tendon transfer. *Instr Course Lect* 2001;50:63–71.
59. Miniaci A, MacLeod M. Transfer of the latissimus dorsi muscle after failed repair of a massive tear of the rotator cuff. A two to five-year review. *J Bone Joint Surg Am* 1999;81: 1120–1127.
60. Gerber C, Hersche O. Tendon transfers for the treatment of irreparable rotator cuff defects. *Orthop Clin North Am* 1997;28:195–203.
61. Harryman DT, Mack LA, Wang KY, Jackins SE, Richardson ML, Matsen FA, III: Repairs of the rotator cuff. Correlation of functional results with integrity of the cuff. *J Bone Joint Surg Am*1991;73:982–989.
62. Gazielly DF, Gleyze P, Montagnon C. Functional and anatomical results after rotator cuff repair. *Clin Orthop Res* 1994;304:43–53.
63. Goutallier D, Postel JM, Bernageau J, Lavau L, Voisin MC. Fatty muscle degeneration in cuff ruptures. Pre- and postoperative evaluation by CT scan. *Clin Orthop* 1994;304:78–83.

64. Jost B, Pfirrmann CW, Gerber C, Switzerland Z. Clinical outcome after structural failure of rotator cuff repairs. *J Bone Joint Surg* Am 2000;82:304–314.
65. Gerber C, Schneeberger AG, Beck M, Schlegel U. Mechanical strength of repairs of the rotator cuff. *J Bone Joint Surg Br* 1994;76:371–380.
66. Warner JP, Krushell RJ, Masquelet A, Gerber C. Anatomy and relationships of the suprascapular nerve: anatomical constraints to mobilization of the supraspinatus and infraspinatus muscles in the management of massive rotator-cuff tears. *J Bone Joint Surg Am* 1992;74:36–45.
67. Woo SL-Y, Akeson W. Ligament, tendon, and joint capsule insertion to bone. In *Injury and Repair of the Musculoskeletal Soft-Tissues.* Woo SL-Y, Buckwalter JA, eds. The American Academy of Orthopaedic Surgeons, Park Ridge, IL, 1988, pp 133–166.
68. Fallon J, Blevins FT, Vogel K, Trotter J. Functional morphology of the supraspinatus tendon. *J Orthop Res* 2002;20:920–926.
69. Fan L, Sarkar K, Franks DJ, Uhthoff HK. Estimation of total collagen and types I and III collagen in canine rotator cuff tendons. *Calcif Tissue Int* 1997;61:223–229.
70. Kumagai J, Sarkar K, Uhthoff HK, Okawara Y, Ooshima A. Immunohistochemical distribution of type I, II and III collagens in the rabbit supraspinatus tendon insertion. *J Anat* 1994;185(Pt 2):279–284.
71. Berenson MC, Blevins FT, Plaas AH, Vogel KG. Proteoglycans of human rotator cuff tendons. *J Orthop Res* 1996;14:518–525.
72. Neer CS2. Anterior acromioplasty for the chronic impingement syndrome in the shoulder: a preliminary report. *J Bone Joint Surg Am* 1972;54:41–50.
73. Neer CS2. Impingement lesions. *Clin Orthop* 1983;70–77.
74. Kumagai J, Sarkar K, Uhthoff HK. The collagen types in the attachment zone of rotator cuff tendons in the elderly: an immunohistochemical study. *J Rheumatol* 1994;21:2096–2100.
75. St Pierre P, Olson E, Elliott J, O'Hair K, McKinney L, Ryan J. Tendon-healing to cortical bone compared with healing to a cancellous trough. A biomechanical and histological evaluation in goats. *J Bone Joint Surg* 1995;77A:1858–1866.
76. Gerber C, Schneeberger AG, Perren SM, Nyffeler RW. Experimental rotator cuff repair. A preliminary study. *J Bone Joint Surg* Am 1999;81:1281–1290.
77. Craft DV, Moseley JB, Cawley PW, Noble PC. Fixation strength of rotator cuff repairs with suture anchors and the transosseous suture technique. *J Shoulder Elbow Surg* 1996;5:32–40.
78. Rossouw DJ, McElroy BJ, Amis AA, Emery RJ. A biomechanical evaluation of suture anchors in repair of the rotator cuff. *J Bone Joint Surg Br* 1997;79:458–461.
79. Reed SC, Glossop N, Ogilvie-Harris DJ. Full-thickness rotator cuff tears. A biomechanical comparison of suture versus bone anchor techniques. *Am J Sports Med* 1996;24:46–48.
80. Burkhart SS, Diaz Pagan JL, Wirth MA, Athanasiou KA. Cyclic loading of anchor-based rotator cuff repairs: confirmation of the tension overload phenomenon and comparison of suture anchor fixation with transosseous fixation. *Arthroscopy* 1997;13:720–724.
81. Caniggia M, Maniscalco P, Pagliantini L, Bocchi L. Titanium anchors for the repair of rotator cuff tears: preliminary report of a surgical technique. *J Orthop Trauma* 1995;9:312–317.
82. Barber FA, Herbert MA. Suture anchors—update 1999. *Arthroscopy* 1999;15:719-25.
83. Soslowsky LJ, Carpenter JE, DeBano CM, Banerji I, Moalli MR. Development and use of an animal model for investigations on rotator cuff disease. *J Shoulder Elbow Surg* 1996;5:383–392.
84. Carpenter JE, Thomopoulos S, Flanagan CL, DeBano CM, Soslowsky LJ. Rotator cuff defect healing: a biomechanical and histologic analysis in an animal model. *J Shoulder Elbow Surg* 1998;7:599–605.
85. Carpenter JE, Flanagan CL, Thomopoulos S, Yian EH, Soslowsky LJ. The effects of overuse combined with intrinsic or extrinsic alterations in an animal model of rotator cuff tendinosis. *Am J Sports Med* 1998;26:801–807.

86. Thomopoulos S, Hattersley G, Rosen V, Mertens M, Galatz L, Williams GR, Soslowsky LJ. The localized expression of extracellular matrix components in healing tendon insertion sites: an in situ hybridization study. *J Orthop Res* 2002;20:454–463.
87. Bjorkenheim JM, Paavolainen P, Ahovuo J, Slatis P. Resistance of a defect of the supraspinatus tendon to intraarticular hydrodynamic pressure: an experimental study on rabbits. *J Orthop Res* 1990;8:175–179.
88. Kumagai J, Sarkar K, Uhthoff HK. Repair process of surgically produced rotator cuff tear—A histological and immunohistochemical study using monoclonal antibodies against collagen type I and III. *Trans Orthop Res Soc* 1993;18:315.
89. Choi HR, Kondo S, Hirose K, Ishiguro N, Hasegawa Y, Iwata H. Expression and enzymatic activity of MMP-2 during healing process of the acute supraspinatus tendon tear in rabbits. *J Orthop Res* 2002;20:927–933.
90. Uhthoff HK, Sarkar K. Surgical repair of rotator cuff ruptures. The importance of the subacromial bursa. *J Bone Joint Surg Br* 1991;73:399–401.
91. Uhthoff HK, Sano H, Trudel G, Ishii H. Early reactions after reimplantation of the tendon of supraspinatus into bone. A study in rabbits. *J Bone Joint Surg Br* 2000;82:1072–1076.
92. Kobayashi K, Hamada K, Gotoh M, Handa A, Yamakawa H, Fukuda H. Healing of full-thickness tears of avian supracoracoid tendons: in situ hybridization of alpha1(I) and alpha1(III) procollagen mRNA. *J Orthop Res* 2001;19:862–868.
93. Koh JL, Szomor Z, Murrell GA, Warren RF. Supplementation of rotator cuff repair with a bioresorbable scaffold. *Am J Sports Med* 2002;30:410–413.
94. Sano H, Kumagai J, Sawai T. Experimental fascial autografting for the supraspinatus tendon defect: remodeling process of the grafted fascia and the insertion into bone. *J Shoulder Elbow Surg* 2002;11:166–173.
95. Kessler KJ, Bullens-Borrow AE, Zisholtz J. LactoSorb plates for rotator cuff repair. *Arthroscopy* 2002;18:279–283.
96. Menetrey J, Kasemkijwattana C, Day C, Bosch P, Fu F, Moreland M, Huard J. Direct-, fibroblast- and myoblast-mediated gene transfer to the anterior cruciate ligament. *Tissue Eng* 1999;5:435–442.
97. Woo S, Suh J, Parsons I, Wang J, Watanabe N. Biological intervention in ligament healing. *Sports Med Arthrosc Rev* 1998;6:74–82.
98. Lattermann C, Baltzer A, Whalen J, Evans C, Robbins P, Fu F. Gene therapy in sports medicine. *Sports Med Arthrosc Rev* 1998;6:83–88.
99. Rubak JM. Osteochondrogenesis of free periosteal grafts in the rabbit iliac crest. *Acta Orthop Scand* 1983;54:826–831.
100. Ritsila V, Alhopuro S. The use of free periosteum for bone formation in congenital clefts of the maxilla. A preleminary report. *Scand J Plast Reconstr Surg* 1972;6:57–60.
101. Uddstromer L, Ritsilia V. Osteogenic capacity of periosteal grafts: a qualitative and quantitative study on membranous and tubular bone periosteum in young rabbits. *Scand J Plast Reconstr Surg* 1978;12:207–214.
102. Youn I, Cohen S, Nauman E, Jones D, Suh J. Stimulative effects of periosteum in tendon-bone attachment: in vivo and in vitro studies. Proceedings from the 48th Annual Meeting of the Orthropaedic Research Society, Dallas, TX. *Trans Orthop Res Soc* 2002;48:150.
103. Chen C, Chen W, Shih C. Enveloping of periosteum of the hamstring tendon graft in anterior cruciate ligament reconstruction. *Arthroscopy* 2002;18:E27.
104. Kyung H, Kim S, Oh C, Kim S. Tendon-to-bone healing in a rabbit model: the effect of periosteum augmentation at the tendon-to-bone interface. Proceedings from the 48th Annual Meeting of the Orthopaedic Research Society, Dallas, TX. *Trans Orthop Res Soc* 2002;48:317.
105. Ohtera K, Yamada Y, Aoki M, Sasaki T, Yamakoshi K. Effects of periosteum wrapped around tendon in a bone tunnel: A biomechanical and histological study in rabbits. *Crit Rev Biomed Eng* 2000;28:115–118.

106. Kobayashi D, Kurosaka M, Yoshiya S, Mizuno K. Effect of basic fibroblast growth factor on the healing of defects in the canine anterior cruciate ligament. *Knee Surg Sports Traumatol Arthrosc* 1997;5:189–194.
107. Sakai T, Yasuda K, Tohyama H, et al. Effects of combined administration of transforming growth factor-beta1 and epidermal growth factor on properties of the in situ frozen anterior cruciate ligament in rabbits. *J Orthop Res* 2002;20:1345–1351.
108. Letson A, Dahners L. The effect of combinations of growth factors on ligament healing. *Clin Orthop* 1994;207–212.
109. Hildebrand K, Woo S, Smith D, et al. The effect of platelet-derived growth factor-BB on healing of the rabbit medial collateral ligament. An in vivo study. *Am J Sports Med* 1998; 26:549–554.
110. Batten M, Hansen J, Dahners L. Influence of dosage and timing of application of platelet-derived growth factor on early healing of the rat medial collateral ligament. *J Orthop Res* 1996;14:736–741.
111. Chan K, Chan B, Fu B. Effect of bFGF on tendon healing: an in vivo model. *Int Soc Arthrosc Knee Surg Orthop Sports Med*, Buenos Aires, 1997
112. Itoh O. An experimental study on effect of bone morphogenetic protein and fibrin sealant in tendon implantation into bone. *Nippon Seigeigeka Gakki Zasshi* 1991;65:580–590.
113. Jeong K, Hatch J, Abbot A, Ying L, McCarthy D, Rodeo S. Identification of the cells that participate in early tendon-to-bone healing. Proceedings from the 47th Annual Meeting of the Orthropaedic Research Society, Dallas, TX. *Trans Orthop Res Soc* 2001;47:742.
114. Weiler A, Scheffler S, Hoher J. Transplant selection for primary replacement of the anterior cruciate ligament. *Orthopäde* 2002;31:731–740.

12
Artificial Ligaments

Andrew A. Amis

INTRODUCTION

The history of artificial ligaments includes possibly more than its fair share of controversy and failures. One main task of this chapter is to review the history to extract the lessons that will be valuable for the future. Although artificial ligaments are presently unpopular, memories of previous disappointments inevitably fade, while at the same time, technology continues, opening up novel approaches to the problem. The second task of this chapter is to look to the future: is there a case for pursuing the development of artificial ligaments at all? If so, how might this be done for the errors of the past to be avoided?

CLINICAL CASE FOR ARTIFICIAL LIGAMENTS

The knee is clearly the main focus for work on ligaments owing to the frequency of ligament injuries at the knee from both sport and other accidental trauma with the disability caused by knee joint instability. Although there are numerous other sites around the body that have clinical applications for this technology, the knee, and particularly the cruciate ligaments, drive the subject forward. This chapter considers the reconstruction of tissues other than ligaments that are primarily collagenous, such as tendon and capsular tissues, as the applications are similar and often have research studies relevant to ligaments. Of the other sites, the rotator cuff is probably the structure affected most frequently and causes sufficient disability for surgery to be considered. However, this disability arises as a result of degenerative changes in the tissues of an older patient population; thus, factors such as healing responses may be different.

There is widespread evidence that ruptured cruciate ligaments do not heal. The stumps usually retract into a tissue mass at the bone attachments and may be resorbed, or sometimes the stump may stick to an adjacent structure. This has been observed with the anterior cruciate ligament (ACL), which may detach from the femur at the proximal end, then become adherent to the side of the posterior cruciate ligament (PCL). Different rupture patterns have been observed that may reflect the injury mechanism and speed of impact. Thus, while the ACL may have peeled off of its femoral attachment relatively intact in many cases observed by the author in the UK, the American literature often describes the ruptured ACL as resembling the fibers of a paintbrush, implying that the ligament has burst open in midsubstance. Regardless of the mechanism, the

From: *Orthopedic Biology and Medicine: Repair and Regeneration of Ligaments, Tendons, and Joint Capsule*
Edited by: W. R. Walsh © Humana Press Inc., Totowa, NJ

remaining ligament structure is predominantly parallel-fibered. This means that sutures can pull out of the ligament stumps at low loads, even when complex suturing methods derived for finger flexor tendon repairs are used *(1)*. As a result, research on ligament repair eventually concludes that this procedure is not reliable for the cruciate ligaments. This conclusion leads the surgeon to reconstruction methods, which require the use of a ligament graft to carry the load for some time.

Although there is now widespread experience of ACL reconstruction using autogenous tissue grafts with reliably good results, factors remain about this procedure that are not optimal. Graft harvest inevitably causes defect pathology that may relate to pain and/or functional deficit, in addition to the problems arising from the initial injury. Furthermore, the harvest and preparation of any graft prolongs the operation. After the operation, many graft fixation methods allow some slippage to occur under the cyclic loads imposed during rehabilitation *(2)*, and the properties of the graft may be reduced significantly during tissue remodeling *(3)*. These circumstances can lead to some return of excess laxity in joints with reconstructed ligaments as time increases postsurgery. These factors are accepted during "isolated" ACL reconstruction, but they become more prominent as injury severity increases. With the rising number of structures to be reconstructed, the surgeon is then faced with searching for autogenous grafts from around the more severely damaged knee and possibly from the other knee as well.

Allogenic tissue grafts offer the surgeon a method to avoid some of these difficult choices, and their use is widespread in North America. However, this is not universal, perhaps because of the lack of organization of tissue banks to supply the grafts in other countries, or because of lingering doubts about disease transmission. Even if grafts are available, the sterilization methods required to minimize the possibility of disease transmission leads to degradation of the graft properties. Gamma irradiation is one particular sterilization method, but the dose of 4 Mrad needed to ensure a sufficiently small rate of organism survival also affects the collagen structure; therefore, there is severe loss of graft strength postoperation as remodeling occurs *(4)*. Generally, it appears that the process of biological remodeling and tissue incorporation entails a greater loss of mechanical properties in allografts than in autografts *(5,6)*.

An artificial ligament is appealing because it could avoid all the drawbacks noted in the problems of auto- and allografts. The devices could be readily available, their design could ensure great strength; their fixation methods could be designed for both strength and resistance to slipping under cyclic loads; and they would not cause any defect pathology. However, the overriding considerations of biocompatibility and durability must be noted. Will the device have any undesirable effects on the surrounding tissues, and will the reconstruction remain intact—both acutely and in the long term? These are the stumbling blocks that have affected virtually all previous work and are the focus of the review.

MECHANICAL CONSIDERATIONS

Although ligaments are innervated and therefore contribute to knee stability via proprioception, their primary role is that of passive tensile restraints to limit the separation distance between their attachments on different bones. Their tensile behavior should be considered with any artificial ligament and is now reviewed briefly.

The loads imposed in use are usually cyclic, based on the activity and joint position. For an artificial structure, this implies a tendency to cause progressive fatigue failure. In addition, cyclic tensile stresses can lead to progressive creep elongation—a phenomenon that will bring a return of joint laxity. Not much data exists on the forces imposed on ligaments, and the most relevant data relates to the knee ligaments when walking. Gait analysis has led to predictions of two load peaks per stride on the ACL of approx 150 N with the implication that this may rise to 600 N when jogging *(7)*. Forces during strenuous athletic activities are largely unknown, despite the aim of most ligament reconstruction surgery to return to such activity levels. This suggests that artificial ligaments should be tested for resistance to cyclic tensile forces in the region of 800 N in an aqueous environment at body temperature. With people taking approx 2×10^6 strides per year, it seems appropriate to run tests for 10^7 load cycles. This level of testing has been rarely used in the development of artificial ligaments, which may explain many of the failures that have been reported. Many publications have included ultimate tensile strength data for artificial ligaments that has been compared to the strength of the natural structures being replaced. However, the above statements show that the strength should actually be much higher than this, as most polymers will creep significantly at a small fraction of their ultimate tensile strength when subjected to cyclic loading at body temperature, leading to the reappearance of joint laxity.

Tensile tests of natural ligaments show nonlinear behavior, where an initial low stiffness is superseded by stiffer linear behavior prior to rupture. This stiffness transition relates to the collagen fibril crimp being straightened out on a microscopic level. At a larger scale, the ligament fibers normally will not all have the same degree of slackness/tightness at any joint position because the ligament fibers attach over an area of bone, rather than at a point. Thus, as the bone attachments pull apart, a progressive tightening of the ligament fibers occurs, and they are recruited sequentially as they pass through the slack–taut transition. It has been hypothesized that this feature of ligament tensile behavior is intended to provide a more gradual arrest of bone–bone displacement, thus reducing impact forces. Regardless of the reason, it is appropriate to try to match the natural tensile characteristics, as this allows the artificial ligament to act in concert with the surrounding tissues, sharing the loads normally between cooperating structures. Clearly, an artificial ligament that has greater stiffness than the natural ligament it has replaced is relatively prominent regarding load sharing, causing it to be subjected to unnecessarily high loads, while other tissues do not experience their normal loads.

There is little evidence available for the strength of natural ligaments in young adults, the typical patients for reconstructive surgery. The ligament that has been studied most is the ACL; it has long been known that the strength declines with advancing age. Woo et al. have shown that the strength declines from approx 3 kN in young adults (20–30 yr old) to approx 0.7–1 kN by 70 yr old *(8)*. This ratio of strength with youth should be noted when reviewing the literature on other ligaments, because almost all such work is based on tissue of the elderly. However, it is not known if other ligaments suffer the same loss of strength with advancing age, and efficient vascularization of surrounding tissues for ligaments that are not intra-articular may possibly reduce this tendency.

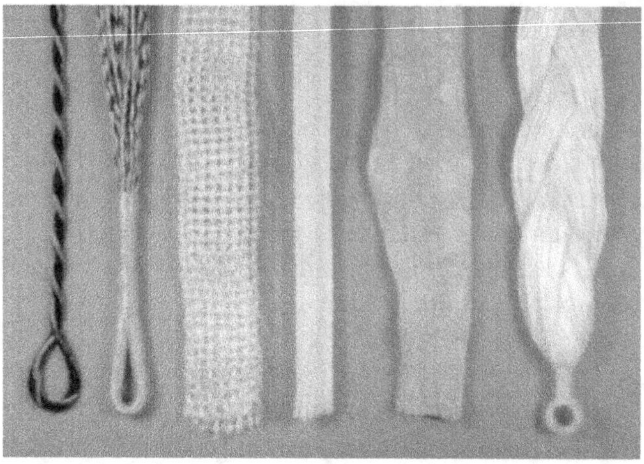

Fig. 1. Artificial ligaments clinically available in the United Kingdom in 1985 (from left to right): carbon (Johnson & Johnson), carbon and polyester (Surgicraft), Leeds-Keio polyester (Neoligaments), Dacron (Stryker-Meadox), bovine glutaraldehyde-fixed xenograft tendon (Xenotech), and Gore-Tex polytetrafluoroethylene (WL Gore).

Although cyclic creep tests imply that the artificial ligament has sufficient fatigue strength, the exact conditions of use and proposed implantation method may indicate additional fatigue testing. This applies particularly to situations where the artificial ligament has to pass over a corner, such as the exit from a femoral bone tunnel, where there could be localized abrasion. Cyclic tensile loads cause the artificial ligament to extend and contract, leading to fretting motion against the bone, which may cause liberation of particulate debris. Along with abrasion against external surfaces, an artificial ligament with multiple fiber strands can suffer internal abrasion between the fibers, if the cyclic loading and/or bending/twisting cause the fibers to rub together. This is most likely to occur if the implant has a braided or woven structure and can lead to progressive loss of strength, as well as chronic liberation of implant particles into the surrounding tissues.

HISTORICAL REVIEW OF ARTIFICIAL LIGAMENTS

The potential of cruciate ligament reconstruction received widespread attention as a result of trauma during World War I, when the first attempts at artificial ligaments appeared. This focus was not revisited until the 1970s, which was followed by a period of intense activity that peaked in the mid-1980s (Fig. 1). A rapid collapse of the use of these devices arose in the early 1990s. Because of the many different approaches pursued during that time, it would be confusing to discuss events in a chronological order; thus, this review describes the individual materials used to fabricate artificial ligaments.

Early Days

Prior to the 1970s, artificial materials were rarely used for reconstruction of ligaments or tendons, but isolated reports included the use of certain materials, such as silver wires or silk sutures *(9)*.

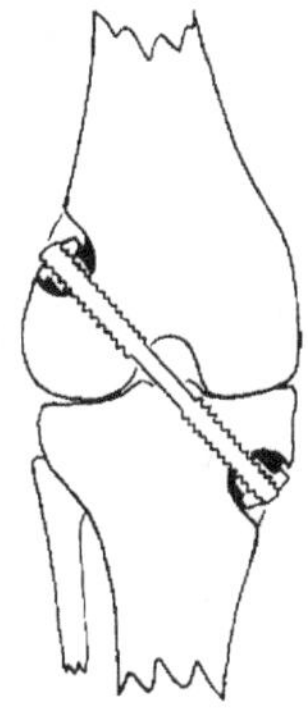

Fig. 2. The polyethylene rod ACL prosthesis, secured by titanium alloy nuts.

There were several attempts to make structures that would reproduce the force-vs-extension characteristics of natural ligaments that are compliant at low loads but stiffen to give quasielastic behavior from approx 4% elongation to failure at about 20% elongation. Typical designs incorporated relatively stiff tapes or cables of Dacron fibers (see following sections for description of this material) that surrounded or took an undulating path among silicone rubber cylinders. The concept was that the rubber would deform easily at low loads, after which the structure would stiffen. While this may sound feasible, the designs were usually not practical.

Polyethylene

The first commercially available device for ACL reconstruction was the polyethylene rod implant. This implant was passed through the knee along the path of the ACL, with tunnels in both the femur and tibia. Then it was secured to the bones using titanium alloy nuts, which were countersunk into the bone surfaces and engaged with threaded ends of the polyethylene rod (Fig. 2). It was not long before these devices started to fail within the knee. They had been designed with little knowledge of the ACL strength, or of the forces and movements within the knee to which it would be subjected. An analysis of these factors showed clearly that the device was susceptible to fatigue failure and was also much weaker than the ACL *(10)*.

Polyethylene is relatively inert and resistant to hydrolytic degradation in vivo, similar to many manmade polymers, and its acceptance for use in joint replacement led to its consideration for ligaments. The polyethylene grade used for artificial joints—ultra-high molecular weight polyethylene—has a tensile yield strength of approx 20 MPa. Thus, to match the 3-kN strength of the ACL in a young adult, a 14-mm diameter rod would be required. Such a device would effectively immobilize the knee owing to its high bending stiffness. In fact, the implant used was 6 mm in diameter and therefore had a failure strength of only 600 N. These implants did not fail because of the lack of tensile strength; the great ductility of polyethylene (approx 200% strain to failure) would require the knee to dislocate if this was the cause. Rather, the reason for failure was fatigue from repetitive bending and torsion of the 6-mm diameter rod at the entrance to the femoral tunnel, along with the cyclic loads during locomotion of about 150 N twice per stride when walking and possibly 6–800 N when running *(7)*.

Bending fatigue is worth considering at this point, because the polyethylene implant has not been the only implant affected by this mode of failure. If a fiber is bent, then the centerline takes a curved path. Reviewing the radius of this curve shows that the fiber surface on the outside of the curve takes a longer path; it is therefore under tension. Similarly, the surface on the inner aspect is under compression, and the stresses act along the fiber. These tensile and compressive stresses balance each other to establish an equilibrium of forces acting across the cross-section of the fibre, and the central point has no bending-induced direct stress. Analysis of the geometry of this curved body reveals that the tensile and compressive stresses build up in proportion to their distance away from the centerline. Hence, for a given imposed curvature, the surface stresses are greater in a larger-diameter fiber. This is the underlying reason why the 6-mm diameter polyethylene rod suffered fatigue failure, with the cracks initiating on the rod surface at the point where it exited the bone tunnel in the femur.

Polypropylene and Nylon

These materials have been employed widely as sutures, which reflects their relatively inert behavior in vivo. With this consideration, the earlier workers experimented with polypropylene and nylon for ligament reconstructions *(11,12)*. However, although these materials can support tissue integration, they lose tensile strength (nylon, *see* ref. *13*) or creep excessively in vivo (polypropylene, *see* ref. *14*) and have consequently faded from use. This property of polypropylene did not stop its brief popularity as a ligament augmentation device—a stent intended to share the load alongside a ligament graft. However, comparative clinical trials failed to show any advantage in its use *(15)*.

Carbon Fibers

Carbon fiber was introduced as a result of pioneering work in the mid-1970s by Jenkins, a surgeon based in Cardiff. The underlying rationale was that our body chemistry is carbon-based; these fibers should be biocompatible. Carbon fibers are made by high-temperature pyrolysis in a hydrocarbon atmosphere of a polymeric precursor fiber, normally polyacrylonitrile, which leaves a carbon residue as a fiber. Contrary to common beliefs in the surgical community at that time, carbon fiber was not pure carbon; approx 1–2% of other material remained to impart some strength and ductility. In addition, the carbon fibers were normally coated with an agent intended to aid the adhesion of polymerizing resins when the fibers were used as reinforcement (e.g., in golf clubs or aircraft structures). Although the fibers are very strong when loaded in tension and embedded within a polymer matrix, they are extremely fragile when exposed to handling or any other outside force. This fragility is due to the brittleness of the material, that has an elongation to failure of only approx 1.5%. The normal commercial production of carbon fiber led to a tow of 10,000 fibers twisted loosely together, each fibre 9 μm in diameter (Fig. 1).

Initial animal experiments led to histological evidence that was claimed to show carbon fiber had been the basis of a "neoligament." Carbon fiber was reported to act as a scaffold on which a new ligament would grow *(16)*—a novel concept that led to further rationalization for the implant design used. This was necessary because the carbon fiber tow supplied for cruciate ligament reconstruction had a tensile strength of approx 900 N, which was much less than the 3-kN strength of the ACL in a young adult.

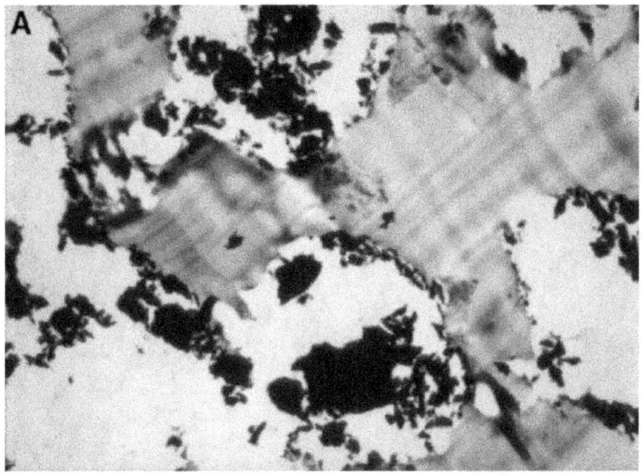

Fig. 3. (**A**) Transmission electron micrograph of transverse section of the middle of a carbon fiber ACL implant at mid-joint space in a rabbit, with very little tissue ingrowth at 36 wk (×3750 magnification). *(Continued on next page.)*

(In fact, at that time, the best data available for ligament strength *(17)* suggested a mean strength of 1.72 kN for the ACL in young adults). It was argued that the progressive breakdown of the carbon fiber implant was actually desirable, as this encouraged the formation of the neoligament tissue. Evidence was presented to show that the strength of the implantation site built up to normal by 6 wk postoperation when implanted as an Achilles tendon replacement in rabbits *(16)*. The early experience in human use was published *(18)*, and carbon fiber implants were then commercially available.

Controversy arose almost immediately when other research groups discovered they could not reproduce the findings from Cardiff. Animal studies found that the carbon fiber tows often disintegrated within the knee joint, leaving large amounts of black debris in the synovium, despite that the implants were of twice the strength of the natural ligament that had been replaced *(19)*. One reaction to this finding was that some groups started to produce the implants with a coating of resorbable biocompatible polymer, such as polylactic acid. This coating was intended to hold the tow together in the postsurgery period while the tissue encapsulation occurred, thus protecting the carbon fiber *(20)*. In addition, development of novel methods to prepare thin tissue slices for histology then allowed the complete cross-section of the carbon fiber tows to be displayed for the first time. Tows were shown to be encapsulated peripherally, but the carbon fibers had not been separated by collagenous tissue ingrowth centrally (Fig. 3A)—this was confined to the periphery of the tows. More detailed examination by electron microscopy showed that the collagen ingrowth was not intimately associated with the carbon fibers, and there was often a multinucleate giant cell reaction to the fibers (Fig. 3B; *21*). These findings, which conflicted with the original reports, led to debate concerning the role of possible coating agents when the fibers were made and of the purity of the carbon fiber, because later clinical implants used a grade of carbon fiber that provided slightly better toughness at the expense of a greater level of residual impurities.

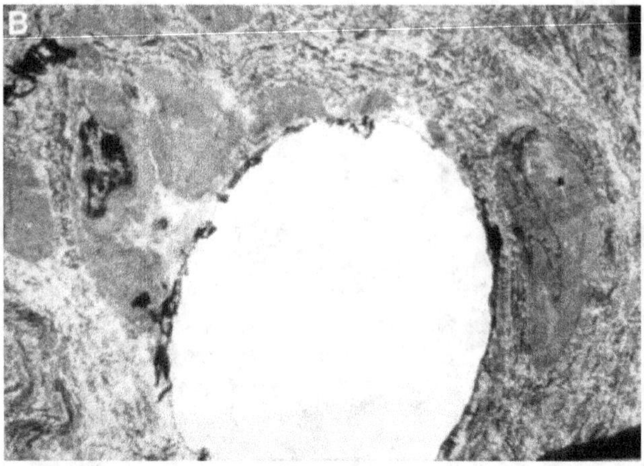

Fig. 3. *(Continued)* **(B)** At the periphery of the implant, carbon fibers were engulfed by multinucleate giant cells; the surrounding tissue included dense collagen fibers (×5200 magnification).

Along with the development of fiber tows, clinical use of carbon fiber led to the first purpose-made ligament anchorage devices. The carbon fiber tow was supplied with a loop at one end, and a toggle was supplied that could be passed through the loop. When the implant was tensioned, the toggle was pulled down to bridge over the entrance to the bone tunnel. At the far end, a bollard device was used. This had a domed head and a shank that was positioned into a drill hole in the bone. When the carbon fiber tow had been tensioned and wound around the shank, the bollard was hammered into the bone, then secured by hammering a central rod through it. The effect of this rod was to spread out the three shank segments, so that they gripped the bone in the same manner as a bolt used for anchorage in concrete. These devices were made of a composite material, with carbon fiber embedded in a polysulfone matrix *(22)*. There were also developments in the surgical instruments, particularly cutters used to remove sharp edges from the entrances to bone tunnels *(23)*.

Despite these developments, the use of carbon fibers was gradually discontinued, as it was recognized that their extreme brittleness was a handicap that could not be overcome. This led to particles being shed that sometimes caused synovitis *(24)*. In the final analysis, it appears that the carbon fiber essentially led to an intense fibrotic reaction, which was attempting to wall-off the implants, rather than the desired goal of benign tissue ingrowth spreading the fibers apart and forming a neoligament.

Polytetrafluoroethylene

Polytetrafluoroethylene (PTFE) is extremely inert when placed in vivo, which led to its use in arterial grafts. This had been noted by Charnley when he developed the first low-friction hip arthroplasty, that used a PTFE acetabular cup. Unfortunately, for Charnley and his patients, although the PTFE implants were inert when placed into the body, the wear particles shed from the hips were not and caused an intense fibrotic reaction. In addition, these cups wore at an unacceptable rate, which increased the volume of wear debris *(25)*. Consequently, all the PTFE cups were revised to polyethylene. It was eventually realized that, despite the inertness of PTFE in bulk and the wear particles'

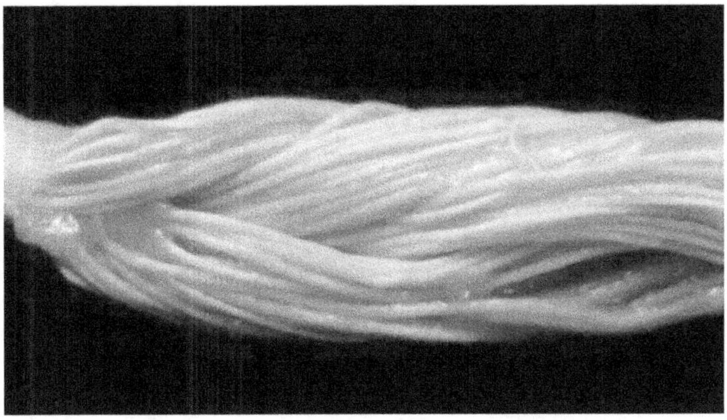

Fig. 4. Gore-Tex PTFE implant retrieved after 6 yr, indicating plaited structure and minimal tissue integration.

chemical inertness, their size and morphology meant that they could not readily be phagocytosed. The resulting cell damage catalyzed a release of enzymes that triggered a chain reaction. This history is relevant because particles from artificial ligaments have caused similar reactions within the knee.

Following the acceptance of PTFE in arterial grafts, Butler reported on a series of dogs and cats that had the ACL replaced by a strip of woven PTFE *(26)*. Histology showed infiltration of the weave by fibroblasts and connective tissue fibers. This gave a smooth glistening structure upon gross examination. However, it was also noted that the implant acted as a reservoir for infection.

In addition to its use as a nonstick surface in cooking utensils (with the brand name Teflon), PTFE is also well known as the basis for Gore-Tex waterproof clothing. The principle by which this fabric works is that it contains numerous pores that are too small to allow passage of water droplets, but are large enough to allow vapor to pass through. The Gore company developed a process in which the PTFE fibers were heated and stretched to form expanded PTFE. This expansion resulted in a microstructure that appeared like a chain of solid polymer nodes that were linked by multiple microfilaments. The water vapor could pass between these microfilaments. This material was used to make the Gore-Tex artificial ligament.

The Gore-Tex artificial ligament had a plaited structure of large-diameter expanded PTFE fibers (Fig. 4). At each end, the PTFE was compressed into an eyelet to take a fixation screw. The plaited structure was intended to provide sufficiently large passages through the implant for bone ingrowth to secure it. The Gore company conducted thorough engineering design and testing, including long-term cyclic creep tests and bending fatigue tests *(27)*. This implant had a tensile strength of 4.4 kN.

Prior to clinical use, there were extensive studies of Gore-Tex ACL reconstruction in sheep, concentrating on the tissue ingrowth and searching for reactions around the knee (stifle) joints. The implants were fixed securely in the bone tunnels by dense fibrocartilagenous tissue (Fig. 5), whereas the intra-articular length was merely covered by a thin film of synovial tissue instead of being incorporated into a neoligament. Thus, the Gore-Tex ligament was unambiguously a permanent prosthesis.

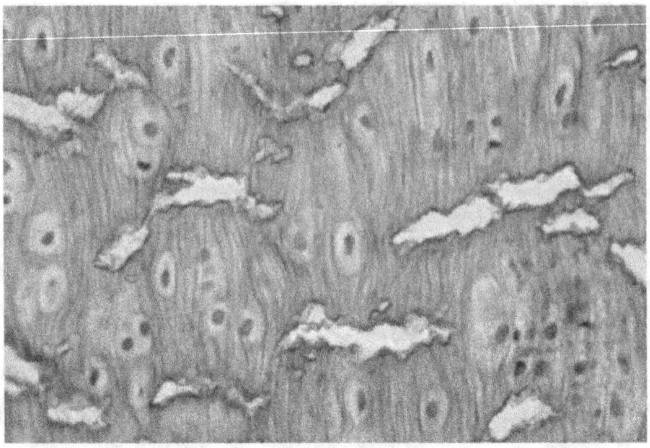

Fig. 5. Longitudinal section of Gore-Tex implant, showing fibrocartilagenous tissue ingrowth between the nodes of PTFE at 15-mo post-implantation (H&E stain, ×570 magnification).

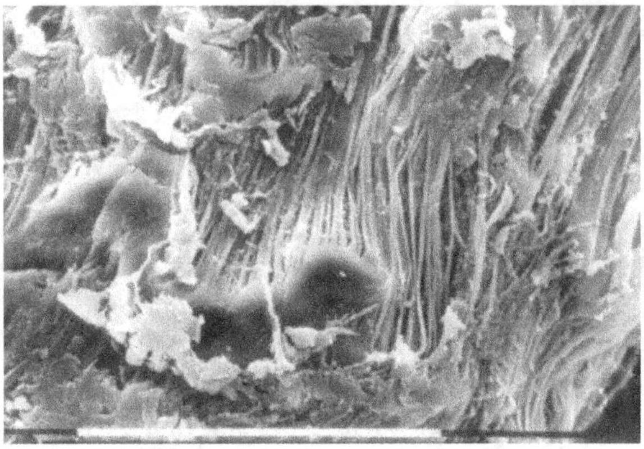

Fig. 6. Scanning electron micrograph of Gore-Tex implant, illustrating microfilaments of PTFE linking the solid nodes (×570 magnification).

The Gore-Tex prosthesis was marketed extensively worldwide, which resulted in large numbers being used in the years around 1990. The solid scientific evidence meant that there was widespread use of an artificial ligament in North America for the first time. However, although the early (2-yr) follow-ups were reporting good results, the 5-yr results showed an increasing number of failures and patients with symptoms related to knee joint effusions and synovitis *(28)*.

An implant retrieved by the author showed the reason why failures from joint effusions occurred. First, the implant shown in Fig. 4 had been removed very easily. It is still intact; it had not been incorporated solidly into the bone tunnels in 6 yr of implantation. When examined by scanning electron microscopy (SEM; Fig. 6), the microstructure of solid nodes of PTFE linked by microfilaments is obvious. Transmission electron microscopy then revealed that the surrounding tissues included numerous needle-like bodies (invisible on light microscopy) within the cells. Their dimensions were similar to the microfilaments of PTFE that crossed the gaps between the solid nodes of the implant fibers. Several mechanisms could explain how these particles were created.

This particular implant had not been integrated into the bone tunnels but was surrounded by a thin coating of soft tissue. Fretting possibly occurred between implant and bone owing to the cyclic loads imposed during locomotion that would abrade the implant surface. Although feasible, this was discounted because other implants that had been solidly fixed also caused effusions. A second related mechanism is intra-articular abrasion caused by the sides of the femoral intercondylar notch rubbing the implant as the knee flexed and the tibia rotated. The third mechanism is fiber fatigue. Each fiber was of comparatively large diameter; thus, as with the polyethylene rods, bending would induce tensile stresses on one side. Individual microfilaments could then be stretched. Whatever the relative contribution of each mechanism, clinical failures appear to have resulted from the implant shedding particulate debris.

The use of artificial ligaments declined drastically after these disappointing results were reported. The Gore company identified the intra-articular abrasion as the cause of the offending particles and so implants were subsequently modified. The mid-length third of the implant within the knee joint space was compressed back to a smaller diameter. The two ends still retained their plaited structure of expanded PTFE fibers to allow bone ingrowth for fixation. The "compact diameter" graft represented a recognition that no significant ingrowth had been found within the knee; the implant was now clearly a permanent prosthesis. In addition, some surgeons recommended the use of a notchplasty procedure when using a Gore-Tex prosthesis to remove the medial aspect of the lateral femoral condyle, thus ensuring that the implant would not be abraded *(29)*. This approach was not suitable for the mood of the time, and Gore withdrew from the market in 1993. These events led to the situation that has since persisted: a lack of artificial ligaments available in North America.

Polyester

Although the term "polyester" consists of a whole family of polymers, there is one specific compound of interest to this review: polyethylene terephthalate, used widely in clothing. In North America, it is often manufactured by duPont, whose brand name for this polymer is Dacron. Similarly, the same material manufactured by ICI in the United Kingdom is known by their brand name as Terylene, and Hoechst in Germany manufacture Trevira fibers. Other manufacturers have other names, but the basic polymer remains the same. Prior to its use in ligament reconstruction, there was a wealth of knowledge of the benign tissue reaction to polyester from the vascular surgery field. Implants constructed by weaving or knitting polyester fibers into tubes have been used extensively as blood vessels since the 1950s, and this work clearly showed that a polyester fabric allowed host tissue invasion and maturation *(30)*. Long-term studies (up to 7 yr) of such grafts revealed that tissue ingrowth took place without adverse reactions *(31)*.

Before polyester was utilized for intra-articular ligament reconstructions, it was investigated for artificial tendons. Much of this work was based on a polyester cord as a central load–carrying core, with a silicone rubber outer layer to provide a smooth gliding function within surrounding tissues *(32)*. Polyester fibers were shown to be unaffected adversely by immersion in tissues and fluids in vivo: there had been no loss of strength or extensibility of the fibres 17 mo after implantation *(33)*. The artificial tendons ends were secured either by suturing or with specific devices, such as screws

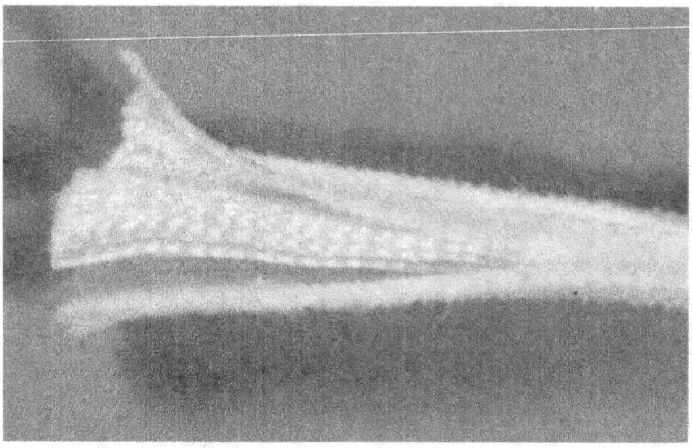

Fig. 7. Stryker-Meadox Dacron implant. The outer velour sheath has been opened to show the dense load-bearing Dacron tapes in the interior.

into bone. This work led to the development of novel ideas for tissue ingrowth anchorage, in which the tendon ends were made into porous fabrics, and these sheets or tabs of fabric were sewn into clefts in the muscles or passed through drill holes in bone. These features then allowed tissue ingrowth to fix the devices *(34,35)*.

Early research on in vivo tissue responses to polyester implants involved a significant rate of mechanical failures within the knee (stifle) joints, along with synovitis that was related to implant particles. However, the implants that had remained intact had been able to act as scaffolds supporting fibrous tissue ingrowth *(12,36)*. The failures were undoubtedly from inadequate implant strength, as no data were available then on the strength of the natural structures being replaced in animals, and the implants were usually based on the woven velour fabrics used as blood vessels. These fabrics were weak and too extensible to duplicate the mechanical behavior of ligaments. As a result, Stryker collaborated with Meadox, a manufacturer of artificial blood vessels, to develop an implant with a Dacron velour tube that contained dense Dacron tapes (Fig. 7). The rationale was that the velour covering would act to trap tissue ingrowth, while the tapes would carry the load and be protected from abrasion by the surrounding sheath *(37)*. This structure resulted in a tissue reaction in which the sheath was invaded by hypercellular fibrous tissue, but the interior contained chondroidal and necrotic tissue *(38)*.

These events showed that tissue reaction depends on many factors in implant design, an issue largely explored during the development of vascular implants. Both Lyman *(39)* and Skelton *(40)* discussed important factors, such as the impact of polymer synthesis and manufacturing on biocompatibility, noting that their effects could arise from numerous sources. These include traces of unpolymerized oligomer or catalyst (often fine particles of heavy metals, e.g., strontium); contaminants collected from dies during fiber drawing; lubricants used during the spinning of fibers into yarn; and other materials within the polymer fibers, such as the delusterants used to remove the shine from fibers intended for clothing (often titanium dioxide particles). Other sources are from the aromatic dyes used to color fibers to make sutures more visible *(39,40)*. Along with these factors, the textile structure has an important role. For example, a woven or

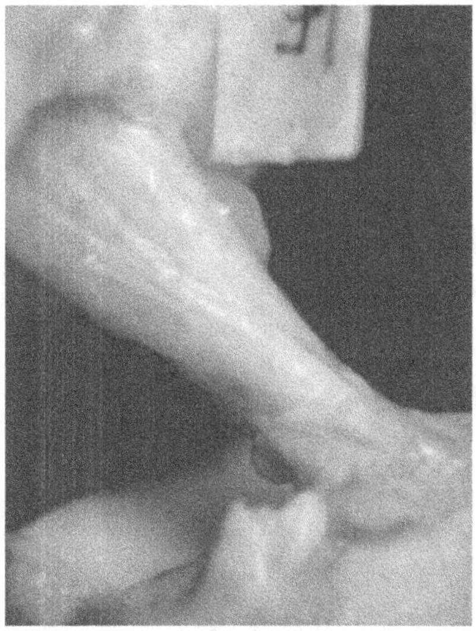

Fig. 8. ACL based on a polyester fiber implant in sheep at 6 mo. The implant has been completely covered by host tissue.

braided structure could lead to the delicate strands of tissue ingrowth within its interstices being strangled when the implant is loaded. Another problematic mechanism is that fibers moving over each other under cyclic loading tend to cause abrasion, and the implant then sheds particulate debris that often triggers an undesirable chronic tissue reaction. Neglect of any of these factors can lead to less than optimal results, and it is unfortunate that much work has had this conflict.

Work on polyester fibers by the present author arose from observations of the development of carbon fiber-based implants by Jenkins et al. Preliminary laboratory work found that the carbon was too stiff to match the elastic behavior of the reconstructed natural structures, and concerns existed about their brittleness that led to fragmentation. Noting the earlier work on polyester fibers for arterial grafts, as well as the problems with polymer fiber biocompatibility, trial implants were made from a grade of ICI Terylene with the following specifications: very low elastic modulus, bright fibers (i.e., without any delusterant particles), undyed, and with the smallest-diameter filaments available (15 μm). These were available as a yarn of 20 filaments twisted loosely together. The low modulus allowed implants to be made with similar strength to the tendon or ligament under study, yet retained physiological structural stiffness with more than 30% elongation to failure.

The biocompatibility of polyester fibers was studied at the calcaneal tendon and ACL in rabbits and sheep in both sites, with up to 24 mo in vivo study. The polyester fibers acted as a template on which collagenous tissue was laid down (Fig. 8). This was a relatively slow process, where tissue ingrowth and subsequent maturation progressed radially inward from the periphery of the cross-section. Thus, the initially delicate cellular ingrowth was followed by progressively more collagen fibers. At the periphery of the implants, the polymer fibers were widely spaced and allowed dense collagenous ingrowth (Fig. 9A). Conversely, the interior initially contained relatively sparse collagen.

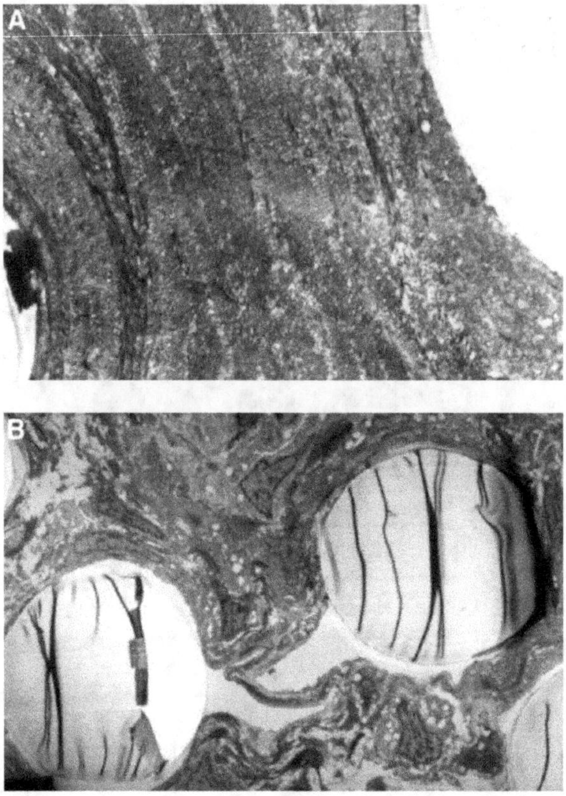

Fig. 9. **(A)** Transmission electron micrograph of transverse section of polyester fiber ACL implant in rabbit at the periphery at mid-joint space at 36 wk. The polyester filaments have been embedded in dense well-organized collagen tissue (×9300 magnification). **(B)** At the center of the implant, the tissue was less mature and still contained many active fibroblasts and areas of collagen fibrils (×2500 magnification).

By 6 mo, transmission electron microscopy of the calcaneal tendons showed a dense well-ordered collagen structure throughout the implants, where most of the collagen fibrils aligned parallel to the implant axis with an ordered array of circumferential fibrils and fibroblasts *(21)*. The tissue ingrowth matured at a slower rate within the knee joint when used to reconstruct the ACL. At 36-wk postsurgery in rabbits, the center of the implant still contained numerous active fibroblasts and pockets of synovial fluid, in addition to bundles of collagen fibers (Fig. 9B; *19*). A preclinical trial in sheep *(41)* found that the entire cross-section of the implants contained mature collagenous tissue by 1 yr postsurgery with a layer of well-organized collagen fibers on its surface. By 2 yr (Fig. 10), this surface layer had proliferated to give bundles of ligament-like tissue.

Although the histological studies had shown proliferation of dense collagenous tissue within and around the polyester fiber implants, this did not necessarily correlate with increased strength. Reconstructions of calcaneal tendons had shown steady increases in strength until the neotendons had the same strength as the normal tendons by 6 mo *(42)*. However, it should be noted that this site heals well, and excision of the

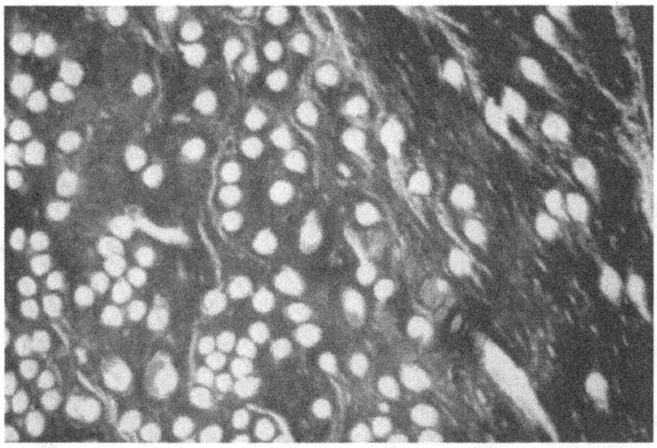

Fig. 10. Transverse section of polyester ACL implant in sheep at 24 mo, at mid-joint space. The cross-section has been filled by dense collagenous tissue similar to ligament that contains some fibroblasts and blood vessels (Martius scarlet-blue stain, ×200 magnification).

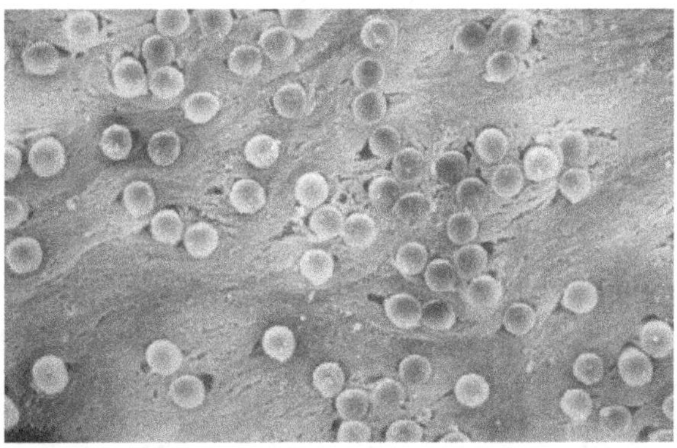

Fig. 11. Scanning electron micrograph of Apex (DePuy-duPont Orthopaedics) polyester implant retrieved from patient at 24 mo. The polyester filaments have been spaced apart by dense tissue ingrowth (×320 magnification).

tendon used as a control led to approx 50% of normal strength owing to a fibrous tissue strand established across a 60-mm defect. When the polyester replaced the ACL in sheep, the strength was significantly less after 2 yr despite the extensive collagenous tissue formation *(41)*. The implants had been linked to the bone tunnel's walls by organized fibrous tissue that bridged the gap from bone trabeculae to the implant, where the fibers were oriented to slant across the gap, thus aligned to resist traction. This resulted in a strength of approx 300 N in the bone tunnel of the tibia at 12 mo.

Human use inevitably had some implants fail, and the retrievals were analyzed *(43)*. Most failed implants had been cut transversely because of impingement by the anterior edge of the femoral intercondylar notch as the knee reached full extension. The others had failed traumatically. It was found that the implants had supported very similar tissue ingrowth to that reported in the animal studies. The implants had been inserted through 6-mm bone tunnels and were approx 13-mm in diameter when retrieved. Thus, the majority of the cross-section was now collagenous tissue (Fig. 11).

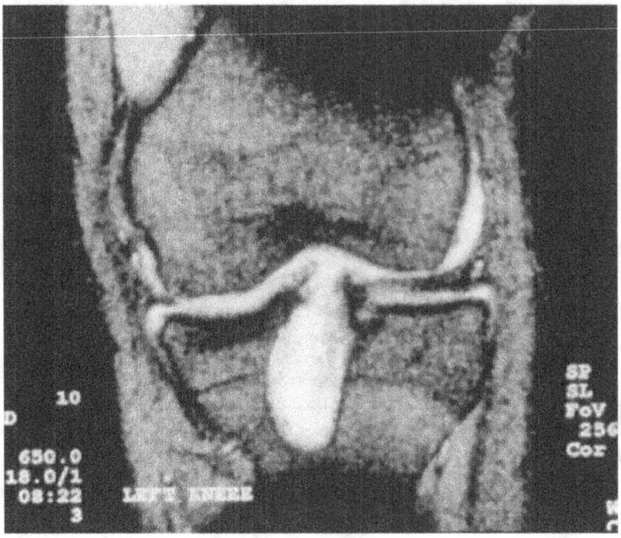

Fig. 12. Magnetic resonance image showing cavity around Apex implant in proximal tibia 5-yr postimplantation.

Given that these early implant failures had explanations unrelated to fundamental problems with the implants themselves, why were these devices withdrawn from clinical use? The immediate answer was that the commercial case collapsed with the loss of confidence associated with the withdrawal of the Gore-Tex implant described earlier. As time increased, however, more fundamental problems arose that gave good scientific reasons to not use polyester fibers within the knee. The phenomenon of bone tunnel widening post ACL reconstruction is well known and affects all types of grafts, including autografts *(44)*. This widening had been measured in the sheep studies with polyester fibers, and the diameter had increased up to 1 yr and then stabilized *(41)*. It had been rationalized as a functional adaptation that allowed a sufficient length of fibrous tissue to accommodate the cyclic elongations of the graft under functional loading that would cause fretting motion between the graft and bone. However, after approx 5 yr in humans, some developed cavities around the implant below the tibial plateau (Fig. 12). At revision surgery, the cavities were found to be filled with a dense fibrous tissue mass and required bone grafting before autogenous graft could be placed. Analysis of the tissue revealed occasional polyester fragments, and these were presumed to have been shed from the implants by an abrasion process, then to have triggered the tissue reaction *(45)*. This failure scenario was supported by SEM of the implant fibers; damage to the polyester filaments was always found. They were often deformed in ways that suggested transverse shearing and compression, along with longitudinal abrasion (Fig. 13). A knee joint test rig was built and run that included a human knee with a polyester ACL. The implant was placed to incur impingement as the knee extended. When the implants were retrieved from the rig and examined by SEM, the fiber damage was identical to that seen on the clinical specimens *(46)*. Although this analysis implies that the implant may still function well long term, provided that abrasion can

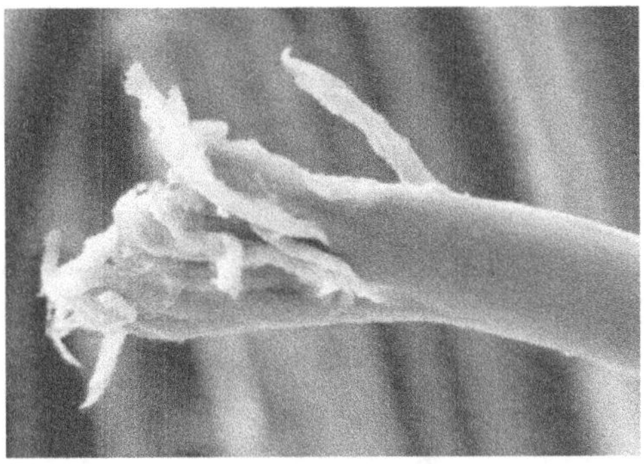

Fig. 13. Scanning electron micrograph of damaged polyester filament from ruptured implant (×1400 magnification).

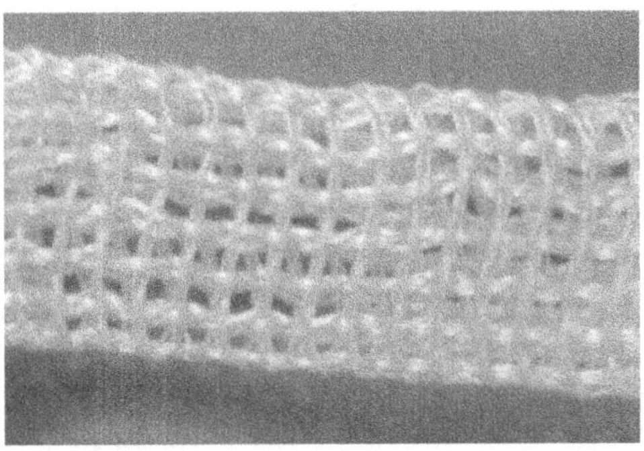

Fig. 14. The structure of the Leeds-Keio polyester ligament, a tubular cross-weave intended to capture tissue ingrowth.

be avoided, further evidence from long-term retrievals suggested otherwise. It was found that these implants usually had extensive areas of tissue deep within them, where the collagenous tissue was acellular and becoming necrotic. Despite the initially healthy appearance of tissue ingrowth, which included vascular structures, the hypertrophy of the collagen structure eventually led to inadequate nutrition. Ingrown tissue may then become weaker with time *(47)*. Of course, this was contrary to the tissue ingrowth philosophy that nearly all fibrous artificial ligaments had been based on.

A similar case relates to the Leeds-Keio polyester ligament (Fig. 14), which also depended on tissue ingrowth to become a collagen–polyester composite structure. Human cases reviewed at arthroscopy showed the appearance of a reformed ACL, and the histology of biopsies showed collagenous tissue was associated with both the surface *(48)* and interior of the grafts *(49)*. However, an animal study *(50)* suggested that the Leeds-Keio implant should be considered as a permanent device, not a scaffold or stent, and the tissue formation associated with the graft did not cause any increase in strength. An independent clinical review concluded that their arthroscopic and histological studies had failed to demonstrate a convincing development of a functional neoligament. Instead, there were instances of synovitis, and the number of complications was greater than expected from a similar series of autogenous grafts *(51)*.

When failings such as this were publicized, along with the sudden withdrawal from use of the Gore-Tex prosthesis, it is not surprising that many surgeons decided not to continue using artificial ligaments on a clinical basis. Even those implants that had extensive testing were eventually subject to abrasion and the tissue reactions from particulate debris. However, this conclusion does not nullify the argument stated earlier, describing the potential appeal of artificial ligaments. How can this clinically desirable aim be approached, while also learning the lessons from the past? It seems that the answer may lay in the realm of resorbable implant technology, augmented by the emerging field of tissue engineering.

RESORBABLE MATRICES AND TISSUE ENGINEERING OF LIGAMENTS: FUTURE POSSIBILITIES

This review has shown that some work on artificial ligaments that used relatively inert polymer fibers as a scaffold was successful in obtaining collagenous tissue ingrowth. Many features of normal ligament development and maturation were observed. Initially, there was a delicate fibroblastic response that left much of the cross-sectional area filled with fluid. As time increased, collagen production and reorganization led to a greater proportion of the cross-section being occupied by tissue presumably similar to an immature ligament but capable of load-bearing function *(43,52)*. This process was an early example of tissue engineering. The implantation of a polymer fiber matrix had provided a template to guide the foundation of a new viable tissue structure, which was intended to reproduce the functions of the damaged structure being reconstructed. In this circumstance, the implanted matrix was intended to be inert; thus, it was only subject to the fibrous tissue encapsulation response expected for an inert foreign body. Fortuitously, this response lays down tissue that is similar to ligament, because it is composed largely of aligned collagen fibrils and includes a population of fibroblasts. As every individual polymer fiber caused a microencapsulation response, the overall effect was to build a substantial collagen structure.

A similar sequence of events has been observed for the revascularization and remodeling of ligament autografts, when a structure, such as patellar tendon, is used to replace a cruciate ligament *(53)*. It has often been questioned whether this process leads to a new ligament. A detailed study by Amiel, Kleiner, and Akeson did show a progressive return toward normal measures for a range of biochemical assays of the neoligaments which introduced the term "ligamentization" *(54)*.

However, studies at the ultrastructural level have shown how attempts to re-form ligaments do not result in collagenous tissue identical to that of a normal mature ligament. Particularly, the collagen fibril population remains dominated by small-diameter fibrils (40–80 nm), rather than including the larger-diameter fibrils that are characteristic of mature ligaments, providing a bimodal distribution curve of occurrence frequency of fibril diameters *(55,56)*. This is important for the mechanical function of the neoligament. Parry, Barnes, and Craig described how the collagen fibril diameters change with increasing age and hypothesized that fibril diameter may relate to tensile strength *(57)*. They later suggested that the large-diameter fibrils that are accumulations of collagen molecules obtain their strength from the increased opportunities for intermolecular crosslinks in these large-diameter, densely-packed bundles *(58)*. They also speculated that the presence of a large number of small-diameter fibrils in immature tissue, such as a maturing ligament scar following trauma (or else a remodeling autograft?) may help to confer creep resistance because of the resulting large surface area available for interaction with the surrounding ground substance. This is particularly important in the period shortly after ligament reconstruction, when the immature structure may elongate irreversibly under the cyclic loads imposed during function and rehabilitation, which would cause a return of joint laxity. Maturing ligament repair tissue has been shown to be more susceptible to creep than a normal ligament *(59)*.

An abnormal collagen fibril population has been observed for cruciate ligament reconstructions based on autogenous grafts *(60)*, where the collagen fibrils remained around 20–60 nm in diameter up to 2-yr postsurgery. In addition, these authors noted that the use of autogenous tissue did not cause restitution of normal profiles for cells, elastic tissue, and proteoglycans. A very similar circumstance has been repeated when the maturation of allogenic ACL grafts has been studied *(6)*, except that the process is more profound and slower than with autografts. The resulting structure is then like that obtained via a polyester fiber scaffold implant, and the collagen fibrils remain at approx 40-nm diameter. None of the studies examining these new tissues have shown that the mechanical properties return to the equivalent of those in the original ligament. Thus, the tissue laid down on an artificial matrix is likely not inferior to that which results from an autogenous graft.

If neoligaments are to be produced for future clinical use, a main difference from earlier experience will be that they must be based on resorbable scaffolds. This new basis is essential to avoid the long-term side effects observed when implant particles are shed chronically into the surrounding tissues. Instead, the aim must be for the resorbable matrix to have resorption characteristics that allow it to maintain its mechanical role for a sufficient time. New tissue ingrowth can then become sufficiently plentiful and strong enough to enable an orderly transfer of function when the matrix degrades.

Although resorbable fibers have been used clinically for many years as sutures, those earlier materials (e.g., chromic catgut, actually based on ovine intestinal mucosa), have a strength retention half-life of 5 d *(30)*, which is too short for a new ligament to be established. An early approach to this problem used a braided polyglycolic acid (PGA) fiber structure (Dexon suture by Davis and Geck) to reinforce repairs of transected ACL in dogs *(61)*. The implant consisted of 30 strands of 2-0 Dexon braided together, giving a strength of 930 N. However, although this experiment appeared to be successful, PGA loses its strength too rapidly to be a basis for ligament reconstruction and has a strength retention half-life of approx 12 d *(30)*. An advantage of PGA, however, is that it degrades harmlessly in vivo, and this is also true for polylactic acid (PLA). Both are excreted as carbon dioxide after the acids are metabolized. Further work led to synthetic degradable sutures with greater strength retention, such as polydioxanone (PDS, Ethicon) and polytrimethylene carbonate (Maxon, Davis and Geck). Bourne et al. found half-lives of 3 and 6 wk, respectively *(62)*. This advantage is added by the finding that these suture materials caused less chronic inflammation than catgut or Polyglactin (PGA-PLA) sutures when used in fascial closure in rats *(63)*. The potential of these degrading fibers to avoid the problems of particulate debris was shown by Claes et al. when their combined reconstructions of anterior cruciate and medial collateral ligaments using PDS showed no capsular changes from normal, whereas the animals with nonresorbing fibers had synovitic inflammatory changes related to particles

(38). The potential for Maxon to retain strength was shown in a study of flexor tendon repairs *(64)*. But this study also showed that degradation products accumulated in the tissue, causing tendon swelling and adhesion. Of the materials currently accepted for clinical use, it appears that PLA or a PLA-PGA copolymer may be best suited for ligament matrices, but other materials are being researched that will not inhibit tissue formation by producing an acidic environment as they degrade.

The term "tissue engineering" usually implies the induction or augmentation of a cellular reaction that brings about the formation and maintenance of a particular type of differentiated tissue. This often requires cells to be grown and expanded under conditions relevant to the expected end-use. The cells can be grown on a relatively inert substrate, as in conventional tissue culture work, or under conditions simulating the organ of interest. In addition, the growth medium must either be replaced regularly or exchanged by a continuous flow process to maintain the optimal cell growth conditions *(65)*. Although it is still early research, work on ligaments and tendons has been reviewed *(66,67)*. One approach was to use growth factors that would stimulate collagen production by uprating the proliferation and activity of fibroblasts. This approach has had promising results. Schmidt et al. found that a range of growth factors uprated the activity of the ACL and medial collateral ligament fibroblasts in vitro (intriguingly, this uprating was not caused by the same factors in each ligament; *68*). Chan et al. have shown that basic fibroblast growth factor (FGF) caused significantly greater patellar tendon fibroblast proliferation in vitro *(69)*. A similar approach has been attempted to augment the healing of tendon grafts into bone tunnels when the grafts were placed with collagen sponge carriers that contained bone morphogenetic proteins, transforming growth factors and FGF *(70)*. Consequently, strength increased by 65% at 8 wk after ACL reconstruction in rabbits.

More recently, it has been recognized that the growth factors must interact with receptors on the cells and that these are present at different stages of the tissue reaction. Such data are becoming available by gene screening of biopsies of healing tissues, which allows active genes to be identified at different times. Work has begun on the introduction of genes to host cells that can upregulate particular factors *(67)*, e.g., decorin, which is associated with collagen fibrillogenesis.

Although the gene and growth factor treatments noted above have already shown promise for enhancing ligament healing or new tissue formation, it should be recognized that a specific growth factor or gene will only accelerate one aspect or phase of this process. A more fundamental approach is to use uncommitted progenitor or pluripotential cells, such as mesenchymal stem cells *(71)*. These cells have the promise of differentiating into fibroblastic ligament or tendon-forming tissue when influenced by appropriate biochemical and mechanical strain effects. Differentiation catalyzes the whole spectrum of genetic events, thereby enhancing all aspects of the host tissue reaction.

A fundamental aspect of ligament behavior is their function as tensile restraints to bone-bone motions, leading to imposition of cyclic tensile strains. The role of joint mobilization after surgery to enhance tissue healing is well recognized. Yet, there is still a lack of essential knowledge about the optimal strain environment in terms of the magnitude, rate of application, or number of strain cycles necessary to obtain the fastest return to normal ligament strength. Zeichen, van Griensven, and Bosch found a biphasic response to increasing application times of 5% strains at 1 Hz to human tendon fibroblasts in vitro *(72)*. There is much scope for further work.

CONCLUSIONS

This chapter has shown that the interior of the knee is a very demanding environment in which to test new materials and that debris from degrading ligament implants causes adverse tissue reactions. Even when a material was used that already had a long history of successful tissue integration elsewhere in the body, in addition to animal studies up to 2 yr, undesirable reactions were still revealed only after years of clinical use. Thus, it appears that artificial ligaments based on permanent, nonresorbing polymeric fibers will inevitably fail eventually. The answer, then, must be to base these reconstructions on novel materials that resorb after a relatively short-term role as a scaffold or matrix on which a new ligament can grow. The emerging knowledge of tissue engineering promises to uprate these cellular proliferation and collagen maturation processes via technologies that are relatively simple, such as cell seeding, to more fundamental manipulation of the genetic environment of the cells. The potential of this approach is still being realized, but manmade constructs may again be offered for clinical use in the future, thus saving the injured joint from further traumatic graft-harvesting insults.

ACKNOWLEDGMENTS

Over the years, the author's work on ligament reconstruction has been funded largely by the Arthritis Research Campaign, a charity based in Chesterfield, England. The microscopy has been done mostly by Dr. Susan Kempson of Edinburgh University Veterinary School.

REFERENCES

1. Radford WJP, Amis AA, Heatley FW. Immediate strength after suturing the anterior cruciate ligament., *J Bone Joint Surg Br* 1994;76:480–484.
2. Guirea M, Zorilla P, Amis AA, Aichroth P. Comparative pull out and cyclic loading strength tests of anchorage of hamstring tendon grafts in anterior cruciate ligament reconstruction. *Am J Sports Med* 1999;27:621–625.
3. Butler DL, Grood ES, Noyes FR, et al. Mechanical properties of primate vascularized versus nonvascularized patellar tendon grafts; changes over time. *J Orthop Res* 1989;7: 68–79.
4. Salehpour A, Butler DL, Proch FS, et al. Dose-dependent response of gamma irradiation on mechanical properties and related biochemical composition of goat bone-patellar tendon-bone allografts. *J Orthop Res* 1995;13:898–906.
5. Jackson DW, Grood ES, Goldstein J, et al. A comparison of patellar tendon autograft and allograft used for anterior cruciate ligament reconstruction in the goat model. *Am J Sports Med* 1993;21:176–185.
6. Jackson DW, Corsetti J, Simon TM. Biologic incorporation of allograft anterior cruciate ligament replacements. *Clin Orthop* 1996;324:126–133.
7. Morrison JB. Function of the knee joint in various activities. *Biomed Eng* 1969;4:573–580.
8. Woo SLY, Hollis JM, Adams DJ, Lyon RM, Takai S. Tensile properties of the human femur-anterior cruciate ligament-tibia complex: the effects of specimen age and orientation. *Am J Sports Med* 1991;19:217–225.

9. Henze CW, Mayer L. An experimental study of silk-tendon plastics with particular reference to the prevention of post-operative adhesions. *Surg Gynecol Obstet* 1914;19:10–24.
10. Chen EH, Black, J. Materials design analysis of the prosthetic anterior cruciate ligament. *J Biomed Mater Res* 1980;14:567–586.
11. Vaughan LC. A study of the replacement of the anterior cruciate ligament in the dog by fascia, skin and Nylon. *Vet Rec* 1963;75:537–541.
12. Meyers JF, Grana WA, Lesker PA. Reconstruction of the anterior cruciate ligament in the dog: comparison of the results obtained with three different porous synthetic materials. *Am J Sports Med* 1979;7:85–90.
13. Leininger RI, Mirkovitch V, Peters A, Hawks WA. Change in properties of plastics during implantation. *Trans Am Soc Artif Organ* 1964;10:320–321.
14. Mendenhall HV, Roth JH, Kennedy JC, Winter GD, Lumb WV. Evaluation of the polypropylene braid as a prosthetic anterior cruciate ligament replacement in the dog. *Am J Sports Med* 1987;15:543–546.
15. Noyes FR, Barber SD. The effect of a ligament augmentation device on allograft reconstructions for chronic ruptures of the anterior cruciate ligament. *J Bone Joint Surg Am* 1992;74:960–973.
16. Jenkins DHR, Forster IW, McKibbin B, Ralis ZA. Induction of tendon and ligament formation by carbon implants. *J Bone Joint Surg Br* 1977;59:53–57.
17. Noyes FR, Grood ES. Strength of the anterior cruciate ligament in humans and rhesus monkeys: age and species-related changes. *J Bone Joint Surg Am* 1976;58:1074–1082.
18. Jenkins DHR, McKibbin B. The role of flexible carbon fibre implants as tendon and ligament substitutes in clinical practice: a preliminary report. *J Bone Joint Surg Br* 1980;62: 497–499.
19. Amis AA, Kempson SA, Campbell JR, Miller JH. Anterior cruciate ligament implants: biocompatibility and biomechanics of polyester or carbon fibre implants in rabbits. *J Bone Joint Surg* 1988;70B:628–634.
20. Alexander H, Parsons JR, Strauchler ID, et al. Canine patellar tendon replacement with a polylactic acid polymer-filamentous carbon degrading scaffold to form new tissue. *Orthop Rev* 1981;10:41–51.
21. Amis AA, Campbell JR, Kempson SA, Miller JH. Comparison of the structure of neotendons induced by implantation of carbon or polyester fibres. *Bone Joint Surg Br* 1984;66;131–139.
22. Amis AA. The strength of artificial ligament anchorages—a comparative experimental study. *J Bone Joint Surg Br* 1988;70:397–403.
23. Strover AE. Technical advances in the reconstruction of knee ligaments using carbon fibre. In Burri C, Claes L, eds. *Alloplastic Ligament Replacement*, Hans Huber, Bern, Switzerland, 1983, pp.127–134.
24. Rushton N, Dandy D, Naylor CPE. The clinical, arthroscopic and histological findings after replacement of the anterior cruciate ligament with carbon fibre. *J Bone Joint Surg Br* 1983;65:308–309.
25. Charnley J. Total hip replacement by low-friction arthroplasty. *Clin Orthop* 1970;72:7–21.
26. Butler HC. Teflon as a prosthetic ligament in repair of ruptured anterior cruciate ligaments. *Am J Vet Res* 1964;25:55–59.
27. Bolton CW, Bruchman WC. The Gore-Tex expanded polytetrafluoroethylene prosthetic ligament: an in vitro and in vivo evaluation. *Clin Orthop* 1985;196:202–213.
28. Paulos LE, Rosenberg TD, Grewe SR. The Gore-Tex anterior cruciate ligament prosthesis: a long-term follow-up. *Am J Sports Med* 1992;20:246–252.
29. Ferkel RD, Fox JM, Wood D, Del Pizzo W, Friedman MJ, Snyder SJ. Arthroscopic "second look" at the Gore-Tex ligament. *Am J Sports Med* 1989;17:147–153.
30. Hoffman AS. Medical applications of polymeric fibres. *J Appl Polymer Sci Appl Polymer Symp* 1977;31:313–314.

31. De Bakey ME, Jordan GL, Abbott JP, Halpert B, O'Neal R. The fate of Dacron vascular grafts. *Arch Surg* 1964;89:757–782.
32. Murray GAW, Semple JC. A review of work on artificial tendons. *J Biomed Eng* 1979;1: 177–184.
33. Levine SN. Survey of biomedical materials and some relevant problems. *Ann NY Acad Sci* 1968;146:3–10.
34. King RN, Dunn HK, Bolstad KE. A single unit digital flexor tendon prosthesis. *J Biomed Mater Res Symp* 1975;6:157–165.
35. King RN, McKenna GB, Statton WO. Novel uses of fibers as tendons and bones. *J Appl Polymer Sci Appl Polymer Symp* 1977;31:335–350.
36. Hinko PJ. The use of a prosthetic ligament in repair of the torn anterior cruciate ligament in the dog. *J Am Animal Hosp Assoc* 1981;17:563–567.
37. Park JP, Grana WA, Chitwood JS. A high-strength Dacron augmentation for cruciate ligament reconstruction: a two-year canine study. *Clin Orthop* 1985;196:175–185.
38. Claes L, Durselen L, Kiefer H, Mohr W. The combined anterior cruciate and medial collateral ligament replacement by various materials: a comparative animal study. *J Biomed Mater Res* 1987;21:319–343.
39. Lyman DJ. Biomedical polymers. *Ann NY Acad Sci* 1968;146:30–48.
40. Skelton J. Textiles in biomedical devices—some unrecognised variables. *Biomater Med Devices Art if Organs* 1974;2:345–352.
41. Amis AA, Camburn M, Kempson SA, Radford WJP, Stead AC. Anterior cruciate ligament replacement with polyester fibre—a long term study of tissue reactions and joint stability in sheep. *J Bone Joint Surg Br* 1992;74:605–613.
42. Amis AA, Campbell JR, Miller JH. Strength of carbon and polyester fibre tendon replacements—variation after operation in rabbits *J Bone Joint Surg Br* 1985;67:829–34.
43. Amis AA, Kempson SA, Hukkanen M. Polyester fiber ACL implants—will they form new ligaments in-vivo? *Trans Orthop Res Soc* 1994;40:617.
44. L'Insalata JC, Klatt B, Fu FH, Harner CD. Tunnel expansion following anterior cruciate ligament reconstruction: a comparison of hamstring and patellar tendon autografts. *Knee Surg Sports Traumatol Arthrosc* 1997;5:234–238.
45. Amis AA, Kempson SA. Bone adaptation to a polyester fiber anterior cruciate ligament replacement. *J Long Term Eff Med Implants* 1999;9:153–168.
46. Amis AA, Kempson SA. Failure mechanisms of polyester fiber anterior cruciate ligament implants—a human retrieval and laboratory study. *J Biomed Mater Res* 1999;48:534–539.
47. Keen CE, Amis AA. Polyester fibre prosthetic anterior cruciate ligament implant rupture: necrosis of ingrown connective tissue. *Histopathology* 1999;35:74–81.
48. Fujikawa K, Iseki F, Seedhom BB. Arthroscopy after anterior cruciate reconstruction with the Leeds-Keio ligament. *J Bone Joint Surg Br* 1989;71:566–570.
49. Zaffagnini S, De Pasquale V, Montanari C, Strocchi R, Marcacci M. Histological and ultrastructural evaluation of Leeds-Keio ligament six years after implant. *Knee Surg Sports Traumatol Arthrosc* 1997;5:89–94.
50. Schindhelm K, Rogers GJ, Milthorpe BK, et al. Autograft and Leeds-Keio reconstructions of the ovine anterior cruciate ligament. *Clin Orthop* 1991;267:278–293.
51. Macnicol MF, Penny ID, Sheppard L. Early results of the Leeds-Keio anterior cruciate ligament replacement. *J Bone Joint Surg Br* 1991;73:377–380.
52. Amis AA. Development of the Apex polyester fibre cruciate ligament implant. *Clin Mater* 1994;15:51–60.
53. Clancy WG, Narechania RG, Rosenberg TD, Gmeiner JG, Wisnefske DD, Lange TA. Anterior and posterior cruciate ligament reconstruction in rhesus monkeys: a histological, microangiographic and biomechanical analysis. *J Bone Joint Surg Am* 1981;63:1270–1284.

54. Amiel D, Kleiner JB, Akeson WH. The natural history of the anterior cruciate ligament autograft of patellar tendon origin. *Am J Sports Med* 1986;14:449–462.
55. Frank C, Bray D, Rademaker A, Chrusch C, Sabiston P, Bodie D, Rangayyan. Electron microscopic quantification of collagen fibril diameters in the rabbit medial collateral ligament: a baseline for comparison. *Connect Tissue Res* 1989;19:11–25.
56. Hart RA, Woo SLY, Newton PO. Ultrastructural morphometry of anterior cruciate and medial collateral ligaments: an experimental study in rabbits. *J Orthop Res* 1992;10:96–103.
57. Parry DAD, Barnes GRG, Craig AS. A comparison of the size distribution of collagen fibrils in connective tissues as a function of age and a possible relation between fibril size distribution and mechanical properties. *Proc Roy Soc Lond* 1978;203:305–321.
58. Parry DAD, Craig AS. Growth and development of collagen fibrils in connective tissue. In Ruggeri A, Motta PM, eds. *Ultrastructure of the Connective Tissue Matrix*, Martinus Nijhoff, Boston, MA, 1984, pp. 34–63.
59. Thornton GM, Leask GP, Shrive NG, Frank CB. Early medial collateral ligament scars have inferior creep behaviour. *J Orthop Res* 2000;18:238–246.
60. Decker B, Bosch U, Kasperczyk W, Oestern HJ, Reale E. Ultrastructural changes of the patellar tendon as a cruciate ligament substitute (one year and two year results). *J Submicrosc Cytol Pathol* 1991;23:9–21.
61. Cabaud HE, Feagin JA, Rodkey WG. Acute anterior cruciate ligament injury and repair reinforced with a biodegradable intraarticular ligament. *Am J Sports Med* 1982;10:259–265.
62. Bourne RB, Bitar H, Andreae PR, Martin LM, Finlay JB, Marquis F. In-vivo comparison of four absorbable sutures: Vicryl, Dexon plus, Maxon and PDS. *Can J Surg* 1988;31:43–45.
63. Sanz LE, Patterson JA, Kamath R, Willett G, Ahmed SW, Butterfield AB. Comparison of Maxon suture with Vicryl, chromic catgut, and PDS sutures in fascial closure in rats. *Obstet Gynecol* 1988;71:418–422.
64. Mashadi ZB, Amis AA. Variation of holding strength of synthetic absorbable flexor tendon sutures with time. *J Hand Surg Br* 1992;17:278–281.
65. Minuth WW, Sittinger M, Kloth S. Tissue engineering: generation of differentiated artificial tissues for biomedical applications. *Cell Tissue Res* 1998;291:1–11.
66. Butler DL, Awad HA. Perspectives on cell and collagen composites for tendon repair. *Clin Orthop Rel Res* 1999;367S:S324–S332.
67. Woo SLY, Hildebrand K, Watanabe N, Fenwick JA, Papageorgiou CD, Wang JHC. Tissue engineering of ligament and tendon healing. *Clin Orthop* 1999;367S:S312–S323.
68. Schmidt CC, Georgescu HI, Kwoh CK, Blomstrom GL, Emgle CP, Larkin LA, et al. Effect of growth factors on the proliferation of fibroblasts from the medial collateral and anterior cruciate ligaments. *J Orthop Res* 1995;13:184–190.
69. Chan BP, Chan KM, Maffulli N, Webb S, Lee KKH. Effect of basic fibroblast growth factor: an in vitro study of tendon healing. *Clin Orthop Rel Res* 1997;342:239–247.
70. Anderson K, Seneviratne AM, Izawa K, Atkinson BL, Potter HG, Rodeo SA. Augmentation of tendon healing in an intraarticular bone tunnel with use of a bone growth factor. *Am J Sports Med* 2001;29:689–698.
71. Young RG, Butler DL, Weber W, Caplan AI, Gordon SL, Fink DJ. Use of mesenchymal stem cells in a collagen matrix for Achilles tendon repair. *J Orthop Res* 1998;16:406–413.
72. Zeichen J, van Griensven M, Bosch U. The proliferative response of isolated human tendon fibroblasts to cyclic biaxial mechanical strain. *Am J Sports Med* 2000;28:888–892.

13

Tendon and Ligament Fixation to Bone

Christopher M. Hill, Yuehuei H. An, and Frank A. Young

INTRODUCTION

For the successful transplantation or transposition of ligaments and tendons, fixation techniques are very important. As most postsurgical rehabilitation protocols emphasize immediate full range of motion and early return to function, fixation must provide adequate strength and stiffness during the early postoperative period. Table 1 lists mechanical properties (failure load, ultimate strength, stiffness, and elastic modulus) of ligament, tendon, or deep fascia of different species. Ideally, fixation strength should meet or exceed the requirements for normal activity on ligaments or tendons. In addition, fixation should not interfere with healing and must be biocompatible for long-term use or easily removable *(1)*. Large animals (goats, dogs, sheep, pigs, and monkeys) are common species for studies of ligament and tendon fixation. Large bone volume of these animals is the most important factor for the facilitation of bone instrumentation (fixations with screws or implants). Selected animal models from the literature to evaluate ligament or tendon fixation to bone are listed in Table 2.

Common fixation techniques include suture, staple, screw/washer, spiked bushing, washer, plate, bone plugs or blocks, and interference screw. Several comparative evaluations of different anchoring techniques have been published *(2–7)*. Recently, a special tension-adjustable artificial ligament anchor has been reported *(8,9)*. Although a distance still exists between the current version and clinical application, it catalyzes a new concept for ligament and tendon anchoring. In recent years, bioabsorbable fixation, along with fixation augmented with bone growth factors, have shown promise in providing stable fixation and rapid biologic incorporation of the grafted tissue *(10–14)*.

HEALING

The normal healing of the grafted tissue and tendon–bone interface has been studied histologically *(27,32,49–52)*. In anterior cruciate ligament (ACL) reconstructions, all autogenous grafts undergo the process of necrosis, revascularization, and maturation. Experimental studies have shown that the intra-articular portion of patellar tendon grafts becomes enveloped by a highly vascular synovial-like tissue during the first 4–6 wk while the core undergoes ischemic necrosis. By 20 wk, revascularization and repopulation of the entire graft with new cells takes place, but the process of remodeling continues. At 1 yr, the transplanted graft can have the histological appearance of a

From: *Orthopedic Biology and Medicine: Repair and Regeneration of Ligaments, Tendons, and Joint Capsule*
Edited by: W. R. Walsh © Humana Press Inc., Totowa, NJ

normal ligament *(32)*. Kasperczyk et al. *(27)* defined a four-stage healing process of autogenic patellar tendon grafts: necrosis, revascularization, collagen formation, and remodeling.

Tendon healing in a bone tunnel may proceed via indirect or direct processes. Rodeo et al. *(51)* found indirect healing with an initial formation of a fibrovascular tissue interface between tendon and bone. This was followed by woven bone in-growth into the interface and progressive organization of collagen fibers, which gradually established continuity between the tendon and bone. Other studies have shown that osseous integration can progress by direct contact healing without the development of a fibrovascular interface *(53)*.

Early in the postoperative period, the graft fixation site is the weakest link of the healing tissue. None of the commonly employed fixation techniques have strength or stiffness comparable to the native tendon or ligament *(54)*. Over time, the graft becomes incorporated into the adjacent bone, and the weakest link shifts to the midsubstance of the graft *(51–53)*. In a canine extra-articular model of tendon healing in a bone tunnel, it was found that all specimens failed by tendon pulling out of the bone tunnel at 8 wk, but by 12 wk all specimens failed by tendon pulling out from the clamp or midsubstance rupture. A progressive increase occurred in the strength of the tendon–bone interface during the first 12 wk, with the most dramatic increase during the first 4 wk. Histologically, this correlated with a progressive rise in the number and organization of collagen fibers extending from the surrounding bone into the implanted tendon. These fibers appeared identical to Sharpey fibers *(51)*. St. Pierre et al *(33)* investigated the healing of tendon attachments in troughs of cancellous bone in comparison to direct cortical attachment. There were 20 goats subjected to a bilateral tenotomy of the infraspinatus tendon. The tendons were attached using sutures either to the cortical surface of bone or to a trough prepared in the cancellous bone. At 6 wk and 12 wk the two techniques were indistinguishable both histologically and biomechanically. The authors found no evidence that one technique was superior to the other.

INTERFERENCE SCREW

Metal Interference Screw

The recent trend toward early motion and aggressive postoperative rehabilitation emphasizes the need for secure initial graft fixation before bony incorporation of the graft *(15,55)*. Interference screw fixation appears to meet the needs for most activities of daily living and rehabilitation programs and has therefore become the standard for bone-tendon-bone graft fixation in ACL repair *(54)*. In 1983, Lambert *(56)* first described interference fixation using a 6.5-mm cancellous screw. Later, Kurosaka et al. *(17)* demonstrated that the 9-mm interference screw (DePuy) had superior initial fixation strength over a 6.5-mm cancellous screw in an in vitro study. Paschal et al. *(42)* compared postfixation (tying to cancellous bone screw) to interference screw fixation in 20 frozen/thawed pig knees using bone-patellar tendon-bone ACL replacement grafts. Displacement of the graft in the bone tunnel by a force of 110 N was measured, as well as the load required to pull the graft out from femurs and tibias separately. Displacements were significantly higher for postfixation than for the interference fixation; however there was no significant difference relating to bone type (tibia vs femur).

Table 1
Selected Mechanical Data of Ligament, Tendon, or Deep Fascia of Different Species

Species	Age	Materials	Failure load (Newton)	Stiffness (N/mm)	Ultimate strength (MPa)	Elastic modulus (MPa)	Reference No.
Human	16 – 26	ACL	1730 ± 660	182 ± 56	—	—	*15*
	48 – 86	ACL	1734 ± 283	129 ± 39	—	—	*15*
	26 ± 6	ACL	1725 ± 269	—	38 ± 4	—	*16*
	59	ACL	559 ± 47	74 ± 3	—	—	*17*
	42	ACL	2195 ± 427	306 ± 80	—	—	*18*
	22 – 35	ACL	2160 ± 157	242 ± 28	—	—	*19*
	40 – 50	ACL	1503 ± 83	220 ± 24	—	—	*19*
	60 – 97	ACL	658 ± 129	180 ± 25	—	—	*19*
	26 ± 6	Bone–PT–bone	2900 ± 260	—	58 + 6	306 ± 59	*3,16*
	44	PT	—	—	47 ± 16	—	*20*
	26 ± 6	Semitendinosus	1216 ± 50	—	89 ± 5	362 ± 22	*3,16*
	26 ± 6	Gracilis	838 + 30	—	111 ± 4	613 ± 41	*3,16*
	26 ± 6	Distal iliotibial band	769 ± 99	—	19 ± 3	—	*16*
	26 ± 6	Fascia lata	628 ± 35	—	79 ± 5	398 ± 17	*3,16*
	44	Fascia lata	—	—	32 ± 14	—	*20*
	44	Achilles tendon	—	—	61 ± 26	—	*20*
Canine	Young adult	ACL (Rottweiler)	1738 ± 476	307 ± 58	63 ± 9	203 ± 10	*21*
	Young adult	ACL (Greyhound)	1781 ± 138	263 ± 17	86 ± 7	221 ± 18	*21*
	Adult	ACL (Mongrel)	1656 ± 125	348 ± 27	147 ± 9	544 ± 36	*22*
	6–180 mo	Whole PT	2080 – 3250	308 ± 66	122 ± 26	474 ± 101	*23*
	Adult	Gluteus tendon	280 ± 55	13 ± 4	—	—	*6*
Rhesus monkey	Young adult	ACL	830 ± 110	194 ± 28	—	—	*15*
	Young adult	Bone–PT–bone	600 ± 132	—	—	—	*24*
Goat	Adult	ACL	1691 ± 209	453 ± 120	—	—	*25*
	Adult	ACL	—	259 ± 7	—	487 ± 28	*26*
Sheep	2-yr	PCL	950	130	—	—	*27*
Pig	?	Toe extensor tendon	—	—	47 ± 5	980	*28*
Rabbit	3.0 + 0.2	ACL	—	—	57 ± 4	600 ± 50	*29*
	3.5 ± 0.2 kg	Bone–PT–bone	300 – 400	—	—	—	*30*
	12 mo	Bone–MCL–bone	—	86 ± 1	—	—	*31*

ACL, anterior cruciate ligament; PT, patellar tendon; PCL, Posterior cruciate ligament; MCL, medial collateral ligament.

Table 2
Selected Animal Models and In Vitro Models Used for Evaluating Ligament or Tendon Fixation to Bone

Method	Device or material	Animal species	Procedure, graft	Initial fixation strength (N)	Strength after in vivo study	Reference no.
Suture	Suture/button	Monkey	ACLR, PCLR, PT	—	300 (1 yr)	*24*
	Stainless steel suture	Dogs	ACLR, PT	—	—	*32*
	Suture/button	Human knee in vitro	ACLR, PT	248 ± 40	—	*17*
	Suture over bone	Human knee in vitro	ACLR, iliotibial band	109 ± 11	—	*17*
	Suture	Goat	Infraspinatus tendon	—	715 – 824 (12 wk)	*33*
Suture anchor	Mitek supperanchor	Human cuboid bone	Tibialis anterior tendon	223	—	*34*
	Absorbable anchor	Rabbit	MCLR	—	—	*35*
Staple	Richard CC1A	Sheep	ACL MCL, artificial ligament	—	160 – 197 (1 yr)	*36*
	Staple	Human knee in vitro	ACLR, PT	129 ± 16	—	*17*
			ACLR, iliotibial band	137 ± 23	—	*17*
	Metal	Goat	ACLR, fascia lata	—	200 – 400	*37*
	Metal	Goat	ACLR, PE	752	1013 – 1233 (3 mo)	*25*
Screw/washer	Cortical screw	Sheep	ACLR, Gore-Tex ligament	369	1380 (7 mo)	*38*
	Screw/bushing	Goat	ACLR, Kennedy LAD	364	841 (24 mo)	*39*
	2-mm cortical screw	Rabbit	ACLR, bone–PT–bone	26 ± 5	51 ± 6 *30*	
	Bicortical screw	Human knee in vitro	ACLR, braided PE	160	—	*40*
	Cancellous screw	Sheep	PCLR, bone–PT–bone	171 ± 16	708 ± 99 (2 yr)	*27*
	AO screw	Goat	ACLR, bone matrix	73 ± 9 (ligament)	474 ± 146 (1 yr)	*41*
Spiked washer, plate,	Plate (Synthes)	Sheep	MCL/ACLR, artificial ligament	—	160 – 197 (1 yr)	*36*
	UHMWPE bushing	Goat	ACLR, fascia lata	—	250 – 400	*37*
	Cancellous screw	Pig bone	ACLR, bone–PT–bone	309	—	*42*

Spiked washer, plate *(Continued)*	Soft tissue plate	Tendon in vitro	Supraspinatus tendon	170–266	—		*43*
	Spiked washer	Tendon in vitro	Supraspinatus tendon	149–514	—		*43*
	Tendon anchor	Tendon in vitro	Supraspinatus tendon	399–729	—		*43*
	AO resin or metal	Human distal femur	Fascia lata	99 ± 35, 149 ± 43	—		*1*
Bone or PLA plug	Press-fit bone	Pig knee in vitro	ACLR, bone–PT–bone	463	—		*44*
	Self-reinforced–PLA	Bovine knee in vitro	ACLR, bone–PT–bone	1100	—		*45*
Interference screw	9-mm	Human knee in vitro	ACLR, PT	476 ± 110	—		*17*
	9 mm (DePuy)	Pig bone	ACLR, bone–PT–bone	535	—		*42*
	7 mm (Acufex)	Bovine bone in vitro	ACLR, bone–PT–bone	1358 ± 348	—		*46*
	7-, 9-mm	Bovine bone in vitro	ACLR,	1161–1198	—		*47*
	7 mm (Linvatec)	Human knee in vitro	ACLR, bone–PT–bone	640 ± 201	—		*48*
	Ti (Arthrex)	Pig knee in vitro	ACLR, bone–PT–bone	769	—		*44*
	AO cancel. screw	Human knee in vitro	ACLR, PT	208 ± 28	—		*17*
	AO cancellous	Bovine bone in vitro	ACLR, bone–PT–bone	1081 ± 331	—		*46*
	Self-reinforced–PLA (Biofix)	Bovine bone in vitro	ACLR, bone–PT–bone	1211 ± 362	—		*46*
	Bioscrew	Same	ACLR, bone–PT–bone	418 ± 118	—		*48*
	PLA (Arthrex)	Pig knee in vitro	ACLR, bone–PT–bone	805	—		*44*
Cylindrical anchor	Titanium	Goat	ACLR, Dacron lines	—	2000 – 4000	(2 mo)	*8,9*

ACLR, anterior cruciate ligament reconstruction; PCLR, posterior cruciate ligament reconstruction; PT, patellar tendon; MCLR, medial collateral ligament reconstruction.

The strength of the postfixation in femurs was 274 N, whereas for interference fixation, it was 543 N. In tibias, the postfixation strength was 343 N, and the interference screw strength 527 N. There was a statistically significant difference between the two types of fixation. All grafts failed at the point of fixation.

Shapiro et al. *(47)* investigated the effect of screw size on the pullout strength of in vitro ACL reconstruction using bovine knees. Results showed no notable difference between 7- and 9-mm interference screws. However, in another study, it was found that a 9-mm tibial interference screw disengaged from the bone tunnel at significantly higher load to failure than a 7-mm screw. This same study also showed that a failed bone plug fixed by a 7-mm screw could be refixed successfully with a 9-mm screw *(57)*. The screw diameter alone may not be as important as its relationship to the gap that exists between the bone block and bone tunnel. A biomechanical study in a porcine model showed that a 7-mm screw in a 1- or 2-mm gap gave equal failure strength to a 9-mm screw in a 3- or 4-mm gap *(58)*. Studies using human cadaver bone yielded similar results *(59)*. Additionally, a study by Brown et al. *(60)* showed that the amount of interference (defined as the screw outer diameter minus the tunnel-bone block gap) correlated with failure load, but gap size alone did not. The metallic interference screw length of 20 mm appears to be sufficient for routine bone plug fixation *(61,62)*.

Screw divergence from the bone plug is commonly seen on postoperative radiographs, particularly with endoscopic placement; however, its clinical relevance remains controversial *(54,63,64)*. A biomechanical study in fresh paired bovine knees showed no variation in strength or stiffness when the femoral screw had a divergence of 15° from the bone plug *(65)*, but Jomha et al. *(66)* demonstrated that there was a significant weakening of fixation for a screw-bone plug angle equal to or greater than 20°. A retrospective study of 73 clinical cases showed no early graft failures despite the presence of screw divergence. The authors suggested that divergence of the femoral screw of less than 30° does not require changing rehabilitation protocols, provided intraoperative stability is achieved *(67)*.

Bioabsorbable Interference Screw

Despite the proven effectiveness of metallic interference screws, bioabsorbable screws offer several significant advantages. These include undistorted magnetic resonance imaging (MRI) views, decreased risk of graft laceration, no release of metallic ions into the surrounding tissue, and no need for hardware removal during revision surgery *(45,48,68–73)*. Biodegradable implants consist mainly of the poly-α-hydroxy acids, polylactide and polyglycolide, including copolymers e.g., poly-(D,L-lactide-coglycolide), and stereopolymers, e.g., poly(L-lactide). These raw materials have different mechanical properties, biocompatibility, and absorption rates that can be further modified by the use of different manufacturing processes *(54, 74)*. Therefore, implants made from the same family of polymers can have vastly different mechanical and biological properties.

In general, biomechanical testing has found the initial fixation strength of bioabsorbable interference screws to be similar to that of metal *(44,46,75–77)*, but a study by Pena et al. reported significantly lower failure loads for absorbable screws *(48)*.

In a study using pig knees, Rupp et al. *(44)* compared press fitting of the bone block in a bone–patellar tendon–bone graft to the use of a biodegradable (polylactic acid [PLA]) interference screw. Titanium interference screw fixation served as a control.

Pull out force to failure was measured. The biodegradable screw fixation yielded a load of 805 N and the titanium screw, 769 N. The press fit yielded a lower load of only 463 N. All specimens failed at the attachment site. In a similar study performed in 1998, Siel et al. examined the failure load of the same three fixation techniques after cyclical loading to duplicate conditions of postoperative physical therapy. Neither of the interference screw fixation groups failed under cyclical loading; however, five of the 10 press fit specimens failed. After 500 loading cycles between 60 and 250 N, the titanium screws failed at a mean load of 945 N, the bioabsorbable screws at 797 N, and the press fit at 708 N. No statistically significant difference was found in ultimate failure loads between the two types of interference screws. They concluded that bioabsorbable screws are a reasonable alternative to titanium screws; however the press fit technique did not provide secure fixation in all cases *(78)*. A more recent study by Kousa et al. examined the effects of cyclical loading at progressively higher loads to a maximum of 100 cycles at 850 N in a porcine knee model. Again, there were no major differences between the titanium screws or absorbable screws regarding displacement, yield load, stiffness, or ultimate load to failure *(12)*.

The exact duration of the resorption process of the different biodegradable screws is not well known, and only few studies have investigated the changes in fixation strength as the implants degrade *(79–82)*. Walton evaluated graft security of titanium and polyglyconate (Acufex, Mansfield, MA) interference screws over a 12-wk healing period in a sheep model. No change in failure strength was found between the titanium screws and the bioabsorbable screws at any time period. Histologically, the bone–patellar tendon–bone grafts showed evidence of bony incorporation at 6 wk, and by 12 wk, the polyglyconate screw had been largely replaced by fibrous tissue *(83)*.

A major disadvantage of biodegradable screws is breakage or drive failure during insertion. Numerous factors can affect screw breakage, including core diameter, outer diameter, drive diameter, drive shape, and molecular weight of the polymer *(13,48,76, 84,85)*. Torsional strength may be more dependent on screw design rather than the type of polymer used to make the implant *(76)*. Concerns also exist about the biocompatibility of certain polymer types used to make bioabsorbable implants. Some studies have shown severe foreign body reactions to polyglycolide implants *(86-88)*. More recently, polylactide materials (including its copolymers and stereopolymers) are used for implants because these are believed to have better biocompatibility *(80,84,89)*. Bioabsorbable polylactide screws are becoming increasingly popular, and studies indicate they provide clinical outcomes comparable to that of metallic screws *(84,90)*.

Interference Screw Fixation of Soft Tissue

Because interference screws have performed reliably well with bone–patellar tendon–bone fixation, surgeons have recently begun to utilize them for soft-tissue fixation of multiple-looped hamstring tendon grafts *(91–94)*. This allows anatomic fixation close to the joint line, which has been shown to increase isometry and stability of the knee *(95–97)*. In addition, anatomic fixation may eliminate the biomechanical disadvantages associated with conventional extra-articular hamstring tendon fixation techniques, such as graft-tunnel motion, graft stretching, and the "windshield wiper" effect. Studies have suggested these create shear forces between the tendon and bone tunnel wall that may lead to tunnel enlargement and delay bony incorporation *(54,98–100)*.

Biomechanical testing has shown interference fixation of soft-tissue grafts to be comparable to conventional hamstring tendon fixation techniques *(101–103)*. The strength of interference screw fixation of soft tissues is affected by many factors. Evidence shows that more precise matching of tunnel size to hamstring graft diameter, i.e., 0.5-mm increments rather than the standard 1-mm increments, will significantly increase fixation strength *(54,102)*. A study by Selby et al. showed that increasing the screw length from 28 to 35 mm will elevate ultimate failure load by 38% *(14)*. Another biomechanical study examining the effect of screw geometry on fixation strength showed that increasing both length and diameter will increase pull out force; of these two, increasing length was more effective *(104)*. Bone mineral density has also been shown to directly affect the ultimate load to failure of interference screws *(105)*. Therefore, it has been suggested that interference screw fixation may be combined with other types of fixation, such as screw and washer, EndoButton (Acufex), or postfixation in instances of poor bone stock *(54)*.

SUTURE ANCHOR

Suture anchors are increasingly being used for a wide variety of orthopedic applications that include rotator cuff repairs, Bankart repairs, and reattachment of various tendons and ligaments to bone *(106–110)*. Recently, different suture anchors have been developed *(111,112)* that are made of metal, nonabsorbable *(34)*, and absorbable materials (e.g., Expanding Suture Plug [Arthrex] *(35,111–114)*.

Shall et al. *(115)* compared failure loads of a metallic suture anchor (SuperAnchor) with either a bioabsorbable staple (Instrument Makar Bioabsorbable Staple) or bioabsorbable tack (Suretac) in a cadaveric model of simulated Bankart repair. The metallic anchor demonstrated almost twice the holding power of either bioabsorbable device, and there was no statistical difference between the staple and tack. Suture breakage was the predominant mode of failure for the anchor, whereas for the staple and tack, it was pullout from bone or implant breakage. An in vivo study in the ram evaluated the change in biomechanical properties over time of several types of suture anchors, including an absorbable expanding suture plug (Arthrex ESP) composed of poly-L-lactic acid (PLLA). At 2 wk, the ESP did not have a pull out strength comparable to the nonabsorbable anchors (17 lb vs 30 lb), but by 6 wk, it had attained the 30-lb failure load that was characteristic of the other anchors tested *(116)*. Histology of the bone–PLLA interface was not performed.

Barber et al. performed a comprehensive series of experiments analyzing the pullout strength and mode of failure of over 30 different types of suture anchors *(111,113,114)*. A fresh porcine femur model was used to test pullout strength in three different environments: the diaphyseal cortex, metaphyseal cortex, and cancellous bone trough created by decortication of the metaphyseal cortex. Whenever possible, the anchors were threaded with wire to test the strength of the implant itself and the implant–bone interface. Overall, it was found that the holding strength of screw type anchors, e.g. Fastak (Arthrex, Naples, FL), PeBA 3, PeBA 5 (Orthopedic Biosystems, Scottsdale, AZ), and AME 5.5 (American Medical Electronics, Richardson, TX), is highly correlated with the size of the screw. This correlation was highly significant in all three bony environments ($p = 0.0001$). With the nonscrew type anchors, e.g., Mitek G2, G3, Superanchor, and Rotator cuff anchor (Mitek Products, Westwood, MA), it was found that larger drill holes were associated with lower mean failure strengths in both the diaphyseal cortex and cancellous bone. Upon examining modes of failure, no correlation was found with drill hole size, anchor type, anchor material, or insertion site *(113)*. With few exceptions, bioabsorbable anchors tend to be larger, presumably to compensate for their lower strength relative to metal, and are available in screw and nonscrew designs. The predominant mode of failure for bioabsorbable screws was wire cutting through the eyelet, whereas for the bioabsorbable nonscrew anchors, it was pullout from the bone. However, both types of bioabsorbable anchors were found to have acceptable initial mechanical strength *(114)*. Overall, the screw designs performed very well and failed at loads higher than the nonscrew designs. Although bioabsorbable implants are generally not as strong as metal implants, they are still stronger than the sutures for which they were designed. It is well recognized that the weakest link with this type of fixation is not the anchor but the suture–soft tissue interface or the suture itself *(113,114,117,118)*. Because of this, all the tested suture anchors should be considered acceptable options.

Rupp et al. showed that loading conditions can have significant effects on failure strength and failure mode *(110)*. They used a porcine tibia model to test failure mechanisms in single maximum loading and cyclical loading to failure for eight different suture anchors, including both metallic and absorbable. In single maximum load to failure, the no. 2 suture was found to be the weakest link for most constructs. The maximum load was equal to the maximum strength of the suture material. Yet, in cyclical loading, the interface between the suture and anchor becomes much more important. In a large number of cases, the suture would wear through at the site where the eyelets of the anchor were roughened and had sharp edges. In this mode of failure, the fatigue strength of the anchor–suture combination was significantly less than the fatigue strength of the suture material alone. In contrast, where the eyelet of the anchor was smooth, as with the bioabsorbable anchors, the usual failure mode was suture failure at the knot, resulting in a fatigue strength that is comparable to the fatigue strength of the suture material alone.

Arthroscopic knot tying is known to be time-consuming to perform and difficult to master in rotator cuff and Bankart repairs. Recently, a Knotless suture anchor (Mitek, Norwood, MA) has been developed that eliminates the need for arthroscopic knot tying and provides direct, secure, low-profile suture anchor repair *(119)*. Biomechanical testing showed it to be comparable to the Mitek G2 suture anchor in both suture strength and bone pull out strength.

Suture

Suture alone, suture tied to a post, or suture-over-button are common techniques for ligament fixation to bone. Common sutures include nonabsorbable suture, bioabsorbable suture, and metal wire. Suture techniques are also commonly used clinically for fixation of tendon to bone, especially in hand surgery. It is used mainly for holding the tendon in place for proper healing of the tendon–bone interface. Because of the relatively low initial fixation strength, early vigorous movement is not encouraged.

Clancy et al. *(24)* studied ACL and posterior cruciate ligament (PCL) replacements in 19 rhesus monkeys. For ACL reconstruction, patellar tendon autografts with bone attached were used. For PCL reconstruction, the medial third of the patellar tendon elongated by attached portions of the patella and tibia were employed. Bone tunnels were drilled in the femur and tibia at a location that corrected for changes in ligament joint space exit location because of the size of the tunnels. Fixation was accomplished by sutures through the ligament and tied over a button. Mechanical testing results showed breaking strengths for control (medial 1/3) patellar tendon specimens to be 300 N. The same setup was used to test the grafted ligaments. Graft pullout strengths, expressed as percentages of the strength of the medial one third of the patellar tendon at 1 yr, were 81% for ACL and 52% for PCL. Test results from earlier time periods indicated lower numbers (e.g., ACL at 2 mo, 34%), and it was concluded that the bone in-growth into the tunnels provided the increased fixation.

Arnoczky et al. *(32)* examined patellar tendon healing in ACL reconstruction in dogs. The proximal tendon end was fixed to bone by stainless steel suturing. The healing process of the graft was reported. No mechanical testing was used for evaluation.

In an in vitro study using human cadaver knees, Kurosaka et al. *(17)* investigated different fixation techniques in ACL reconstruction using bone–patellar tendon–bone grafts, iliotibial band grafts, and semitendinosus grafts. Fixation strength by the suture-over-button technique was found equivalent to that by staples but was lower than that by cancellous screws and interference screws. The constructs failed by breakage of the button, suture cutting through the bone pegs, or grafts slipping out from under the staples. Other studies have found contradicting results. Matthews et al. *(120)* found that the fixation strength of a no. 2 or 5 nonabsorbable suture tied over a screw/washer was equivalent to that of interference screw fixation. But Rowden et al. *(18)* demonstrated hamstring grafts fixed with no. 5 braided polyester secured to a titanium button proximally and a screw distally were actually stronger and just as stiff as patellar tendon-bone grafts fixed with interference screws.

The elongation or stretching that can occur before failure of suture fixation is a significant concern *(2,42,121)*. A report by Robertson et al. *(2)* showed that suture fixation of soft tissue to bone had a failure load that was equal or superior to staple fixation. However, the suture techniques allowed the soft tissue to pull away from the bone long before failure occurred. If cyclical tension will be applied at the fixation site, the authors recommended against suture fixation. This concern was addressed by Jassem et al. *(122)*, who found that by increasing the pitch of the popular Krackow stitch (from 0.5 to 1.0 cm), stiffness could be increased by 16%.

STAPLE

Many brands of commercial fixation staples are currently available, such as the Richards type CC1A XSMO staple (spiked; *36*). Single staples are convenient to use, but recorded fixation strengths are consistently lower than that of other fixation forms *(2,6,17)*. Studies testing single staples in single or cyclic loading show them to be no stronger or stiffer than direct tendon-to-tendon attachment using suture *(2,6)*.

Graft-tunnel length mismatch is considered one of the primary indications for staple fixation in ACL repairs. The use of doubled staples to fix a bone plug in a shallow trough has been shown to provide strength and stiffness (588 N, 86 N/mm) comparable to that of interference screw fixation (506–758 N, 49–55 N/mm) in a young human cadaveric model. However bone block breakage was significantly greater for staples than for interference screws (27% vs 1%; *123*). When using staples to secure tendon without a bone block, looping the graft over the first staple and securing it again with a second, referred to as the "belt-buckle" technique, has been shown to significantly improve fixation in a porcine model *(121)*. Holden et al. *(37)* measured the strength of fascia lata autograft ACL replacements in 50 goats for a period ranging from 0 to 8 wk. The objective was to compare stapled grafts with the belt-buckle technique, to those fixed with a cancellous bone screw and spiked bushing. The control ACL had an average tensile failure load of 2748 N, a value which significantly exceeds that found by other investigators. At time 0, the failure force for the screw/bushing fixed specimens exceeded that for staple fixation. Other time periods yielded no major variations in strength between the two techniques. The graft failure values were reported only as percentages of the control. At 8 wk, the value for staple fixation was 15%, and the screw/bushing fixation was 9% of the control value.

Other studies have used staples to successfully secure artificial ligaments to bone. In 1991, Powers et al. *(25)* performed anatomical reconstruction of the ACL in goats using two tunnels each in the femur and tibia and two ligament strands to simulate the anteromedial and posterolateral bands. Long-chain polyethylene fibers were used for the ligaments, and staples were used to fix them to bone. The increased strength obtained in the 3-mo specimens was deemed to be the result of bone in-growth into the tunnels, providing increased resistance to pullout. Failure modes were not reported.

POSTFIXATION

Cancellous screws and cortical screws with or without washers have been used as posts, around which suture is tied to secure fixation of a tendon or ligament graft *(40,121,124)*. Studying cadaver knees, Steiner et al. have shown that hamstring tendons fixed to bone with no. 2 Ethibond (Ethicon, Summerville, NJ) placed in a whipstitch and tied around a post have a strength of 335 ± 87 N and stiffness of 16 ± 16 N/mm. When the graft was doubled to produce four tendons and no. 5 Ethibond was used, the strength and stiffness increased to 573 ± 109 N and 18 ± 5 N/mm, respectively *(124)*. Paschal et al. *(42)* examined postfixation and interference screw fixation in a porcine knee model. AO 6.5-mm cancellous screws with washers and the no. 5 Ticron (Davis and Geck, Wayne, NJ) suture were compared to 9 ×20-mm interference screws in securing bone–patellar tendon–bone grafts. A statistically significant difference was found in ultimate failure load between postfixation (309 N) and interference fixation (535 N). In addition, displacement at 110 N was significantly greater for postfixation (2.21 mm) than for the interference fixation (0.32 mm). Although postfixation is generally inferior to spiked washers or interference screws, suture and postfixation may prove to be the most reliable method in cases where a short graft or poor bone quality preclude the use of these devices *(122)*.

Bolton and Bruchman *(38)* evaluated the performance of PTFE (Gore-Tex) artificial ACL replacements in 17 sheep for periods ranging from 0 to 369 d. Cortical bone screws placed through eyelets built into the prosthesis were employed to fix the ligament and were placed in bone tunnels using the "over-the top" technique. Pull out tests were conducted, and the 0-time implants yielded a mean failure strength of 1814 N. The 90-d implants with bone screws in place yielded a failure value of 2445 N. Screws were removed from one group that had an average of 218-d residence and a failure strength of 1379 N. Testing a control group of ACL specimens yielded a failure strength of 1912 N. Fixation screws were pulled out of the bone for the time-0 implants, and the increased strengths observed in the experimental groups were attributed to bone growth fixation in the tunnels.

In a sheep model of PCL reconstruction, Kasperczyk et al. *(27)* investigated the healing of patellar tendon autograft over a 2 yr period. The graft was fixed to the femur with no. 0 suture tied around a cancellous screw and to the tibia with a cancellous screw/washer through the graft. They defined a four-stage healing process of autogenic patellar tendon graft—necrosis, revascularization, collagen formation, and remodeling. The biomechanical data were correlated with the morphological phases of healing. Beginning at 2 wk after surgery, biomechanical testing showed all grafts failed at the ligament portion during all time periods, which demonstrated the efficacy of the screw fixation.

In a goat model, Jackson et al. *(41)* attempted to improve fixation by selecting an ACL replacement material that would foster bone formation in the femoral and tibial tunnels. Demineralized bone matrix was used as the ligament and was connected to a screw/washer by sutures. Biomechanical and histological evaluations were performed at 6 mo and 1 yr postsurgery. Seven animals were sacrificed at 1 yr, and accelerated bone formation was noted in the tunnels. The mean ultimate force to failure for the reconstructed ligament at 1 yr was 474 ± 146 N when compared with the time–0 strength of the matrix graft of 73 ± 9 N.

SPIKED WASHER, BUSHING, OR PLATE

Currently, several brands of commercial spiked washers or plates are available, such as the Synthes type 65.00.11 soft-tissue fixation plate *(36)*, the AO polyacetal resin-spiked washer, and AO soft-tissue fixation plate *(1)*.

Robertson et al. compared the immediate holding strength of various types of soft-tissue fixation, including spiked washer, soft-tissue plate, staples, and suture techniques. Holding strength and stiffness was tested in three different types of soft tissue using cyclical loading with progressively greater loads until failure. Testing was performed on human cadaveric tissue. Overall, the screws with the spiked washer and soft-tissue plate proved to be superior in all three tissue types. The screw and washer was best in securing broad, thin, capsular tissue (joint capsule) and wider, thicker, extensor-type tendons (patellar tendon). The soft-tissue plate proved best for narrow, cord-like tissue (semitendinosus) *(2)*. Markel et al. contrasted various methods of gluteus medius attachment in a canine cadaver model. The spiked washer and screw were found to be stronger than the staple but equal in stiffness. This study found no difference in strength or stiffness when comparing the spiked washer with four different suture apposition techniques *(6)*.

Holden et al. studied the effect of a spiked bushing (with a 5-mm diameter shaft) on the fixation of fascia lata graft for ACL reconstruction in a goat model. Results showed that at time 0, the spiked bushing was superior to staples. However, by 8 wk the strength of the graft was only 9% of the control value, vs 15% achieved by belt-buckle staple fixation *(37)*. McPherson et al. *(39)* also used a goat model to examine the effect of a 6-mm polyethylene ligament augmentation device on ACL reconstruction, consisting of a portion of the rectus femoris tendon, prepatellar tissue, and the central one third of the patellar tendon. Tensioning was secured by attaching the ligament with a bushing and cortical bone screw to the lateral surface of the femur. The augmented ligaments had an initial failure strength of 364 N. After 2 yr, the augmented grafts had a strength of 841 N and for the unaugmented grafts, 528 N. These strengths were compared to a natural goat ACL estimated at 2023 N. Graft failure was typically found to occur by pullout of the device from the tibia.

Claes et al. *(36)* tested combined replacements of ACL and medial collateral ligament (MCL) of four ligament replacement materials in 30 sheep for 1 yr. Carbon fiber (Lafil), polydioxanone strand, Dacron, and a bovine tendon xenograft were employed. The combined replacement technique utilized three bone tunnels and a continuous ACL-MCL replacement. Both prosthesis ends were anchored on the lateral surface of the femur using either a staple or spiked fixation plate with a screw (Table 2). Tensile tests were conducted for MCL and ACL separately with the staples or fixation plates removed. No ligaments were fractured during the tensile tests, and all failures occurred by pulling the ligament out of the bone tunnel. The fixation technique was not found to have any effect on strength of fixation or ligament healing.

Gottsauner-Wolf et al. *(43)* researched different fixation methods of tendons to metal prostheses using a soft-tissue fixation plate (Synthes), a spiked polyacetal washer (Synthes), and a new Enhanced Tendon Anchor (ETA; a device with spikes designed to interlock both prosthesis and tendon and held in place by two screws). Each method was used to attach a canine supraspinatus tendon using a bone block technique and a direct tendon attachment technique. There were no differences in strength or stiffness between the plate and washer with the direct tendon attachment technique; however, the ETA had a higher ultimate pullout strength. The ETA was stronger and just as stiff as the washer in the bone block fixation technique. The plate was not as strong or stiff as either method with the bone block technique. The authors concluded that the soft-tissue fixation plate was unsuitable as a bone attachment method. Overall, the use of a tendon with an attached bone block significantly increased the fixation strength, but none of the methods proved to be as strong as the intact muscle-tendon unit.

An in vivo canine study by Hulse et al. used a screw and spiked washer to secure a patellar tendon–fascia lata graft in an over-the-top procedure to replace the ACL. Biomechanical testing performed at 0 wk and 4 wk showed that all grafts failed by the ligament slipping out from underneath the washer. Failure strengths were 169 ± 32 N and 309 ± 109 N, respectively. At 12 wk and 26 wk, post operative failure strengths had increased to 454 ± 83 N and 584 ± 108 N, respectively. Only one specimen (12 wk) had failure by slippage beneath the washer; all other failures were from interstitial graft tears or tibial bone fracture *(22,125)*.

Straight et al. performed a biomechanical analysis of spiked washers to determine the most important design considerations for effective soft-tissue fixation. Washers with two different prototype designs were evaluated and compared to the AO polyacetal resin spiked washer and the AO soft-tissue fixation plate (Synthes USA, Paoli, PA). Freeze-dried and ethylene oxide–sterilized human fascia lata was used as the soft tissue and fixed to the distal femur using each device. Results showed that a six-spike design had superior holding strength vs a three-spike design when a 19-mm diameter washer was used. When smaller diameter washers were used, there was no difference between the two designs. Fixation provided by the six-spike design was comparable to both AO devices. The authors concluded that the design, number, and position of the spikes are the most important factors in determining holding strength of the device. They also suggested that washers should be available in different diameters and spike lengths to accommodate tissues of different thickness *(1)*.

BONE OR ABSORBABLE PLUG

Bioabsorbable plugs and "press fitting" of bone plugs are used to avoid the pitfalls of interference screw fixation, i.e., thread damage to the graft or suture, possible complicated hardware removal, disturbed MRI, or breakage of the absorbable screw *(126)*. Bone plugs may be used with either artificial ligaments or biological grafts *(44,127)*. Rupp et al. used a porcine model to compare fixation strengths of bone-patellar tendon-bone grafts using a titanium interference screw, bioabsorbable interference screw, or press fit technique. The bone plug used for press fit was trimmed to 11-mm diameter and 30-mm length, with a slightly tapered tip. The plug was driven into a 10-mm diameter tibial tunnel from the articular surface using a pusher and hammer. The mean ultimate failure loads for the titanium screw and absorbable screw were 769 N and 805 N, respectively. There was no statistical difference between these two modes of fixation. The press fit technique had a significantly lower mean ultimate failure load of 463 N *(44)*. When the same three techniques were tested in cyclical loading of 500 cycles between 60 and 250 N, half of the press fit specimens failed by bone plug pullout, whereas none of the interference screw fixations failed *(78)*. Reinforcing a press fit bone plug with sutures tied to a bone bridge or bone button may significantly increase pullout strength *(52,128)*.

Ligament fixation using a self-reinforced (SR) PLA expansion plug was reported by Tuompo et al. *(45)* in a bovine bone model. The maximum tensile strength of the SR-PLA plug was above 1100 N, and it seems that the initial strength of the absorbable plug is strong enough for clinical use. Similarly, Kousa et al. compared the fixation strength of an absorbable poly-L-lactide/D-lactide copolymer plug to conventional titanium interference screws. No significant differences in strength or stiffness were found between the two groups when the specimens were tensioned to failure in both monotonic and cyclical loading. The authors concluded that the new plugging technique is a reasonable method for fixation of the femoral site of a bone-patellar tendon-bone graft in ACL reconstruction *(126)*.

YOUNG'S LIGAMENT ANCHOR

Young and An reported a new adjustable screw anchor to secure artificial ACL prosthesis to the femur and tibia *(8,9)*. Fixation was provided by screw threads on the exterior surface of a hollow cylinder that was placed in the bone tunnels created in the femoral condyle and tibial plateau. The artificial ACL was attached to a sliding portion inside the threaded cylinder, which was adjusted for tension by a screw accessed from outside of the exterior bone surfaces. Push-out tests of anchors retrieved after 2-mo implantation in goats indicated values of approx 2000–4000 N.

CONCLUSION

In the early postoperative period, the site of graft fixation remains the weak link whenever tendon or ligament is affixed to bone. It is imperative that the chosen method of fixation is able to withstand the demands of postoperative rehabilitation. Motion at the bone–graft interface may cause delayed healing or nonhealing with eventual failure of the repair. Over a period of months, the graft will become progressively incorporated into bone, and the strength of the repair will become more dependent on the substance of the grafted tissue. Ideally, the fixation technique should facilitate the biological incorporation of the graft. Future research will likely focus on anatomic and isometric reconstruction to reduce stress on the tissues, as well as manipulation of the biological environment with growth factors to speed the healing process. Refinements in bioabsorbable implants may allow them to serve as carriers for growth factors and provide predictable degradation and replacement with normal osseous tissue.

REFERENCES

1. Straight CB, France EP, Paulos LE, Rosenberg TD, Weiss JA. Soft tissue fixation to bone. A biomechanical analysis of spiked washers. *Am J Sports Med* 1994;22:339–343.
2. Robertson DB, Daniel DM, Biden E. Soft tissue fixation to bone. *Am J Sports Med* 1986; 14:398–403.
3. Butler DL, Grood ES, Noyes FR, Zernicke RF, Brackett K. Effects of structure and strain measurement technique on the material properties of young human tendons and fascia. *J Biomech* 1984;17:579–596.
4. Amis AA. The strength of artificial ligament anchorages. A comparative experimental study. *J Bone Joint Surg Br* 1988;70:397–403.
5. Good L, Tarlow SD, Odensten M, Gillquist J. Load tolerance, security, and failure modes of fixation devices for synthetic knee ligaments. *Clin Orthop* 1990;253:190–196.
6. Markel MD, Rock MG, Bergenthal DS, Young DR, Vanderby R Jr, Chao EY. A mechanical comparison of gluteus medius attachment methods in a canine model. *J Orthop Res* 1993;11: 457–461.
7. Letsch R. Comparative evaluation of different anchoring techniques for synthetic cruciate ligaments. A biomechanical and animal investigation. *Knee Surg Sports Traumatol Arthrosc* 1994;2:107–117.
8. Young FA, An Y, inventor. *Adjustable Ligament Anchor*. US patent no. 5,458,601, 1995.
9. Young FA, AnYH. A new artificial ACL anchor. *Material Research Society Symposium Proceeding*, vol. 394. Orthopaedic Research Society, Pittsburgh PA, 1995, pp. 31–34.
10. Anderson K, Seneviratne AM, Izawa K, Atkinson BL, Potter HG, Rodeo SA. Augmentation of tendon healing in an intraarticular bone tunnel with use of a bone growth factor. *Am J Sports Med* 2001;29:689–698.
11. Rodeo SA, Suzuki K, Deng XH, Wozney J, Warren RF. Use of recombinant human bone morphogenetic protein-2 to enhance tendon healing in a bone tunnel. *Am J Sports Med* 1999;27:476–488.
12. Kousa P, Jarvinen TL, Kannus P, Jarvinen M. Initial fixation strength of bioabsorbable and titanium interference screws in anterior cruciate ligament reconstruction. Biomechanical evaluation by single cycle and cyclic loading. *Am J Sports Med* 2001;29:420–425.
13. Costi JJ, Kelly AJ, Hearn TC, Martin DK. Comparison of torsional strengths of bioabsorbable screws for anterior cruciate ligament reconstruction. *Am J Sports Med* 2001; 29:575–580.
14. Selby JB, Johnson DL, Hester P, Caborn DN. Effect of screw length on bioabsorbable interference screw fixation in a tibial bone tunnel. *Am J Sports Med* 2001;29:614–619.
15. Noyes FR, Grood ES. The strength of the anterior cruciate ligament in humans and Rhesus monkeys. *J Bone Joint Surg Am* 1976;58:1074–1082.
16. Noyes FR, Butler DL, Grood ES, Zernicke RF, Hefzy MS. Biomechanical analysis of human ligament grafts used in knee-ligament repairs and reconstructions. *J Bone Joint Surg Am* 1984;66:344–352.

17. Kurosaka M, Yoshiya S, Andrish JT. A biomechanical comparison of different surgical techniques of graft fixation in anterior cruciate ligament reconstruction. *Am J Sports Med* 1987;15:225–229.
18. Rowden NJ, Sher D, Rogers GJ, Schindhelm K. Anterior cruciate ligament graft fixation. Initial comparison of patellar tendon and semitendinosus autografts in young fresh cadavers. *Am J Sports Med* 1997;25:472–478.
19. Woo SL, Hollis JM, Adams DJ, Lyon RM, Takai S. Tensile properties of the human femur-anterior cruciate ligament-tibia complex. The effects of specimen age and orientation. *Am J Sports Med* 1991;19:217–225.
20. France EP, Paulos LE, Rosenberg TD, Harner CD. The biomechanics of anterior cruciate allografts. In: Friedman MJ, Ferkel RD, eds. *Prosthetic Ligament Reconstruction of the Knee*. Saunders, Philadelphia, PA, 1988.
21. Wingfield C, Amis AA, Stead AC, Law HT. Comparison of the biomechanical properties of rottweiler and racing greyhound cranial cruciate ligaments. *J Small Anim Pract* 2000;41: 303–307.
22. Butler DL, Hulse DA, Kay MD, Grood ES, Shires PK, D'Ambrosia R, Shoji H. Biomechanics of cranial cruciate ligament reconstruction in the dog. *Vet Surg* 1983;112:113–118.
23. Haut RC, Lancaster RL, DeCamp CE. Mechanical properties of the canine patellar tendon: some correlations with age and the content of collagen. *J Biomech* 1992;25:163–173.
24. Clancy WG, Jr., Narechania RG, Rosenberg TD, Gmeiner JG, Wisnefske DD, Lange TA. Anterior and posterior cruciate ligament reconstruction in rhesus monkeys. *J Bone Joint Surg Am* 1981;63:1270–1284.
25. Powers DL, Jacob PA, Drews MJ. Anatomical reconstruction of the anterior cruciate ligament in goats. *J Invest Surg* 1991;4:191–202.
26. Ng GY, Oakes BW, McLean ID, Deacon OW, Lampard D. The long-term biomechanical and viscoelastic performance of repairing anterior cruciate ligament after hemitransection injury in a goat model. *Am J Sports Med* 1996;24:109–117.
27. Kasperczyk WJ, Bosch U, Oestern HJ, Tscherne H. Staging of patellar tendon autograft healing after posterior cruciate ligament reconstruction. A biomechanical and histological study in a sheep model. *Clin Orthop* 1993;286:271–282.
28. Smith CW, Young IS, Kearney JN. Mechanical properties of tendons: changes with sterilization and preservation. *J Biomech Eng* 1996;118:56–61.
29. Ishizue KK, Lyon RM, Amiel D, Woo SL. Acute hemarthrosis: a histological, biochemical, and biomechanical correlation of early effects on the anterior cruciate ligament in a rabbit model. *J Orthop Res* 1990;8:548–554.
30. Ballock RT, Woo SL, Lyon RM, Hollis JM, Akeson WH. Use of patellar tendon autograft for anterior cruciate ligament reconstruction in the rabbit: a long-term histologic and biomechanical study. *J Orthop Res* 1989;7:474–485.
31. King GJ, Edwards P, Brant RF, Shrive NG, Frank CB. Intraoperative graft tensioning alters viscoelastic but not failure behaviours of rabbit medial collateral ligament autografts. *J Orthop Res* 1995;13:915–922.
32. Arnoczky SP, Tarvin GB, Marshall JL. Anterior cruciate ligament replacement using patellar tendon. An evaluation of graft revascularization in the dog. *J Bone Joint Surg Am* 1982;64:217–224.
33. St. Pierre P, Olson EJ, Elliott JJ, O'Hair KC, McKinney LA, Ryan J. Tendon-healing to cortical bone compared with healing to a cancellous trough. A biomechanical and histological evaluation in goats. *J Bone Joint Surg Am* 1995;77:1858–1866.
34. Fennell CW, Ballard JM, Pflaster DS, Adkins RH. Comparative evaluation of bone suture anchor to bone tunnel fixation of tibialis anterior tendon in cadaveric cuboid bone: a biomechanical investigation. *Foot Ankle Int* 1995;16:641–645.

35. Ono K, Williams GR, Clem M, Hwa JL, Wirth MA, Aufdemorte TB, et al. Repair of soft tissue to bone using a biodegradable suture anchor. *Orthopedics* 1997;20:1051–1055.
36. Claes L, Durselen L, Kiefer H, Mohr W. The combined anterior cruciate and medial collateral ligament replacement by various materials: a comparative animal study. *J Biomed Mater Res* 1987;21(Suppl A3):319–343.
37. Holden JP, Grood ES, Butler DL, Noyes FR, Mendenhall HV, Van Kampen CL, et al. Biomechanics of fascia lata ligament replacements: early postoperative changes in the goat. *J Orthop Res* 1988;6:639–647.
38. Bolton CW, Bruchman WC. The GORE-TEX expanded polytetrafluoroethylene prosthetic ligament. An in vitro and in vivo evaluation. *Clin Orthop* 1985;196:202–213.
39. McPherson GK, Mendenhall HV, Gibbons DF, Plenk H, Rottmann W, Sanford JB, et al. Experimental mechanical and histologic evaluation of the Kennedy ligament augmentation device. *Clin Orthop* 1985;196:186–195.
40. Gillquist J, Good L. Load and length changes in an artificial ligament substitute. 10 cases of anterior cruciate ligament reconstruction. *Acta Orthop Scand* 1993;64:575–579.
41. Jackson DW, Simon TM, Lowery W, Gendler E. Biologic remodeling after anterior cruciate ligament reconstruction using a collagen matrix derived from demineralized bone. An experimental study in the goat model. *Am J Sports Med* 1996;24:405–414.
42. Paschal SO, Seemann MD, Ashman RB, Allard RN, Montgomery JB. Interference fixation versus postfixation of bone-patellar tendon-bone grafts for anterior cruciate ligament reconstruction. A biomechanical comparative study in porcine knees. *Clin Orthop* 1994; 300:281–287.
43. Gottsauner-Wolf F, Egger EL, Markel MD, Schultz FM, Chao EY. Fixation of canine tendons to metal. *Acta Orthop Scand* 1994;65:179–184.
44. Rupp S, Krauss PW, Fritsch EW. Fixation strength of a biodegradable interference screw and a press-fit technique in anterior cruciate ligament reconstruction with a BPTB graft. *Arthroscopy* 1997;13:61–65.
45. Tuompo P, Partio EK, Jukkala-Partio K, Pohjonen T, Helevirta P, Rokkanen P. Strength of the fixation of patellar tendon bone grafts using a totally absorbable self-reinforced poly-L-lactide expansion plug and screw. An experimental study in a bovine cadaver. *Arthroscopy* 1996;12:422–427.
46. Kousa P, Jarvinen TL, Pohjonen T, Kannus P, Kotikoski M, Jarvinen M. Fixation strength of a biodegradable screw in anterior cruciate ligament reconstruction. *J Bone Joint Surg Br* 1995;77:901–905.
47. Shapiro JD, Jackson DW, Aberman HM, Lee TQ, Simon TM. Comparison of pullout strength for seven- and nine-millimeter diameter interference screw size as used in anterior cruciate ligament reconstruction. *Arthroscopy* 1995;11:596–599.
48. Pena F, Grontvedt T, Brown GA, Aune AK, Engebretsen L. Comparison of failure strength between metallic and absorbable interference screws. Influence of insertion torque, tunnel-bone block gap, bone mineral density, and interference. *Am J Sports Med* 1996;24:329–334.
49. Ishibashi Y, Toh S, Okamura Y, Sasaki T, Kusumi T. Graft incorporation within the tibial bone tunnel after anterior cruciate ligament reconstruction with bone-patellar tendon-bone autograft. *Am J Sports Med* 2001;29:473–479.
50. Greis PE, Burks RT, Bachus K, Luker MG. The influence of tendon length and fit on the strength of a tendon-bone tunnel complex. A biomechanical and histologic study in the dog. *Am J Sports Med* 2001;29:493–497.
51. Rodeo SA, Arnoczky SP, Torzilli PA, Hidaka C, Warren RF. Tendon-healing in a bone tunnel. A biomechanical and histological study in the dog. *J Bone Joint Surg Am* 1993;75: 1795–1803.
52. Papageorgiou CD, Ma CB, Abramowitch SD, Clineff TD, Woo SL. A multidisciplinary study of the healing of an intraarticular anterior cruciate ligament graft in a goat model. *Am J Sports Med* 2001;29:620–626.

53. Weiler A, Hoffmann RF, Bail HJ, Rehm O, Sudkamp NP. Tendon healing in a bone tunnel. Part II: Histologic analysis after biodegradable interference fit fixation in a model of anterior cruciate ligament reconstruction in sheep. *Arthroscopy* 2002;18:124–135.
54. Brand J, Jr., Weiler A, Caborn DN, Brown CH, Jr., Johnson DL. Graft fixation in cruciate ligament reconstruction. *Am J Sports Med* 2000;28:761–774.
55. Shelbourne KD, Nitz P. Accelerated rehabilitation after anterior cruciate ligament reconstruction. *Am J Sports Med* 1990;18:292–299.
56. Lambert KL. Vascularized patellar tendon graft with rigid internal fixation for anterior cruciate ligament insufficiency. *Clin Orthop* 1983;172:85–89.
57. Kohn D, Rose C. Primary stability of interference screw fixation. Influence of screw diameter and insertion torque. *Am J Sports Med* 1994;22:334–338.
58. Butler JC, Branch TP, Hutton WC. Optimal graft fixation—the effect of gap size and screw size on bone plug fixation in ACL reconstruction. *Arthroscopy* 1994;10(5):524–529.
59. Matthews LS, Parks BG, Sabbagh RC. Determination of fixation strength of large-diameter interference screws. *Arthroscopy* 1998;14:70–74.
60. Brown GA, Pena F, Grontvedt T, Labadie D, Engebretsen L. Fixation strength of interference screw fixation in bovine, young human, and elderly human cadaver knees: influence of insertion torque, tunnel-bone block gap, and interference. *Knee Surg Sports Traumatol Arthrosc* 1996;3:238–244.
61. Brown CH, Jr., Hecker AT, Hipp JA, Myers ER, Hayes WC. The biomechanics of interference screw fixation of patellar tendon anterior cruciate ligament grafts. *Am J Sports Med* 1993;21:880–886.
62. Hulstyn M, Fadale PD, Abate J, Walsh WR. Biomechanical evaluation of interference screw fixation in a bovine patellar bone-tendon-bone autograft complex for anterior cruciate ligament reconstruction. *Arthroscopy* 1993;9:417–424.
63. Lemos MJ, Albert J, Simon T, Jackson DW. Radiographic analysis of femoral interference screw placement during ACL reconstruction: endoscopic versus open technique. *Arthroscopy* 1993;9:154–158.
64. Fineberg MS, Zarins B, Sherman OH. Practical considerations in anterior cruciate ligament replacement surgery. *Arthroscopy* 2000;16:715–724.
65. Lemos MJ, Jackson DW, Lee TQ, Simon TM. Assessment of initial fixation of endoscopic interference femoral screws with divergent and parallel placement. *Arthroscopy* 1995;11:37–41.
66. Jomha NM, Raso VJ, Leung P. Effect of varying angles on the pullout strength of interference screw fixation. *Arthroscopy* 1993;9:580–583.
67. Dworsky BD, Jewell BF, Bach BR, Jr. Interference screw divergence in endoscopic anterior cruciate ligament reconstruction. *Arthroscopy* 1996;12:45–49.
68. Brown CH, Jr., Carson EW. Revision anterior cruciate ligament surgery. *Clin Sports Med* 1999;18:109–171.
69. Jacobs JJ, Gilbert JL, Urban RM. Corrosion of metal orthopaedic implants. *J Bone Joint Surg Am* 1998;80:268–282.
70. Safran MR, Harner CD. Technical considerations of revision anterior cruciate ligament surgery. *Clin Orthop* 1996;325:50–64.
71. Suh JS, Jeong EK, Shin KH, Cho JH, Na JB, Kim DH, et al. Minimizing artifacts caused by metallic implants at MR imaging: experimental and clinical studies. *AJR Am J Roentgenol* 1998;171:1207–1213.
72. Matthews LS, Soffer SR. Pitfalls in the use of interference screws for anterior cruciate ligament reconstruction: brief report. *Arthroscopy* 1989;5:225–226.
73. Shellock FG, Mink JH, Curtin S, Friedman MJ. MR imaging and metallic implants for anterior cruciate ligament reconstruction: assessment of ferromagnetism and artifact. *J Magn Reson Imaging* 1992;2:225–228.
74. Chambat P. Letters to the editor. *Am J Sports Med* 2001;29:266–267.

75. Abate JA, Fadale PD, Hulstyn MJ, Walsh WR. Initial fixation strength of polylactic acid interference screws in anterior cruciate ligament reconstruction. *Arthroscopy* 1998;14: 278–284.
76. Weiler A, Windhagen HJ, Raschke MJ, Laumeyer A, Hoffmann RF. Biodegradable interference screw fixation exhibits pull-out force and stiffness similar to titanium screws. *Am J Sports Med* 1998;26:119–126.
77. Caborn DN, Urban WP, Jr., Johnson DL, Nyland J, Pienkowski D. Biomechanical comparison between BioScrew and titanium alloy interference screws for bone-patellar tendon-bone graft fixation in anterior cruciate ligament reconstruction. *Arthroscopy* 1997;13: 229–232.
78. Seil R, Rupp S, Krauss PW, Benz A, Kohn DM. Comparison of initial fixation strength between biodegradable and metallic interference screws and a press-fit fixation technique in a porcine model. *Am J Sports Med* 1998;26:815–819.
79. Bostman OM, Pihlajamaki HK. Late foreign-body reaction to an intraosseous bioabsorbable polylactic acid screw. A case report. *J Bone Joint Surg Am* 1998;80:1791–1794.
80. Stahelin AC, Weiler A, Rufenacht H, Hoffmann R, Geissmann A, Feinstein R. Clinical degradation and biocompatibility of different bioabsorbable interference screws: a report of six cases. *Arthroscopy* 1997;13:238–244.
81. Powers DL, Sonawala M, Woolf SK, An YH, Hawkins R, Pietrzak WS. Comparison of the biomechanics and histology of two soft-tissue fixators composed of bioabsorbable copolymers. *J Biomed Mater Res* 2001;58:486–495.
82. An YH, Friedman RJ, Powers DL, Draughn RA, Latour RA, Jr. Fixation of osteotomies using bioabsorbable screws in the canine femur. *Clin Orthop* 1998:300–311.
83. Walton M. Absorbable and metal interference screws: comparison of graft security during healing. *Arthroscopy* 1999;15:818–826.
84. Barber FA, Elrod BF, McGuire DA, Paulos LE. Preliminary results of an absorbable interference screw. *Arthroscopy* 1995;11:537–548.
85. Stahelin AC, Feinstein R, Friederich NF. Clinical experience using bioabsorbable interferende screw for ACL reconstruction. *Ortho Trans* 1995;19:287–288.
86. Bostman OM. Intense granulomatous inflammatory lesions associated with absorbable internal fixation devices made of polyglycolide in ankle fractures. *Clin Orthop* 1992;278: 193–199.
87. Friden T, Rydholm U. Severe aseptic synovitis of the knee after biodegradable internal fixation. A case report. *Acta Orthop Scand* 1992;63:94–97.
88. Weiler A, Helling HJ, Kirch U, Zirbes TK, Rehm KE. Foreign-body reaction and the course of osteolysis after polyglycolide implants for fracture fixation: experimental study in sheep. *J Bone Joint Surg Br* 1996;78:369–376.
89. Bucholz RW, Henry S, Henley MB. Fixation with bioabsorbable screws for the treatment of fractures of the ankle. *J Bone Joint Surg Am* 1994;76:319–324.
90. Marti C, Imhoff AB, Bahrs C, Romero J. Metallic versus bioabsorbable interference screw for fixation of bone-patellar tendon-bone autograft in arthroscopic anterior cruciate ligament reconstruction. A preliminary report. *Knee Surg Sports Traumatol Arthrosc* 1997; 5:217–221.
91. Corry IS, Webb JM, Clingeleffer AJ, Pinczewski LA. Arthroscopic reconstruction of the anterior cruciate ligament. A comparison of patellar tendon autograft and four-strand hamstring tendon autograft. *Am J Sports Med* 1999;27:444–454.
92. Fu FH, Bennett CH, Ma CB, Menetrey J, Lattermann C. Current trends in anterior cruciate ligament reconstruction. Part II. Operative procedures and clinical correlations. *Am J Sports Med* 2000;28:124–130.
93. Fu FH, Bennett CH, Lattermann C, Ma CB. Current trends in anterior cruciate ligament reconstruction. Part 1: Biology and biomechanics of reconstruction. *Am J Sports Med* 1999;27:821–830.

94. Stahelin AC, Weiler A. All-inside anterior cruciate ligament reconstruction using semitendinosus tendon and soft threaded biodegradable interference screw fixation. *Arthroscopy* 1997;13:773–779.
95. Morgan CD, Kalmam VR, Grawl DM. Isometry testing for anterior cruciate ligament reconstruction revisited. *Arthroscopy* 1995;11:647–659.
96. Ishibashi Y, Rudy TW, Livesay GA, Stone JD, Fu FH, Woo SL. The effect of anterior cruciate ligament graft fixation site at the tibia on knee stability: evaluation using a robotic testing system. *Arthroscopy* 1997;13:177–182.
97. Scheffler SU, Sudkamp NP, Gockenjan A, Hoffmann RF, Weiler A. Biomechanical comparison of hamstring and patellar tendon graft anterior cruciate ligament reconstruction techniques: the impact of fixation level and fixation method under cyclic loading. *Arthroscopy* 2002;18:304–315.
98. Hoher J, Livesay GA, Ma CB, Withrow JD, Fu FH, Woo SL. Hamstring graft motion in the femoral bone tunnel when using titanium button/polyester tape fixation. *Knee Surg Sports Traumatol Arthrosc* 1999;7:215–219.
99. L'Insalata JC, Klatt B, Fu FH, Harner CD. Tunnel expansion following anterior cruciate ligament reconstruction: a comparison of hamstring and patellar tendon autografts. *Knee Surg Sports Traumatol Arthrosc* 1997;5:234–238.
100. Nebelung W, Becker R, Merkel M, Ropke M. Bone tunnel enlargement after anterior cruciate ligament reconstruction with semitendinosus tendon using Endobutton fixation on the femoral side. *Arthroscopy* 1998;14:810–815.
101. Weiler A, Hoffmann RF, Stahelin AC, Bail HJ, Siepe CJ, Sudkamp NP. Hamstring tendon fixation using interference screws: a biomechanical study in calf tibial bone. *Arthroscopy* 1998;14:29–37.
102. Steenlage E, Brand JC, Caborn D, et al. Interference screw fixation of a quadrupled hamstring graft is improved with precise match of tunnel to graft diameter. *Arthroscopy* 1999; 15:59.
103. Caborn DN, Coen M, Neef R, Hamilton D, Nyland J, Johnson DL. Quadrupled semitendinosus-gracilis autograft fixation in the femoral tunnel: a comparison between a metal and a bioabsorbable interference screw. *Arthroscopy* 1998;14:241–245.
104. Weiler A, Hoffmann RF, Siepe CJ, Kolbeck SF, Sudkamp NP. The influence of screw geometry on hamstring tendon interference fit fixation. *Am J Sports Med* 2000;28:356–359.
105. Brand JC, Jr., Pienkowski D, Steenlage E, Hamilton D, Johnson DL, Caborn DN. Interference screw fixation strength of a quadrupled hamstring tendon graft is directly related to bone mineral density and insertion torque. *Am J Sports Med* 2000;28:705–710.
106. Burkhart SS, Diaz Pagan JL, Wirth MA, Athanasiou KA. Cyclic loading of anchor-based rotator cuff repairs: confirmation of the tension overload phenomenon and comparison of suture anchor fixation with transosseous fixation. *Arthroscopy* 1997;13:720–724.
107. Martinez FD, Morgan WJ, Wright AL, Holberg C, Taussig LM. Initial airway function is a risk factor for recurrent wheezing respiratory illnesses during the first three years of life. Group Health Medical Associates. *Am Rev Respir Dis* 1991;143:312–316.
108. Berlet GC, Johnson JA, Milne AD, Patterson SD, King GJ. Distal biceps brachii tendon repair. An in vitro biomechanical study of tendon reattachment. *Am J Sports Med* 1998;26: 428–432.
109. Kato H, Minami A, Takahara M, Oshio I, Hirachi K, Kotaki H. Surgical repair of acute collateral ligament injuries in digits with the Mitek bone suture anchor. *J Hand Surg [Br]* 1999;24:70–75.
110. Rupp S, Georg T, Gauss C, Kohn D, Seil R. Fatigue testing of suture anchors. *Am J Sports Med* 2002;30:239–247.
111. Barber FA, Herbert MA, Click JN. The ultimate strength of suture anchors. *Arthroscopy* 1995;11:21–28.

112. Barber FA, Deck MA. The in vivo histology of an absorbable suture anchor: a preliminary report. *Arthroscopy* 1995;11:77–81.
113. Barber FA, Herbert MA, Click JN. Suture anchor strength revisited. *Arthroscopy* 1996;12: 32–38.
114. Barber FA, Herbert MA, Click JN. Internal fixation strength of suture anchors—update 1997. *Arthroscopy* 1997;13:355–362.
115. Shall LM, Cawley PW. Soft tissue reconstruction in the shoulder. Comparison of suture anchors, absorbable staples, and absorbable tacks. *Am J Sports Med* 1994;22:715–718.
116. Barber FA, Cawley P, Prudich JF. Suture anchor failure strength—an in vivo study. *Arthroscopy* 1993;9:647–652.
117. Shea KP, O'Keefe RM, Jr., Fulkerson JP. Comparison of initial pull-out strength of arthroscopic suture and staple Bankart repair techniques. *Arthroscopy* 1992;8:179–182.
118. Hughes PJ, Hagan RP, Fisher AC, Holt EM, Frostick SP. The kinematics and kinetics of slipknots for arthroscopic Bankart repair. *Am J Sports Med* 2001;29(6):738-45.
119. Thal R. A knotless suture anchor. Design, function, and biomechanical testing. *Am J Sports Med* 2001;29:646–649.
120. Matthews LS, Lawrence SJ, Yahiro MA, Sinclair MR. Fixation strengths of patellar tendon-bone grafts. *Arthroscopy* 1993;9:76–81.
121. Magen HE, Howell SM, Hull ML. Structural properties of six tibial fixation methods for anterior cruciate ligament soft tissue grafts. *Am J Sports Med* 1999;27:35–43.
122. Jassem M, Rose AT, Meister K, Indelicato PA, Wheeler D. Biomechanical analysis of the effect of varying suture pitch in tendon graft fixation. *Am J Sports Med* 2001;29:734–737.
123. Gerich TG, Cassim A, Lattermann C, Lobenhoffer HP. Pullout strength of tibial graft fixation in anterior cruciate ligament replacement with a patellar tendon graft: interference screw versus staple fixation in human knees. *Knee Surg Sports Traumatol Arthrosc* 1997;5:84–88.
124. Steiner ME, Hecker AT, Brown CH, Jr., Hayes WC. Anterior cruciate ligament graft fixation. Comparison of hamstring and patellar tendon grafts. *Am J Sports Med* 1994;22: 240–247.
125. Johnson SG, Hulse DA, Hogan HA, Nelson JK, Boothe HW. System behavior of commonly used cranial cruciate ligament reconstruction autografts. *Vet Surg* 1989;18:459–465.
126. Kousa P, Jarvinen TL, Kannus P, Ahvenjarvi P, Kaikkonen A, Jarvinen M. A bioabsorbable plug in bone-tendon-bone reconstruction of the anterior cruciate ligament: Introduction of a novel fixation technique. *Arthroscopy* 2001;17:144–150.
127. Fujikawa K. Clinical study of anterior cruciate ligament reconstruction with the Leeds-Keio artificial ligament. In: Friedman MJ, Ferkel RD, eds. *Prosthetic Ligament Reconstruction of the Knee*. Saunders, Philadelphia, PA, 1988.
128. Boszotta H, Anderl W. Primary stability with tibial press-fit fixation of patellar ligament graft: An experimental study in ovine knees. *Arthroscopy* 2001;17:963–970.

14

Tissue Engineering Strategies for Regeneration of the Anterior Cruciate Ligament

Michael G. Dunn

INTRODUCTION: THE CHALLENGE OF ACL REGENERATION

The anterior cruciate ligament (ACL) is a primary stabilizer of the knee joint that is frequently injured, compromising knee stability and leading to degeneration of other joint structures. Because the ACL has a poor intrinsic healing capacity, surgical reconstruction is required to restore knee function in young active patients. Biological grafts are the gold standard for ACL reconstruction, resulting in formation of scar-like tissue, which remodels but remains structurally and biomechanically inferior to the normal ACL. The ultimate challenge of ACL reconstruction is ACL regeneration: reestablishing the unique structure, function, and mechanical properties of the normal ACL. Despite significant recent advances *(1)*, existing ACL reconstruction techniques do not result in ACL regeneration *(2)*. In fact, regeneration of the musculoskeletal soft tissues, including ligament, tendon, meniscus, disc, and cartilage, remains an elusive goal.

Rather than review the current state-of-the-art in ACL reconstruction surgery, strategies and tools needed to ultimately achieve ACL regeneration are considered. With this focus on tissue engineering, there is an essential emphasis on the author's preclinical studies. as clinical results are not yet available. The introductory sections detail three major challenges in ACL regeneration: (1) the complex structure and function of the ACL; (2) inadequate healing in the ACL and the "race" between repair and regeneration; and (3) limitations of the grafts and biomaterials that are currently available to the surgeon. With these challenges in mind, the second section (Tissue Engineering Strategies for ACL Regeneration) explores the potential of the tissue engineering approach, specifically the use of implantable scaffolds, cells, and cell signals to induce ACL regeneration. Finally, the last section (Technical, Regulatory, and Social Issues) examines critical issues associated with taking this technology from the "bench to the bedside," involving manufacturing issues and potential difficulties with regulation and reimbursement of tissue-engineered medical devices.

Complex Structure and Function of the ACL

Ligaments are strong flexible bands of collagen-rich tissue that connect bone to bone, providing a delicate balance of stability and flexibility to the joints of the body. The

From: *Orthopedic Biology and Medicine: Repair and Regeneration of Ligaments, Tendons, and Joint Capsule*
Edited by: W. R. Walsh © Humana Press Inc., Totowa, NJ

largest joint in the body—the knee—is stabilized by pairs of collateral and cruciate ligaments. The ACL is considered the primary stabilizer of the knee and is frequently injured in athletic maneuvers and accidents. The ACL does not usually heal spontaneously; therefore, surgical intervention is often required to restore knee function. In fact, approx 125,000 ACL reconstruction surgeries are performed worldwide each year, most often using biological grafts (autografts or allografts).

The ACL is part of a bone-ligament-bone complex that includes bone, fibrocartilage, and a soft-tissue midsubstance (the ACL proper), consisting largely of type I collagen (to provide high strength), a sheath for protection, vascularity for nourishment, and nerves for proprioception *(3)*. Clearly, such a complex structure is very difficult, if not impossible to replicate using traditional biomaterials approaches and/or biological grafts *(4)*. Despite significant progress in understanding ACL anatomy, structure, biomechanics, and healing, there is still no biological graft or prosthesis ideally suited for ACL reconstruction.

The primary function of the ACL is mechanical: to limit anterior translation and twisting of the tibia with respect to the femur. Its mechanical properties are well suited to its function, and these properties are mostly a consequence of the hierarchical arrangement of type I collagen. The ultimate tensile strength of the human ACL is 38 MPa in young donors and decreases with age *(5)*. Other important mechanical properties are elasticity, resistance to creep, and resistance to fatigue failure.

The ACL attaches to the posteromedial aspect of the lateral femoral condyle and to the tibia, anterolateral to the tibial spine *(6)*. Gross dissection reveals that the human ACL averages 31 mm in length *(7)* and twists approx 130–140° from origin to insertion with the knee in full flexion *(8)*. Two distinct functional units are in the ACL: an anteromedial band (tightest during flexion) and a posterolateral band (tightest during extension) *(9)*. The largest well-defined structural unit is the fascicle, which is 20–400 μm in diameter and surrounded by the paratenon, a connective tissue sheath. The fascicles are composed of subfascicles *(10)* or fiber bundles of 1–20-μm diameter *(11)*, and collagen fibrils of 25–150-nm diameter. The fibers are crimped with a period of 45–60 μm and an amplitude of less than 5 μm *(12)*. The extracellular matrix of the ACL is composed primarily of collagen (80% of the tissue dry weight) with 88% type I collagen and 12% type III collagen *(12)*.

The collagenous matrix of the ACL is synthesized and maintained by fibroblasts. These fibroblasts are ovoid or round in shape, contrasting to other tendon or ligament fibroblasts, which are typically elongated and spindle-shaped *(13)*. ACL fibroblasts are relatively large (5–8 by 12–15 μm) and are arranged in columns between the collagen fibers, resembling fibrocartilage near the bony insertion sites.

The ACL is intra-articular, but extrasynovial because of a surrounding protective sheath. The vascular supply originates from soft tissues (mainly the middle genicular artery), not from bone junctions *(14)*. The dominant function of the synovial sheath is to protect the ACL from synovial fluid. When the sheath is compromised, the ACL begins to break down via exposure to proteinases *(15)* and inflammatory cytokines found in the synovial fluid.

Fibrocartilage is present at both bone insertion sites, providing a transitional tissue that may reduce local stress concentrations *(16)*. Like cartilage, fibrocartilage is characterized by a higher proteoglycan and type II collagen content *(17)* when compared to the ligament proper, and seems to develop in response to compressive loads *(18)*. Within the fibrocartilage there are two regions: a nonmineralized region interfacing with the soft tissue and a mineralized region interfacing with the bone. Obviously, proper integration within the bone tunnel attachment sites is a prerequisite for a graft or neoligament tissue to function; reestablishment of a fibrocartilagenous interface is most desirable. Rodeo's group has focused on this interface during healing and recently reviewed tissue engineering approaches toward establishing a normal bone–ligament interface following ACL reconstruction *(19)*.

Mechanoreceptors in the ACL provide sensory feedback to help position the joint and protect it from damage due to overloading *(20)*. Thus, regeneration of proprioceptive structures should be an additional goal of ACL reconstruction *(21)*.

In summary, the ACL is part of a bone-ligament-bone complex that includes various tissue types, such as the ACL proper, surrounded by a protective sheath, with vascularity for nourishment, nerves for proprioception, fibrocartilagenous transition zones, and the bone ends that are linked together by the ligament. To date, it has been impossible to accurately reconstruct or regenerate such a complex structure using traditional biomaterial prostheses and/or biological grafts. New approaches, e.g., tissue engineering (possibly coupled with genetic engineering) may be needed to induce regeneration of complex tissues like the ACL. In addition to the complexity of the structure, however, there is another major biological problem: musculoskeletal injuries tend to mount a rapid and fibrotic heading response that may interfere with attempts to regenerate the tissue.

Repair vs Regeneration of Musculoskeletal Tissues

The ultimate goal of ACL reconstruction is to regenerate a fully functional ACL with the same structure and mechanical properties as the normal ACL. "Regeneration" is a frequently misused term in the biomaterials literature, often interchanged with "repair" or "reconstruction," which are altogether different processes. Regeneration mimics embyronic development, resulting in nearly complete reconstitution of the original structure, function, and mechanical properties of the tissue. For example, phylogenetically lower vertebrates (e.g., urodeles) can regenerate entire limbs by forming a blastema at the injury site *(22)*. The blastema is a population of mesenchymal progenitor cells derived from cells that are liberated by enzymatic breakdown of local stump tissues. This blastema grows and eventually redifferentiates to replace the lost tissue with a nearly exact copy of the original.

In adult humans, spontaneous regeneration is limited to bone and liver; regeneration of other tissues can also occur in fetuses and newborns. Human bone regenerates by maintaining a reserve of embryonic stem cells throughout adulthood. Liver regenerates in a different manner, via local dedifferentiation of cells, similar to blastema formation in urodeles.

In contrast to bone and liver, which can regenerate after injury, musculoskeletal soft tissues tend to heal through formation of relatively weak, disorganized scar tissue. Severe ligament sprains can be particularly problematic; even in the best case, there is a fibrotic repair response that remodels over several years, causing scar tissue that is structurally and biomechanically inferior to the normal tissue. For most soft tissues, the fibrotic repair process is thought to interfere with the possibility of regeneration; i.e., there is a “race” between repair and regeneration, and repair wins. This makes sense from an evolutionary standpoint: rapid repair renders functionality to the injured tissue, enhancing chances for survival in the wild. On the contrary, the repair tissue is disorganized and weak and does not necessarily restore full function.

Soft tissues typically heal by fibrosis, potentially impairing regeneration, but the ACL presents a worst-case scenario regarding to healing. Following complete rupture, the torn ends of the ACL retract toward the bone, leaving a large gap that is difficult to close by natural healing or primary surgical repair. Thus, surgical reconstruction is recommended to restore ACL function. However, currently available grafts and biomaterials are not completely satisfactory for this purpose.

Limitations in Currently Available Grafts and Biomaterials

ACL reconstruction has been performed using various collagenous tissues *(23)*, including fascia lata, semitendinosus, meniscus, iliotibial band, and the mid-third patellar tendon, which remains the gold standard *(24)*. Biological grafts undergo four phases after implantation: necrosis, repopulation by cells and blood vessels, remodeling, and maturation *(2)*. Necrosis occurs rapidly postimplantation, even for vascularized autografts. After the necrosis period, extrinsic cells and blood vessels gradually repopulate the graft. The gradual breakdown of the graft tissue during remodeling causes a significant loss of tensile strength. Finally, during maturation, deposition and rearrangement of new collagen occurs, causing a gain in strength.

Although the repopulated graft matures in response to its new mechanical and nutritional environment, a process termed “ligamentization” *(25)*, the tensile strength and collagen fibril diameter distribution of the normal ACL are not reestablished *(26)*. In fact, preclinical studies show that even at 1 yr postimplantation, the breaking load of the graft ranges from only 11 to 52% of the normal ACL *(27,28)*. The scar tissue that forms is inferior to normal ACL tissue; biological grafts do not restore normal joint function and biomechanics. Presently, efforts are being made to improve the efficacy of allografts or xenografts using tissue modifications *(29)*, such as cryopreservation, decellularization *(30)*, protein engineering, and genetic engineering. These graft-enhancing technologies are promising but beyond the scope of this chapter.

Because of the problems and complications associated with biological grafts, great interest exists in developing synthetic substitutes to replace a torn ACL. Synthetic polymeric ACL prostheses have several potential advantages over biological grafts: preserving local autogenous structures, avoiding potential disease transmission related to allografts, high initial strength, and ease of fabrication, sterilization, and storage. For several decades, there were major research efforts to develop a completely prosthetic ACL from traditional biomaterials, but these efforts failed, and there is currently no synthetic ACL prosthesis approved by the US Food and Drug Administration (FDA) for primary ACL reconstruction *(31)*. Synthetic polymers clinically evaluated for ACL reconstruction included polytetrafluoroethylene (Gore-Tex), polyethylene terephthalate (Dacron; Stryker-Meadox and Leeds-Keio ligaments), carbon fibers (Integraft), and braided polypropylene (Kennedy Ligament Augmentation Device). Clinical ACL reconstruction studies using prostheses have generally shown poor long-term results because of persistent pain, synovitis, sterile effusions, arthritis, and mechanical breakdown of the synthetic polymers.

In conclusion, there are at least three major challenges associated with ACL regeneration: (1) the complex structure and function of the ACL; (2) the poor healing response of the ACL, coupled with the natural tendency for fibrotic repair instead of regeneration; and (3) the limitations of currently available grafts and biomaterials. Can a tissue engineering strategy be designed and implemented to overcome these significant challenges?

TISSUE ENGINEERING STRATEGIES FOR ACL REGENERATION

Tissue engineering is an emerging discipline that blends the fields of biomaterials, bioengineering, and cell biology and has the goal of inducing tissue repair or regeneration. What differentiates this from more traditional biomaterials fields is that implants are designed to induce a response from the recipient and provide a biological tissue replacement. Typically, a temporary biomaterial scaffold, cells, and/or cell signals are combined in vitro or in vivo to elicit the desired response. This approach sharply contrasts the use of permanent prostheses, which are intended to remain inert over long periods of time. Tissue engineering is being explored for virtually all fields of medicine and surgery, and it is likely that as this field develops, the need for biological grafts and traditional prostheses will be greatly diminished.

The success of tissue-engineered ACL regeneration depends on three principal factors, each with several variables: the characteristics of the implant (scaffolds, cells, and cell signals), surgical procedure (multivariate), and the postsurgery rehabilitation protocol. One logical approach to ACL regeneration is to mimic "spontaneous regeneration" that occurs in limbs of lower vertebrate species and certain tissues in adult humans. In these cases, regeneration recapitulates embryonic development to a certain extent. Examples include limb regeneration in urodeles via local cell dedifferentiation to form a blastema *(22)* and bone regeneration in humans via reserves of embryonic stem cells. Taking cues from nature, our group and other investigators are combining resorbable scaffolds, cells, and cell signals to form a "blastema-like" template for tendon *(32)* or ACL regeneration. To reiterate, the feasibility of this tissue engineering approach has been established *(33,34)*, but true ACL regeneration has not yet been realized.

Resorbable Polymeric Scaffolds for ACL Regeneration

Similar to a scaffold erected around a building under repair, tissue engineering scaffolds are designed to provide temporary mechanical support and serve as a substratum for the attachment, migration, and activities of the "workers" (cells). The success of a scaffold-based implant depends on the well-coordinated timing of implant resorption and new tissue in-growth. Scaffolds for ligament reconstruction are typically biomimetic, designed to be similar to normal ligaments: complex composite materials with continuous fibers aligned in parallel within a deformable matrix. Various textile configurations, e.g., yarns or braids, also provide constructs with different mechanical and biological properties.

Scaffold Design Criteria

Tissue engineering scaffolds for ACL reconstruction can be of natural or synthetic origin but must satisfy diverse design criteria. The criteria involves mechanical properties, biocompatibility, and a "moderate" resorption rate to gradually transfer mechanical loads to in-growing neoligament tissue. As in all engineering designs, there are trade-offs with optimizing scaffold performance, and it is difficult, if not impossible, to satisfy all the design criteria. For example, currently available synthetic materials are generally deficient relevant to tissue interactions, whereas for natural materials, the mechanical properties and resorption rates are difficult to reproducibly control.

Clearly, there are special mechanical considerations for tissue engineering applications in the musculoskeletal system, because these tissues (and their replacements) must bear significant mechanical loads. In fact, several early attempts to develop tissue-engineered tendons or ligaments failed because the biomaterial scaffold had inadequate strength and stiffness. Examples include the use of relatively weak collagen gels seeded with cells in vitro. Although these constructs appeared to be "ligament-like" based on histology and/or biochemical markers, they lacked the key ingredient required for a ligament: mechanical strength.

Recently, the concept of functional tissue engineering emerged, emphasizing the need to consider the role of biomechanics in tissue engineered constructs *(35)*. How these principles are important in the design of ACL regeneration scaffolds is briefly discussed. The first four principles involve understanding the mechanical state of the normal tissue: (1) measuring stress/strain histories in vivo; (2) measuring the mechanical properties under subfailure and failure conditions; (3) selecting and prioritizing a subset of these mechanical properties; and (4) setting standards to evaluate surgical outcomes. For ACL regeneration scaffolds, it is critical to consider these mechanical factors.

Several studies have determined actual stresses and/or strains generated in the ACL during knee loading in animals *(36)* or humans *(37,38)*. The loads generated during normal usage are well below the failure load of the ACL and vary within the anteromedial and posterolateral bundle as a function of loading conditions. The mechanical properties of isolated femur-ACL-tibia complexes have also been studied under subfailure and failure conditions. The structural properties (breaking load, stiffness, and extensibility) and material properties (ultimate strength, modulus, and ultimate strain) of various tendons and ligaments have been determined from uniaxial constant strain rate failure testing *(39,40)*. The ACL is anisotropic, nonlinear, and viscoelastic (experiences creep and stress relaxation), making it even more difficult to match its properties. To obtain design criteria, these mechanical properties must be prioritized, according to the most important to restore normal knee function and mechanics. The stiffness certainly is critical because it influences load sharing between the implant and neoligament tissue. If the implant is too stiff, the neoligament tissue will not bear significant loads, and may atrophy from stress-shielding. Viscoelastic properties are also significant because the knee is loaded cyclically. Finally, standards should be set to evaluate surgical outcomes; these must be based largely on mechanical performance and, in clinical studies, patient satisfaction. Again, the reader is referred to the excellent seminal article by Butler, Goldstein, and Guilak for a more complete treatment of this topic *(35)*.

Another level of difficulty is that the tissue-engineered ACL is designed to gradually degrade, lose strength, and transfer mechanical loads to newly formed neoligament tissue. The optimal rate of scaffold strength loss is not known, but two extreme cases are unsatisfactory. If the implant remains too stiff for too long, stress shielding will occur, and the neoligament tissue may not mature owing to lack of mechanical loading. At the other extreme, if the implant is initially too weak, or resorbs too rapidly, mechanical failure will occur before neoligament tissue can form and bear loads. Ideally, the mass resorption of the implant would coincide with the strength loss so that a "nonfunctional implant" would not take up space needed for neoligament tissue formation.

It is important to note that biological properties are also critical to the scaffold design. The scaffold must be biocompatible and capable of supporting or inducing tissue in-growth and remodeling. Thus, only scaffolds containing biocompatible polymers were investigated, including collagen and various synthetics.

Collagen Fiber-Based Scaffolds

Type I collagen is a candidate biomaterial for this application because of its unique physical, chemical, and biological properties. Collagen is a triple-helical protein that self-assembles into strong rope-like fibers that provide mechanical stability to all tissues of the body. Collagen is the major structural component of connective tissues *(41)*, especially the tendon and ligament *(12)*. Collagen can be extracted from tissues and processed into high-strength fibers *(42)* and scaffolds with mechanical behavior similar to that of autografts *(43)*. Collagen is widely used in cell culture studies because fibroblasts attach, proliferate, and secrete matrix on collagen scaffolds. Collagen has numerous biological functions, serving as the natural scaffold supporting cell attachment, proliferation, and matrix synthesis within the body. The resorption rate of collagen can be controlled by the extent of crosslinking *(44–46)*. Collagen is not highly antigenic *(47)* and is chemotactic for fibroblasts and other cells involved in tissue repair *(48)*. Several groups have explored the use of tissue-derived biomaterials and/or purified collagen for reconstruction of tendon *(32)*, meniscus *(49)*, or ACL *(50–52)*; this section focuses on efforts from the author's laboratory.

In our studies, collagen fibers (50–100 μm diameter) for ACL reconstruction scaffolds are made by extruding a 1% (w/v) acid-insoluble bovine dermal collagen dispersion into saline solution, rinsing, and drying under tension. Fibers are crosslinked to improve the mechanical properties and control the resorption rate after implantation. The wet tensile strength of individual extruded collagen fibers (40–80 MPa) is comparable to that of native ligament tissue. Composite collagen scaffolds for implantation are made by embedding several hundred to several thousand (depending on the animal model) parallel continuous collagen fibers within a collagen or synthetic polymeric matrix.

Feasibility studies demonstrated that collagen fiber–based scaffolds can induce tissue ingrowth and gain strength (similar to biological grafts) following reconstruction of the Achilles tendon *(43)* or ACL *(53)*. Collagen scaffolds for ACL reconstruction were made by aligning 225 crosslinked type I collagen fibers (60-μm diameter) in an uncrosslinked type I collagen matrix. The ACL was removed in skeletally mature rabbits and reconstructed using an acellular collagen scaffold implanted through the anatomic ACL attachment sites. Polymethylmethacrylate cement was used to secure the scaffolds within the femoral and tibial bone tunnels.

In our initial study *(53)*, about 50% of the collagen scaffold implants ruptured before adequate neoligament tissue was formed, partly because of surgical and rehabilitation factors. Most failures were likely a result of unrestricted knee motion postsurgery (animals were not immobilized), which cut the device at the sharp bone tunnel interface.

The other half of the implanted scaffolds induced formation of functional, intact neoligament tissue connecting the femur and tibia. At 4-wk postimplantation, neoligament tissue was composed of newly deposited collagen, fibroblasts, and inflammatory cells within the implanted collagen fiber scaffold. At 20-wk postimplantation, the dehydrothermal-cyanamide crosslinked scaffolds appeared to be completely resorbed (based on light microscopic observations) and were completely replaced by aligned functional neoligament tissue. The strength of the neoligament at 4-wk postimplantation was less than that of an unimplanted collagen scaffold. However, at 20 wk, the neoligament strength had increased to 17 MPa, exceeding the strength of the unimplanted scaffold. Acellular collagen scaffolds initially lost strength, then strength increased from tissue ingrowth and remodeling, similar to the behavior of biological grafts.

The bone tunnel attachment sites contained new bone at the periphery of the surgical drill holes, approaching the fibrous neoligament. In a follow-up study, we further evaluated the bone tissue response to acellular collagen fiber scaffolds. Results suggest that bone and fibrocartilage tissue in-growth or "biological fixation' might effectively secure the scaffolds within the surgical bone tunnels *(54)*.

Collagen fiber-based scaffolds have the potential to be developed into ACL regeneration scaffolds, but further work is needed. The use of proteinase inhibitors may improve control of the collagen degradation rate. For example, when matrix metalloproteinases are inhibited in dermal wounds, the wound strength increases *(55)*. Our laboratory has explored various crosslinking methods to improve collagen fiber scaffold performance for ACL reconstruction, including chemical methods (carbodiimides and glutaraldehyde; *56,57*) and so-called "physical" methods (dehydrothermal treatment and ultraviolet light; *45,46*). Typically, chemical crosslinkers compromise biocompatibility to some extent, whereas physical methods can partially denature collagen, leading to a more rapid resorption rate.

Collagen-based materials have many advantages, but they are difficult to reproducibly fabricate, and there are no ideal sterilization methods for collagen *(58)*. Thus, we are also exploring the use of synthetic polymeric fiber–based scaffolds and collagen-synthetic hybrid scaffolds for ACL regeneration.

Synthetic Polymeric Fiber-Based Scaffolds

Synthetic resorbable polymeric fibers are appealing for this application because critical properties, e.g., strength, strength retention, and degradation rate, can be tailored during processing. We are evaluating both the polyarylate and polycarbonate families of tyrosine-derived polymers *(59)*. By making small variations in the backbone structure and pendant chain length, a broad series of physical properties (strength, stiffness, degradation rate, Tg, and surface tension) can be customized within these families of polymers. Polycarbonates and polyarylates are typically amorphous polymers, soluble in a wide selection of organic solvents. Both have glass transition temperatures (<100°C) significantly lower than their decomposition temperature (>300°C), allowing for various processing modes, such as conventional solvent casting, evaporation techniques, extrusion, compression molding, and fabrication into complex shapes by injection molding.

Poly(DTE adipate), one of the polyarylates, was initially selected based on favorable mechanical and resorption properties found previously for rods and films *(60)*. Fibers of these polymers had not been made previously. As a first screening test for these new polymeric fibers, we evaluated the strength retention, mass loss, and molecular weight (MW) loss of poly(DTE adipate) fibers as a function of time in vitro. Poly(DTE adipate) polymer (100 kDa = initial MW) was spun into 150-μm diameter fibers. Fibers had an initial strength of 48.1 ± 7.4 MPa with a MW of 88 ± 2 kDa. Fibers ($n = 8$ per group) were incubated in phosphate-buffered saline at 37°C for 0, 1, 2, 4, 8, 16, and 32 wk. After 1 wk of incubation, the strength decreased to about half of the initial value. By wk 16, strength decreased to 10 MPa. Mechanical integrity was lost by 32 wk. There was a continuing decrease in MW throughout the experiment but no mass loss. Poly(DTE adipate) fibers had slightly higher initial strength and degradation rate than reported for films. The mechanical properties and degradation rate of poly(DTE adipate) fibers were within the range suitable for use in an ACL reconstruction device.

Based on these in vitro results, our next step was to evaluate in vivo strength retention and the tissue response to poly(DTE adipate) fibers. Because this polymer degrades hydrolytically, rather than enzymatically, similar degradation behavior was expected in vivo. Scaffold implants (4-cm length) were made by aligning 100 poly(DTE adipate) fibers in parallel. Scaffolds were sterilized by cold ethylene oxide. The implants were placed subcutaneously in five mature male rats that were sacrificed at 2, 4, or 8 wk. At all time periods, there was significant fibrous tissue in-growth surrounding individual fibers. No unusual inflammatory response was observed throughout the length of the study. The poly(DTE adipate) scaffolds had 73% MW retention at 4 wk in vivo. By 8 wk, MW retention significantly decreased to 36% of the initial value.

The initial mechanical properties of synthetic tyrosine-derived polyarylate and polycarbonate fibers are in the same range as those of collagen fibers; however, the synthetics have improved strength retention in comparison to collagen. The synthetic fiber scaffolds have also shown excellent biocompatibility and tissue in-growth in a subcutaneous implantation model. Based on our preliminary results and previous work by Kohn's group *(60)*, we selected tyrosine-derived polyarylates (intermediate-strength retention) and polycarbonates (prolonged-strength retention) as model polymer systems to test the effects of scaffold strength retention on neoligament formation. The strength retention of these polymers can be tailored by subtle changes in the polymer backbone and pendant chain. These groups of synthetic resorbable polymers are currently being investigated for use as ACL regeneration scaffolds *(61)*. Other groups have used polylactide-glycolide polymer-based fibers *(62)* and silk fibers *(63)* as experimental ACL reconstruction scaffolds.

Hybrid (Natural-Synthetic) Scaffolds

Another strategy to improve the properties of fibrous composites is to combine natural and synthetic fibers and/or modify the matrix surrounding the fibers. We fabricated hybrid (natural-synthetic) composites by embedding parallel collagen fibers within a polylactic acid (PLA) matrix *(64)*. PLA was applied by dipping 500 collagen fibers in a 10% solution of L-PLA in chloroform and drying overnight under vacuum.

The mechanical properties, resorption rates, and subcutaneous tissue reactions were determined for collagen–PLA and collagen–collagen composites. The tensile strength and modulus of collagen–PLA composites were twice that of collagen–collagen composites. Subcutaneous fibrous tissue in-growth was improved, and implant resorption was slightly delayed in the collagen–PLA composites.

ACL reconstruction surgeries were also performed in rabbits using collagen–PLA composite implants. After 4 wk, neoligament tissue was observed in seven of eight implants; however, four neoligaments had ruptured either in the midsubstance ($n = 2$) or at the bone tunnel interface ($n = 2$). These results and our previous work suggest that resorbable polymeric composite scaffolds are potentially useful for ACL reconstruction. Again, these resorbable implants must be protected from excessive mechanical loading during the formation of host neoligament tissue.

We are currently investigating various types of synthetic polymeric matrices and fibers as scaffolds for ACL reconstruction. Others developed a hybrid tissue-engineered ACL device, consisting of a poly(L-lactic acid) fiber braid filled with collagen *(65)*.

In summary, scaffolds for ACL regeneration must meet rigorous mechanical and biological design criteria. Natural and synthetic fibers are potentially useful as scaffolds, and a combination of the two may be needed to satisfy the design criteria. Of course, scaffolds should interact with cells and cell signals to form new tissue and enable ACL regeneration.

Cells and Cell Signals to Promote ACL Regeneration

Although scaffolds provide temporary mechanical support, the long-term success of tissue-engineered devices depends on cells to deposit and remodel new matrix; cell signals are critical to this process. Growth factors have tremendous potential to improve tissue repair or induce regeneration, but these soluble factors may need to be incorporated into delivery vehicles (scaffolds) with appropriate release rates. Mechanical loads provide critical signals that influence normal musculoskeletal tissue development, growth, remodeling, and repair. When deprived of mechanical loads, musculoskeletal tissues atrophy; increased loads cause hypertrophy. Yet, until very recently, mechanical loads were not routinely applied to developing tissue analogs in vitro. Our laboratory is investigating cell seeding and various cell signals, including delivery of growth factors, genes, and mechanical loads to enhance ligament analog formation in vitro and ligament regeneration in vivo.

Development of Cell-Seeded "Ligament Analogs"

Toward the long-term goal of providing an embryonic or regenerative environment, a blastema-like structure or supply of locally active cells, we hypothesized that neoligament formation can be influenced by preseeding a scaffold with autogenous fibroblasts in vitro, creating a viable "ligament analog" for ACL reconstruction. Similar "tissue analogs" have been developed by others to repair large defects in skin and cartilage. In theory, preseeding a scaffold with autogenous cells might improve neoligament formation in the short term by controlling extracellular matrix deposition and the recruitment of local cells and may improve in the long term by influencing scaffold resorption and neoligament remodeling.

We fabricated ligament analogs in vitro by seeding high-strength resorbable collagen fiber scaffolds with intra-articular (ACL) or extra-articular (patellar tendon [PT]) fibroblasts *(66)*. Fibroblasts explanted from rabbit or human tissues were cultured and seeded onto collagen scaffolds. Fibroblasts attached and proliferated on collagen fiber bundles and deposited new collagen within the ligament analogs in vitro. The cells adhered rapidly to the collagen scaffolds, spread along the long axis of the collagen fibers, proliferated, and remained viable for weeks in vitro. Fibroblast function was a mechanism of the culture substratum (ligament analog vs tissue culture plate) and the origin of the fibroblasts (ACL vs PT). PT fibroblasts proliferated more rapidly than ACL fibroblasts when cultured on ligament analogs. Collagen synthesis by ACL and PT fibroblasts was approximately tenfold greater on ligament analogs than tissue culture plates. The composition, structure, and geometry of the collagen fiber scaffolds may promote collagen synthesis within ligament analogs in vitro. These findings suggest that collagen fiber scaffolds influence cell behavior and collagen deposition, which is potentially beneficial following implantation.

However, possible benefits depend on sustained viability of the seeded cells following implantation into the knee joint. In ACL reconstruction surgery, implants are placed intra-articularly, surrounded by synovial fluid. Because the joint environment is relatively avascular, and nutrition may be compromised, the viability and function of a fibroblast-seeded ligament analog implanted in this environment is of particular interest.

The next question we addressed was whether these living ligament analogs would remain viable after implantation *(67)*. We examined the fate of autogenous ACL and skin fibroblasts that were seeded on ligament analogs and implanted into the knee joint space. ACL and skin fibroblasts that were harvested, cultured, labeled, seeded on collagen fiber scaffolds in vitro, and implanted into the autogenous knee joint remained viable for at least 4–6 wk postimplantation. Thus, fibroblast-seeded ligament analogs may impact neoligament formation and remodeling. Studies are in progress to compare the efficacy of acellular scaffolds vs fibroblast-seeded ligament analogs in a load-bearing ACL reconstruction surgery model.

These results indicate that synovial fluid provides sufficient nutrition to sustain ACL or skin cells transplanted into the joint space. We selected skin as a possible source of fibroblasts because it is easily accessible in a clinical setting, and it has a robust healing potential. Although skin fibroblasts normally reside in an extrasynovial environment, they survived transplantation into the relatively harsh environment of the synovial joint. ACL fibroblasts also survived in the knee joint space, but their potential to improve neoligament formation may be limited by a poor intrinsic healing capacity. For example, relative to fibroblasts of the medial collateral ligament (MCL), ACL fibroblasts have decreased rates of migration, adhesion, proliferation, and collagen synthesis. Thus, it may be necessary to seed with a different type of fibroblast or to use cells genetically modified to optimize neoligament formation.

This preliminary work established the feasibility of harvesting, culturing, seeding, implanting, and tracking fibroblasts on viable ligament analogs grown in the laboratory. This approach would not specifically result in ACL regeneration, but it might enhance repair or formation of neoligament tissue. However, these studies establish the foundation for future studies, such as seeding a high-strength scaffold with pluripotential mesenchymal cells to create an ACL regeneration blastema. Autogenous mesenchymal stem cell–seeded collagen gels appear to enhance healing of Achilles tendon defects *(68)*. Prockop recently reviewed the potential uses of marrow stem cells for nonhematopoietic tissues, including tissue engineering applications for musculoskeletal tissues *(69)*.

Local Delivery of Growth Factors and Genes

Growth factors are soluble peptides that influence normal tissue morphogenesis, repair, and regeneration. Platelet-derived growth factor (PDGF) and transforming growth factor β (TGF-β) are present in the normal healing response of the MCL and ACL. PDGF or a combination of TGF-β and epidermal growth factor administered locally in a soluble form can improve MCL healing *(70,71)*. In vitro research implies that growth factors may enhance repair by increasing ligament fibroblast proliferation *(72–75)* and matrix synthesis *(76,77)*.

A potential problem with these soluble growth factors is rapid diffusion away from the site where activity is required in vivo. The duration of growth factor activity may be prolonged by incorporating these soluble factors within a scaffold delivery vehicle, e.g., bone morphogenetic protein delivered via a collagen sponge enhanced tendon healing in a bone tunnel *(78)*.

Finally, genetic alteration of seeded cells, including stem cells *(79)* and other gene therapies, are rapidly emerging technologies that will complement and expand tissue engineering methods to tissue repair. Gene delivery may be advantageous when compared to protein delivery. Tendon–bone integration was improved by bone morphogenetic protein gene delivery *(80)*; therapeutic genes can also be delivered directly to ligaments using various vectors *(81,82)*. Like growth factors, genes should be delivered locally over some period of time to maximize efficacy. The concept of sustained local gene delivery from biomaterials is in its infancy. A "gene activated matrix," a polylactic-glycolic acid or collagen scaffold soaked with plasmid DNA prior to implantation *(83)* is potentially useful to encourage repair of various tissues. However, it is difficult to control the rate and duration of gene delivery, and delivery vehicles generally have poor mechanical properties *(84)*.

Mechanical Loads and Postoperative Rehabilitation

Mechanical loads provide critical signals that influence cells *(85,86)* and help control musculoskeletal tissue development, growth, remodeling, and repair *(87,88)*. Mechanical loads can increase collagen production by ligament fibroblasts and interact synergistically with growth factors to influence fibroblast behavior *(89)*. Yet, until recently, mechanical loads were not routinely used to influence tissue analog development in vitro.

Note the concept of functional tissue engineering *(35)*, and its first four principles, as discussed in the Scaffold Design Criteria section. The last two principles of functional tissue engineering involve interactions between mechanical signals and cells: physical regulation of cells on matrices in vivo and physical stimulation of cell-scaffold constructs in vitro *(35)*. It is now well accepted that mechanical loads have a major role in regulating cell behavior in vitro and in vivo. For example, mechanical loads cause morphological changes in fibroblast-seeded collagen lattices *(90)* and influence collagen gene expression by ACLs in vitro *(91)*. Mechanical loading also affects graft remodeling and biological fixation of ACL grafts in vivo *(92)*. Therefore, patients undergoing

ACL reconstruction who receive grafts are typically exposed to protected loading or continuous passive motion shortly after surgery *(93)*. Early motion prevents excessive scar formation in the joint and stimulates healing and remodeling of tissues. However, postoperative rehabilitation protocols will likely need to be redesigned for tissue-engineered ligament regeneration devices, because their initial mechanical properties and changes in properties postoperatively are not necessarily similar to biological grafts. The process of tissue regeneration may be prolonged in comparison to rapid scar formation; thus, prolonged rehabilitation may be a prerequisite for ACL regeneration.

Technical, Regulatory, and Social Issues

There are important issues that need to be resolved as the field of tissue engineering transforms from the bench to the bedside *(94)*. The first generation of tissue-engineered products (primarily for skin repair) have successfully overcome many of these challenges *(95)*. Many concerns remain regarding the development, clinical use, and safety of tissue-engineered devices *(96)*.

From a technical standpoint, there are many unknowns about interactions between scaffolds, cells, and cell signals. Can a scaffold meet mechanical and biological requirements? Does cell seeding improve implant performance? If so, by what mechanisms? Are the effects of cells short term, or are there long-term benefits? Implantation studies comparing acellular vs cell-seeded scaffolds are required. Should autogenic (self), allogenic (human donor), or xenogenic (animal) tissues *(97)* or cells be used? Can stem cells be led to differentiate into various tissue types? How can gene therapy be incorporated into designs? Is gene therapy safe? What are the optimal conditions to harvest, grow, sterilize, store, and ship cells and cell-seeded implants? It is difficult enough to make a few functional devices for ACL reconstruction in the laboratory; imagine the complexity associated with scale-up and manufacture of a tissue-engineered ligament device.

In addition to the technical and manufacturing obstacles, there are challenges with federal regulation of tissue-engineered implants. Regulation of tissue-engineered devices by the FDA in the United States is still in development *(98)*, and there are serious regulatory concerns in Europe *(99,100)*. Are these new implants categorized as tissues, drugs, devices, or combination of these designations? The regulatory pathways for these categories are quite different. Can the same safety and efficacy tests used to evaluate traditional inert biomaterials be used for tissue-engineered devices?

Finally, there are political and socioeconomic issues, including government funding of research, corporate liability, medical insurance reimbursement, and ethical concerns. Currently, the use of embryonic stem cells is controversial *(101)*, and research funding is limited by the US government. Companies may be reluctant to develop novel tissue-engineered implants because of liability issues. Furthermore, a new implant must have significant advantages over the existing standard of care to be considered for reimbursement by medical insurers.

SUMMARY

Tissue engineering strategies may provide alternatives to biological grafts and permanent prostheses by improving repair or inducing regeneration of soft connective tissues, such as skin, cartilage, meniscus, and ligaments. The success of the musculoskeletal soft-tissue reconstruction procedure depends on three major factors: implant characteristics (scaffolds, cells, and signals), surgical procedure, and the postsurgery rehabilitation protocol. Tissue-engineered implants combine three dominant components: scaffolds, cells, and signals. Scaffold design generally involves trade-offs between biocompatibility and other physical–mechanical properties. The mechanical properties, resorption rate, and strength retention requirements vary according to the type of tissue being replaced. It is likely that natural and synthetic material properties must be combined to achieve the ideal ligament reconstruction scaffold.

Surgery and rehabilitation protocols must be carefully designed for tissue-engineered implants that may not behave the same as grafts or permanent prostheses. Many other technical, regulatory, and business challenges should be addressed in the development of tissue-engineered ACL devices. Nonetheless, over the next several decades, the use of biological grafts and traditional prostheses will probably diminish as tissue engineering gradually moves from the bench to the bedside.

ACKNOWLEDGMENTS

The author's research on tissue-engineered ligaments has been funded by grants from the National Institutes of Health-NIAMS (R01-AR42230 and R29-AR42230), the Whitaker Foundation, the Orthopaedic Research and Education Foundation, the Musculoskeletal Transplant Foundation, the International Foundation for Ethical Research, the New Jersey Commission on Science and Technology, the Foundation of UMDNJ, and the New Jersey Center for Biomaterials.

REFERENCES

1. Jaureguito JW, Paulos LE. Why grafts fail. *Clin Orthop* 1996;325:25–41.
2. Corsetti JR, Jackson DW. Failure of anterior cruciate ligament reconstruction: the biologic basis. *Clin Orthop* 1996;325:42–49.
3. Petersen W, Tillmann B. Structure and vascularization of the cruciate ligaments of the human knee joint. *Anat Embryol (Berl)* 1999;200:325–334.
4. Dodds JA, Arnoczky SP. Anatomy of the anterior cruciate ligament: a blueprint for repair and reconstruction. *Arthroscopy* 1994;10:132–139.
5. Noyes FR, Grood ES. The strength of the anterior cruciate ligament in humans and Rhesus monkeys. *J Bone Joint Surg Am* 1976;58:1074–1082.
6. Arnoczky SP. Anatomy of the anterior cruciate ligament. *Clin Orthop* 1983;172:19–25.
7. Odensten M, Gillquist J. Functional anatomy of the anterior cruciate ligament and a rationale for reconstruction. *J Bone Joint Surg Am* 1985;67:257–262.
8. Fuss FK. Anatomy of the cruciate ligaments and their function in extension and flexion of the human knee joint. *Am J Anat* 1989;184:165–176.
9. Girgis FG, Marshall JL, Monajem A. The cruciate ligaments of the knee joint. Anatomical, functional and experimental analysis. *Clin Orthop* 1975;106:216–231.
10. Danylchuk KD, Finlay JB, Krcek JP. Microstructural organization of human and bovine cruciate ligaments. *Clin Orthop* 1978;131:294–298.
11. Clark JM, Sidles JA. The interrelation of fiber bundles in the anterior cruciate ligament. *J Orthop Res* 1990;8:180–188.
12. Amiel D, et al. Tendons and ligaments: a morphological and biochemical comparison. *J Orthop Res* 1984;1:257–265.
13. Nagineni CN, et al. Characterization of the intrinsic properties of the anterior cruciate and medial collateral ligament cells: an in vitro cell culture study. *J Orthop Res* 1992;10: 465–475.

14. Arnoczky SP. Blood supply to the anterior cruciate ligament and supporting structures. *Orthop Clin North Am* 1985;16:15–28.
15. Amiel D, Billings Jr E, Harwood FL. Collagenase activity in anterior cruciate ligament: protective role of the synovial sheath. *J Appl Physiol* 1990;69:902–906.
16. Cooper RR, Misol S. Tendon and ligament insertion. A light and electron microscopic study. *J Bone Joint Surg Am* 1970;52:1–20.
17. Visconti CS, et al. Biochemical analysis of collagens at the ligament-bone interface reveals presence of cartilage-specific collagens. *Arch Biochem Biophys* 1996;328:135–142.
18. Benjamin M, Ralphs JR. Fibrocartilage in tendons and ligaments—an adaptation to compressive load. *J Anat* 1998;193:481–494.
19. Koski JA, Ibarra C, Rodeo SA. Tissue-engineered ligament: cells, matrix, and growth factors. *Orthop Clin North Am* 2000;31:437–452.
20. Friden T, et al. Proprioception after an acute knee ligament injury: a longitudinal study on 16 consecutive patients. *J Orthop Res* 1997;15:637–644.
21. Goertzen M, et al. Neurohistological findings after experimental anterior cruciate ligament allograft transplantation. *Arch Orthop Trauma Surg* 1992;111:126–129.
22. Brockes JP. Amphibian limb regeneration: rebuilding a complex structure. *Science* 1997; 276:81–87.
23. Miller SL, Gladstone JN. Graft selection in anterior cruciate ligament reconstruction. *Orthop Clin North Am* 2002;33:675–683.
24. Johnson RJ, et al. The treatment of injuries of the anterior cruciate ligament. *J Bone Joint Surg Am* 1992;74:140–151.
25. Amiel D, et al. The phenomenon of "ligamentization": anterior cruciate ligament reconstruction with autogenous patellar tendon. *J Orthop Res* 1986;4:162–172.
26. Bosch U, Kasperczyk WJ. Healing of the patellar tendon autograft after posterior cruciate ligament reconstruction—a process of ligamentization? An experimental study in a sheep model. *Am J Sports Med* 1992;20:558–566.
27. Ballock RT, et al. Use of patellar tendon autograft for anterior cruciate ligament reconstruction in the rabbit: a long-term histologic and biomechanical study. *J Orthop Res* 1989; 7:474–485.
28. Clancy Jr WG, et al. Anterior and posterior cruciate ligament reconstruction in rhesus monkeys. *J Bone Joint Surg Am* 1981;63:1270–1284.
29. Black KS, Goldstein S, Ollerenshaw J. Tissue modifications. *Transplant Proc* 1998;30: 2729–2731.
30. Cartmell JS, Dunn MG. Effect of chemical treatments on tendon cellularity and mechanical properties. *J Biomed Mater Res* 2000;49:134–140.
31. Dunn MG. Biomechanics of ligament reconstruction. In Tria AJ, ed., *Ligaments of the Knee*. Churchill Livingstone, New York, NY, 1995.
32. Butler DL, Awad HA. Perspectives on cell and collagen composites for tendon repair. *Clin Orthop* 1999;367:S324–332.
33. Dunn MG, et al. The tissue engineering approach to ligament reconstruction. *Mater Res Soc Symp Proc* 1994;331:13–16.
34. Dunn MG. Tissue engineering strategies for ligament reconstruction. *MRS Bulletin* 1996; 21:43–46.
35. Butler DL, Goldstein SA, Guilak F. Functional tissue engineering: the role of biomechanics. *J Biomech Eng* 2000;122:570–575.
36. Holden JP, et al. In vivo forces in the anterior cruciate ligament: direct measurements during walking and trotting in a quadruped. *J Biomech* 1994;27:517–526.
37. Sakane M, et al. In situ forces in the anterior cruciate ligament and its bundles in response to anterior tibial loads. *J Orthop Res* 1997;15:285–293.
38. Livesay GA, et al. Evaluation of the effect of joint constraints on the in situ force distribution in the anterior cruciate ligament. *J Orthop Res* 1997;15:278–284.

39. Butler DL, et al. Biomechanics of ligaments and tendons. *Exerc Sport Sci Rev* 1978;6: 125–181.
40. Butler DL, et al. On the interpretation of our anterior cruciate ligament data. *Clin Orthop* 1985;196:26–34.
41. Burgeson RE, Nimni ME. Collagen types. Molecular structure and tissue distribution. *Clin Orthop* 1992;282:250–272.
42. Kato YP, et al. Mechanical properties of collagen fibres: a comparison of reconstituted and rat tail tendon fibres. *Biomaterials* 1989;10:38–42.
43. Kato YP, et al. Regeneration of Achilles tendon with a collagen tendon prosthesis. Results of a one-year implantation study. *J Bone Joint Surg Am* 1991;73:561–574.
44. Weadock K, Olson RM, Silver FH. Evaluation of collagen crosslinking techniques. *Biomater Med Devices Artif Organs* 1983;11:293–318.
45. Weadock KS, Miller EJ, Bellincampi LD, Zawadsky JP, Dunn MG. Physical crosslinking of collagen fibers: comparison of ultraviolet irradiation and dehydrothermal treatment. *J Biomed Mater Res* 1995;29:1373–1379.
46. Weadock KS, Miller EJ, Keuffel EL, Dunn MG. Effect of physical crosslinking methods on collagen-fiber durability in proteolytic solutions. *J Biomed Mater Res* 1996;32: 221–226.
47. DeLustro F, et al. Immune responses to allogeneic and xenogeneic implants of collagen and collagen derivatives. *Clin Orthop* 1990;260:263–279.
48. Postlethwaite AE, Seyer JM, Kang AH. Chemotactic attraction of human fibroblasts to type I, II, and III collagens and collagen-derived peptides. *Proc Natl Acad Sci USA* 1978; 75:871–875.
49. Cook JL, et al. Kinetic study of the replacement of porcine small intestinal submucosa grafts and the regeneration of meniscal-like tissue in large avascular meniscal defects in dogs. *Tissue Eng* 2001;7:321–334.
50. Kemp PD, Cavallaro JF, Hastings DN. Effects of carbodiimide crosslinking and load environment on the remodeling of collagen scaffolds. *Tissue Eng* 1995;1:71–79.
51. Badylak S, et al. Naturally occurring extracellular matrix as a scaffold for musculoskeletal repair. *Clin Orthop* 1999;367 Suppl:S333–343.
52. Yamada T. Bone-demineralized bone-bone graft for ligament reconstruction in rats. *J Med Dent Sci* 2004;51:45–52.
53. Dunn MG, et al. Anterior cruciate ligament reconstruction using a composite collagenous prosthesis. A biomechanical and histologic study in rabbits. *Am J Sports Med* 1992;20: 507–515.
54. Dunn MG, Maxian SH, Zawadsky JP. Intraosseous incorporation of composite collagen prostheses designed for ligament reconstruction. *J Orthop Res* 1994;12:128–137.
55. Witte MB, et al. Metalloproteinase inhibitors and wound healing: a novel enhancer of wound strength. *Surgery* 1998;124:464–470.
56. Dunn MG, Avasarala PN, Zawadsky JP. Optimization of extruded collagen fibers for ACL reconstruction. *J Biomed Mater Res* 1993;27:1545–1552.
57. Caruso AB, Dunn MG. Functional evaluation of collagen fiber scaffolds for ACL reconstruction: cyclic loading in proteolytic enzyme solutions. *J Biomed Mater Res* 2004;69A: 164–171.
58. Ohan MP, Dunn MG. Glucose stabilizes collagen sterilized with gamma irradiation. *J Biomed Mater Res* 2003;67A:1188–1195.
59. Bourke SL, Kohn J. Polymers derived from the amino acid L-tyrosine: polycarbonates, polyarylates and copolymers with poly(ethylene glycol). *Adv Drug Deliv Rev* 2003;55: 447–466.
60. Fiordeliso J, Bron S, Kohn J. Design, synthesis, and preliminary characterization of tyrosine-containing polyarylates: new biomaterials for medical applications. *J Biomater Sci Polym Ed* 1994;5:497–510.

61. Bourke SL, Kohn J, Dunn MG. Preliminary development of a novel resorbable synthetic polymer fiber scaffold for anterior cruciate ligament reconstruction. *Tissue Eng* 2004;10: 43–52.
62. Lin VS, et al. Ligament tissue engineering using synthetic biodegradable fiber scaffolds. *Tissue Eng* 1999;5:443–452.
63. Altman GH, et al. Silk matrix for tissue engineered anterior cruciate ligaments. *Biomaterials* 2002;23:4131–4141.
64. Dunn MG, et al. Preliminary development of a collagen-PLA composite for ACL reconstruction. *J Appl Poly Sci* 1997;63:1423–1428.
65. Ide A, et al. Collagen hydridization with poly(L-lactic acid) braid promotes ligament cell migration. *Mater Sci Eng C* 2001;17:95–99.
66. Dunn MG, et al. Development of fibroblast-seeded ligament analogs for ACL reconstruction. *J Biomed Mater Res* 1995;29:1363–1371.
67. Bellincampi LD, et al. Viability of fibroblast-seeded ligament analogs after autogenous implantation. *J Orthop Res* 1998;16:414–420.
68. Awad HA, et al. Autologous mesenchymal stem cell-mediated repair of tendon. *Tissue Eng* 1999;5:267–277.
69. Prockop DJ. Marrow stromal cells as stem cells for nonhematopoietic tissues. *Science* 1997;276:71–74.
70. Letson AK, Dahners LE. The effect of combinations of growth factors on ligament healing. *Clin Orthop* 1994;308:207–212.
71. Batten ML, Hansen JC, Dahners LE. Influence of dosage and timing of application of platelet-derived growth factor on early healing of the rat medial collateral ligament. *J Orthop Res* 1996;14:736–741.
72. Schmidt CC, et al. Effect of growth factors on the proliferation of fibroblasts from the medial collateral and anterior cruciate ligaments. *J Orthop Res* 1995;13:184–190.
73. DesRosiers EA, Yahia L, Rivard CH. Proliferative and matrix synthesis response of canine anterior cruciate ligament fibroblasts submitted to combined growth factors. *J Orthop Res* 1996;14:200–208.
74. Scherping SC Jr, et al. Effect of growth factors on the proliferation of ligament fibroblasts from skeletally mature rabbits. *Connect Tissue Res* 1997;36:1–8.
75. Meaney Murray M, et al. The effect of selected growth factors on human anterior cruciate ligament cell interactions with a three-dimensional collagen-GAG scaffold. *J Orthop Res* 2003;21:238–244.
76. Deie M, et al. The effects of age on rabbit MCL fibroblast matrix synthesis in response to TGF-beta 1 or EGF. *Mech Ageing Dev* 1997;97:121–130.
77. Marui T, et al. Effect of growth factors on matrix synthesis by ligament fibroblasts. *J Orthop Res* 1997;15:18–23.
78. Rodeo SA, et al. Use of recombinant human bone morphogenetic protein-2 to enhance tendon healing in a bone tunnel. *Am J Sports Med* 1999;27:476–488.
79. Gafni Y, et al. Stem cells as vehicles for orthopedic gene therapy. *Gene Ther* 2004;11:417–426.
80. Martinek V, et al. Enhancement of tendon-bone integration of anterior cruciate ligament grafts with bone morphogenetic protein-2 gene transfer: a histological and biomechanical study. *J Bone Joint Surg Am* 2002;84:1123–1131.
81. Woo SL, et al. Functional tissue engineering for ligament healing: potential of antisense gene therapy. *Ann Biomed Eng* 2004;32:342–351.
82. Hildebrand KA, et al. Early expression of marker genes in the rabbit medial collateral and anterior cruciate ligaments: the use of different viral vectors and the effects of injury. *J Orthop Res* 1999;17:37–42.
83. Bonadio J. Tissue engineering via local gene delivery: update and future prospects for enhancing the technology. *Adv Drug Deliv Rev* 2000;44:185–194.

84. Wallace DG, Rosenblatt J. Collagen gel systems for sustained delivery and tissue engineering. *Adv Drug Deliv Rev* 2003;55:1631–1649.
85. Ruoslahti E. Stretching is good for a cell. *Science* 1997;276:1345–1346.
86. Banes AJ, et al. Mechanoreception at the cellular level: the detection, interpretation, and diversity of responses to mechanical signals. *Biochem Cell Biol* 1995;73:349–365.
87. Wren TA, Beaupre GS, Carter DR. A model for loading-dependent growth, development, and adaptation of tendons and ligaments. *J Biomech* 1998;31:107–114.
88. Benjamin M, Hillen B. Mechanical influences on cells, tissues and organs. Mechanical morphogenesis. *Eur J Morphol* 2003;41:3–7.
89. Banes AJ, et al. PDGF-BB, IGF-I and mechanical load stimulate DNA synthesis in avian tendon fibroblasts in vitro. *J Biomech* 1995;28:1505–1513.
90. Eastwood M, et al. Effect of precise mechanical loading on fibroblast populated collagen lattices: morphological changes. *Cell Motil Cytoskeleton* 1998;40:13–21.
91. Hsieh AH, Sah RL, Paul Sung KL. Biomechanical regulation of type I collagen gene expression in ACLs in organ culture. *J Orthop Res* 2002;20:325–331.
92. Sakai H, et al. Biological fixation of the graft within bone after anterior cruciate ligament reconstruction in rabbits: effects of the duration of postoperative immobilization. *J Orthop Sci* 2000;5:43–51.
93. Kvist J. Rehabilitation following anterior cruciate ligament injury: current recommendations for sports participation. *Sports Med* 2004;34:269–280.
94. Longley D, Lawford P. Engineering human tissue and regulation: confronting biology and law to bridge the gaps. *Med Law Int* 2001;5:101–115.
95. Naughton GK. From lab bench to market: critical issues in tissue engineering. *Ann N Y Acad Sci* 2002;961:372–385.
96. Galbraith DN. Regulatory and microbiological safety issues surrounding cell and tissue engineering products. *Biotechnol Appl Biochem* 2004.
97. Badylak SF. Xenogeneic extracellular matrix as a scaffold for tissue reconstruction. *Transpl Immunol* 2004;12:367–377.
98. Dornish M, Kaplan D, Skaugrud O. Standards and guidelines for biopolymers in tissue-engineered medical products: ASTM alginate and chitosan standard guides. American Society for Testing and Materials. *Ann N Y Acad Sci* 2001;944:388–397.
99. Schutte E. Regulatory barriers to tissue-engineered products. *Med Device Technol* 2002; 13:27–29.
100. Cox M. Progress on regulations for human-derived therapeutic products. *Med Device Technol* 2003;14:32–34.
101. Cogle CR, et al. An overview of stem cell research and regulatory issues. *Mayo Clin Proc* 2003;78:993–1003.

15

Gene Therapy and Ligament Healing

Norimasa Nakamura

INTRODUCTION

Although there has been substantial progress in operative techniques, surgical instrumentation, and rehabilitation programs, based on the wealth of knowledge about the biology and biomechanics of articular joints, the clinical outcomes following ligament injury are often still far from ideal. Ligaments take longer to heal than other connective soft tissues, and the repaired ligament tissue is scarlike and inferior to normal ligament tissue both biologically and biomechanically *(1)*. Furthermore, some ligament-deficient joints subsequently become unstable and can lead to lifelong disability with osteoarthritis *(2)*. Therefore, a novel therapeutic approach to accelerate and improve ligament repair is needed. One option could be the biological manipulation of ligament healing by the controlled delivery of biological reagents.

PROBLEMS IN LIGAMENT HEALING

Animal studies on ligament healing have revealed that the same sequence of events appears to occur in the ligament as observed in skin wound healing. The healing processes consist of inflammation (days to weeks), repair/proliferation (weeks), and remodeling (months to years; *see* Fig. 1). Through these biological processes, ligaments heal with scarring that is inferior to normal tissue biologically and biomechanically. In addition, owing to their relative hypocellularity and hypovascularity, ligaments generally have a lower healing potential than other soft tissues, e.g., skin. In fact, the tensile strength of injured skin recovers by 10 wk following injury *(3)*, whereas gap-healing rabbit medial collateral ligament (MCL) of the knee reaches only about 30% of the normal ligament strength on a material basis (i.e., per square cross-section of material) at even 1-yr postinjury *(4)*. Even a completely remodeled ligament at over 2 yr postinjury remains scar-like *(5)*. Such ligament scar remains different from normal tissue in many aspects: elevated glycosaminoglycan content, decreased collagen content, abnormal collagen crosslinking different collagen types, and specifically, different ultrastructure *(1,4,5)*. Ligament scar has predominantly small-diameter collagen fibrils when compared with the bimodal distribution (large and small diameter) found in normal ligament *(5)*. Such differences collectively seem to contribute to the inferior biomechanical properties of the ligament. Considering that the major role of ligaments is to mechanically stabilize joints, ignoring inferior quality of scar material can lead to seri-

From: *Orthopedic Biology and Medicine: Repair and Regeneration of Ligaments, Tendons, and Joint Capsule*
Edited by: W. R. Walsh © Humana Press Inc., Totowa, NJ

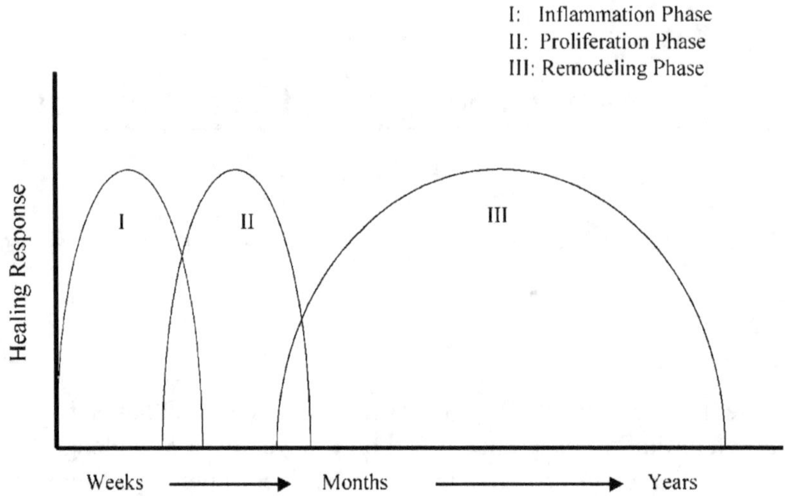

Fig. 1. The healing processes of inflammation, repair/proliferation, and remodeling.

ous clinical problems, such as functional deficits and/or osteoarthritis. Furthermore, recent investigation has revealed that healing ligaments show inferior creep behavior (increase in strain under constant or repetitive stress) under low stress *(6)*. As recent evidence suggests that ligaments are subject to repetitive low loads in vivo *(7)* and that irrecoverable creep may result in a permanent stretching out of the ligament over time *(6,8)*, such inferior creep behavior of the healing ligament might have significant clinical implications.

STRATEGIES TO IMPROVE LIGAMENT HEALING

Exogenous Addition of Biological Factors Involved in Tissue Repair

Researchers have tried to develop strategies to improve and speed up the healing process of injured ligaments. To this end, biological manipulation of scar-tissue formation has predominantly focused on the overexpression of growth factors, which have been revealed as an important influence to cutaneous wound healing. As described previously, this is because the healing process of the ligament is basically analogous to that of skin tissue.

Normal wound healing begins with the accumulation of fibrin and platelet degranulation, the latter event involving the release of transforming growth factor-β (TGF-β), platelet-derived growth factor (PDGF), epidermal growth factor (EGF), and insulin-like growth factor 1 (IGF-1), which are chemotactic and mitogenic for inflammatory cells. Accordingly, neutrophils and macrophages accumulate during the inflammatory phase of wound healing with the latter cell type secreting more TGF-β, basic fibroblast growth factor (bFGF), and vascular endothelial growth factor (VEGF). These growth factors stimulate fibroblasts and endothelial cells to proliferate, then fibroblasts and other reparative cells accumulate at the injured site and continue to synthesize and secrete extracellular matrix (ECM) components. Hepatocyte growth factor (HGF) is a

Table 1
Application of Biological Factors to Promote Wound Healing

Factor	Biological effects	References
TGF-β	Influx of mononuclear cells and fibroblasts	*11*
	Enhanced collagen deposition	*12*
	Increase in wound tensile strength	*13*
EGF	Proliferation of fibroblasts	*14*
	Enhanced collagen deposition	
	Increase in wound tensile strength	
PDGF-B	Influx of mononuclear cells and fibroblasts	*15*
	Enhanced angiogenesis	*12*
	Enhanced collagen deposition	*3*
	Increase in wound tensile strength	
bFGF	Proliferation of fibroblasts	*16*
	Enhanced collagen deposition	
	Increase in wound tensile strength	
VEGF	Enhanced angiogenesis	*17*
	Enhanced granulation deposition	*18*
HGF/SF	Enhanced angiogenesis	*9*
	Enhanced collagen deposition	
EGR-1	Overexpression of TGF-β, PDGF, HGF, and VEGF	*33*
	Enhanced angiogenesis	*34*
	Enhanced collagen deposition	

mesenchyme-derived pleiotropic factor that regulates cell growth, cell motility, and morphogenesis of various cells and is thus considered a humoral mediator of epithelial–mesenchymal interactions, including wound healing *(9)*. Recent research has revealed that HGF is expressed in wound fibroblasts, and its expression peaks at 7-d postwounding, suggesting the importance of this growth factor in early wound repair *(10)*. The early phase of tissue repair is then followed by tissue maturation, remodeling, and reorganization. Collectively, the early phases of wound healing depend on the transient and coordinated expression of various growth factors within wounds. Therefore, application of these factors may potentially accelerate and improve wound repair. Based on these findings, various experimental studies have investigated the effect of these growth factors on the improvement of wound healing. Positive results with the administration of TGF-β *(11–13)*, EGF *(14)*, PDGF-B *(3,15)*, bFGF *(16)*, VEGF *(17,18)*, and HGF *(9)* in wound repair have been demonstrated (*see* Table 1).

Regarding to ligaments, some studies have begun to characterize growth factors and their receptors during healing. Transcripts for TGF-β1, EGF, bFGF, IGF-1, IGF-2, as well as insulin and IGF-2 receptors, have been detected in normal and injured ligaments *(19)*. Immunohistochemical studies demonstrated the expression of TGF-β *(20, 21)*, EGF *(22)*, bFGF *(21,22)*, PDGF 2, and VEGF *(23,24)* during the early healing phases of the ligaments. All these findings have led to the experimental use of exogenous growth factors to enhance ligament healing. Hart et al. investigated the effect of TGF-β1 on rabbit MCL healing. Delivery of TGF-β into the MCL scar by direct injection or infusion pump methods resulted in excessive scar formation; however, it did not improve the biomechanical material properties of the ligament scar *(25)*. TGF-β1 and 2 may promote scarring of healing cutaneous tissue, but on the contrary, TGF-β3 is likely more involved in "scarless" healing *(26)*. In this regard, TGF-β1 administration appears to accelerate tissue repair by scarring, whereas TGF-β3 might be more beneficial to improve tissue quality through "scarless" healing mechanisms. Therefore, the effect of TGF-β3 therapy on wound repair needs to be elucidated. The in vivo impact of PDGF-BB has been evaluated in a healing rat and rabbit MCL healing model *(27,28)*. Both studies showed increased mechanical strength of healing ligaments. Administration of bFGF to the healing ligament has also been conducted, and some positive effects on matrix formation with enhanced angiogenesis have been demonstrated *(29,30)*. But, both studies have shown that the response is very dose-dependent and that excess growth factor could interfere with the healing process. Alternatively, growth and differentiation factors (GDFs) 5, 6, and 7 (identical to bone morphogenic protein [BMP]-12, -13, and -14), members of the TGF-β gene superfamily, were found to induce neotendon/ligament-like tissue formation when implanted at ectopic sites in vivo. In addition, comparative *in situ* localizations of the GDF-5, -6, and -7 mRNAs suggest that these molecules might be important regulatory components of synovial joint morphogenesis *(31)*. Their chondrogenic action to mesenchymal cells has also been reported *(32)*. Further characterization of these molecules for proper differentiation of mesenchymal stem cells into neotendon/ligament tissue will be needed.

Along with these growth factors, the potential feasibility of other biological molecules to improve tissue repair has been suggested. Effective tissue repair results from a rapid, temporally orchestrated series of events. At the site of local tissue injury, the production of many growth factors and cytokines is partly stimulated by the early growth response transcription factors, which are expressed minutes after acute injury. A recent study has revealed that early growth response factor 1 (EGR-1), a transcription factor, stimulates the production of many growth factors involved in early tissue repair, such as PDGF-AB, HGF, TGF-β1, and VEGF *(33)*. It also promotes angiogenesis in vitro and in vivo, increases collagen production, and accelerates wound closure (*34*; Table 1). These results indicate the potential use for this therapeutic transcription factor, EGR-1, to improve tissue repair. Thus far, this strategy has not been adopted in a ligament-healing study.

Alteration of Scar Tissue Composition Involved in Tissue Repair

This subsection introduces a strategy to improve scar-tissue quality by altering the matrix composition and organization. Not many experimental studies have been conducted to date using this approach. Because collagen (especially type I) is the main tensile element in the ligament, this matrix molecule is focused on as a target of this strategy. Collagen is a major constituent of all ECM, and it is defined as having a lengthy triple-helical domain and as aggregating in an extracellular space to function as a "supporting element" of the tissue. At present, more than 20 genetically distinct types of collagens have been identified. According to the supramolecular forms within ECM, well-characterized collagens are subgrouped into classes: fibrillar (types I, II,

Table 2
Matrix Molecules Implicated in Regulating Collagen Fibril Size

		References
Collagens	Collagen III	*38*
	pNcollagen III	*39*
	Collagen V	*40,41*
	Collagen VI	*42*
Proteoglycans	Decorin	*43–46*
	Fibromodulin	*47,48*
	Lumican	*48,49*
Other matrix molecules	Thrombospondin-2	*50*
	Osteopontin	*51*

III, V, and XI), fibril-associated (IX and XII), network-forming (IV), filamentous (VI), short-chain (VIII and X), and long-chain (VII; *35*). Among these classes, the fibrillar collagens are thought to be chiefly responsible for the mechanical properties of the tissues. Collagen type I appears to be the major collagen in both normal and injured ligaments, providing the leading component of the millions of collagen fibers (seen on light microscopy) and their component, microfibrils (seen by transmission electron microscopy [TEM]; *1*). Of the various attributes of collagen (amount, concentration, alignment, type, and so on.), many investigators have suggested that collagen fibril thickness may best correlate with the mechanical properties of connective tissues *(36,37)*. Specifically, collagen fibril diameters seen on TEM may have a relationship to tissue strength; apparently, larger fibrils are required for greater strength and stiffness. Ligament wounds, even over 2 yr after injury, contain mainly a homogenous population of small-collagen fibrils as commonly observed in scar tissues, with a few patches of normal larger fibrils being observed *(5)*. Also, as noted above, these ligaments never achieve their original biomechanical properties *(4)*. Accordingly, production of larger-diameter collagen fibrils could potentially improve the material strength of the ligament scar. Relating to growth factor/cytokine therapy, however, there have been no growth factor cytokines identified that directly promote collagen fibrillogenesis in vitro or in vivo. Therefore, another approach is required to achieve this purpose. The interaction of collagen microfibrils with other matrix molecules is one of the mechanisms implicated in the regulation of collagen fibril diameters. Regarding collagens, collagen III, procollagen III with aminopropeptides (pN collagen III), collagen V, and collagen VI have been revealed to regulate collagen fibril diameters. In addition, members of the small leucine-rich proteoglycans (SLRPs), decorin, fibromodulin, and lumican may inhibit the lateral growth of collagen fibrils. Furthermore, involvement of adhesion molecules, thrombospondin-2 and osteopontin in collagen fibrillogenesis has been indicated by knockout mice studies. All these studies are listed in Table 2 *(38–51)*. Collectively, these observations suggest that the alteration of the molar ratio of these molecules to collagen microfibrils in ligament scar might result in changes in the lateral growth of collagen fibrils and thus potentially improve the mechanical properties of the ligament scar.

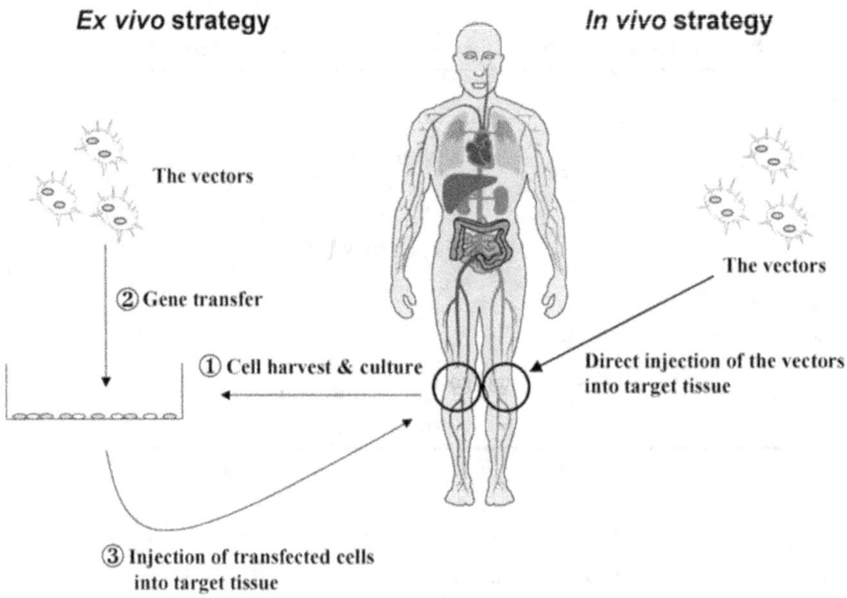

Fig. 2. Gene transfer into somatic cells.

METHODS FOR GENE THERAPY

Gene therapy involves the transfer of a gene or genes to tissues within an individual for a therapeutic purpose. This technology offers the ability to manipulate the expression of key molecules in tissue repair by the introduction of genes or gene antagonists directly into the affected tissues. Gene therapy not only allows an unprecedented ability to quantify the contributions of various crucial molecules during the healing of joint injuries, but it also offers ways to control local tissue repair processes in a unique manner.

Generally, there are two strategies for gene transfer. The first strategy involves isolation of cells from an organism, establishment of the cells in tissue culture, transfer of specific genes into the cells, and subsequent reengraftment of the cells back into the patient. This strategy is termed "ex vivo gene transfer" and has been successful with cells that adapt well to culture and reengraftment. The second strategy is to perform the gene transfer directly into somatic cells in the patient, termed "in vivo gene transfer" (Fig. 2).

Considerable effort in developing gene therapies has historically focused on gene delivery systems. With few exceptions, naked DNA is not well taken up and expressed by most cells. Agents that enable the cellular uptake and expression of genetic material are known as "vectors." Vector characteristics have been reviewed in detail in other comprehensive sources *(52–55)*. Viral vectors (retrovirus, adeno-associated virus [AAV], and adenovirus [AV]) have been most extensively investigated. Their goal is to infect target cells and to deliver the virally contained genetic material to the nuclei of cells without permitting viral replication or viral pathology. Each vector has certain strengths and weaknesses in achieving this goal (Table 3). Because retroviruses insert

Table 3
Advantages and Disadvantages of Common Vectors for Gene Transfer

Vector		Advantages	Disadvantages
Viral	• Retrovirus	• Low toxicity • Low immunogenicity • High persistence of gene expression	• Low gene-insert capacity • Infection only of dividing cells • Oncogenesis
	• Adenovirus	• High efficiency of transfection • Infection of nondividing cells	• Toxicity • Immunogenicity
	• Adeno-associated virus	• Low toxicity • Low immunogenicity • High persistence of gene expression • Infection of nondividing cells	• Low gene-insert capacity
	• Herpes simplex virus	• Large insert capacity • High efficiency of transfection • Infection of nondividing cells	• Immunogenicity
Nonviral	• Liposomes	• Low toxicity	• Low efficiency of transfection
	• DNA–ligand complexes	• Low immunogenicity	• Low efficiency of transfection
	• Colloidal gold (gene gun)	• Easy preparation	• Transient gene expression
Hybrid	• HVJ liposomes	• Large-insert capacity • High efficiency of transfection • Infection of nondividing cells	• Transient gene expression

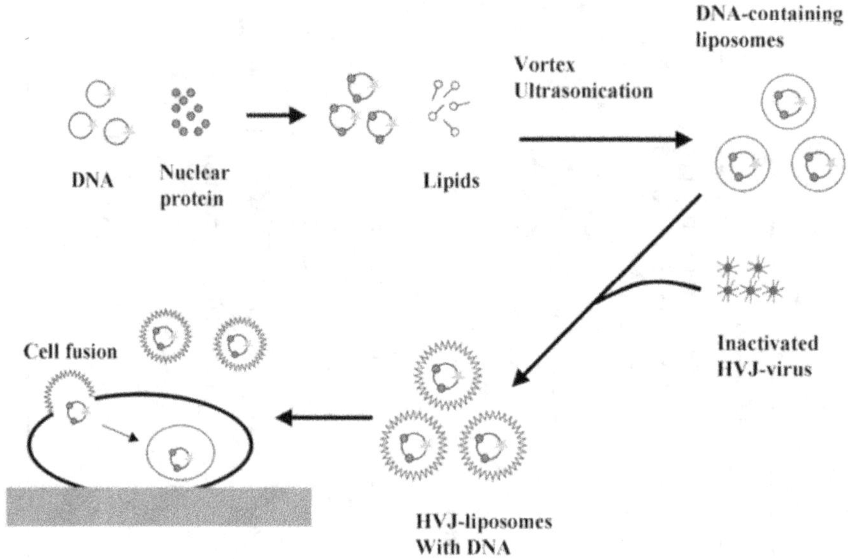

Fig. 3. Fusigenic viral liposome developed for direct introduction of macromolecules into the cytoplasm through cell fusion mediated.

into the cellular genome at random locations, there are safety concerns regarding the possibility of insertional mutagenesis that leads to cell transformation. AAVs insert DNA at a site-specific location at the tip of chromosome 19 and, unlike retroviruses, can infect nondividing cells. Furthermore, they generally enable high persistence of transgene expression; they only accommodate 4 kb of carrier DNA. In addition, recombinant AAV is difficult to produce in high titer and may not retain the site specificity of the wild-type virus. On the contrary, AV can be produced in very high titers. They can infect both dividing and nondividing cells, and they have high infectivity rates. However, their transgene expression is transient and the persistent expression of AV protein can lead to a high incidence of antibody production, which can then influence infected cells or subsequent reexposure. Thus, this vector does not appear to be suitable for repetitive delivery. Furthermore, infection with high titers of virus can sometimes give rise to cytopathic effects.

As a result of these potential problems, other nonviral vectors have been developed, such as liposomes, DNA–ligand complexes, and colloidal gold (gene gun). Although the alteration of gene expression is more transient, and their efficiency is generally recognized to be lower than that of viral vectors, these nonviral options are potentially safer than viral vectors. The general concept of these techniques is that the carrier agent and plasmid DNA forms complexes that are transported into cells by endocytosis, or in the case of the gene gun, by mechanical pressure. Among these vectors, liposomes are most widely used. In fact, certain cationic liposome preparations are currently in clinical use. Recently, a unique fusigenic viral liposome has been developed for direct introduction of macromolecules into the cytoplasm through cell fusion mediated by Sendai virus (hemagglutinating virus of Japan [HVJ]; Fig. 3; *56,57*). With this cell fusion mechanism, HVJ liposomes have proved to be 100–10,000 times more efficient

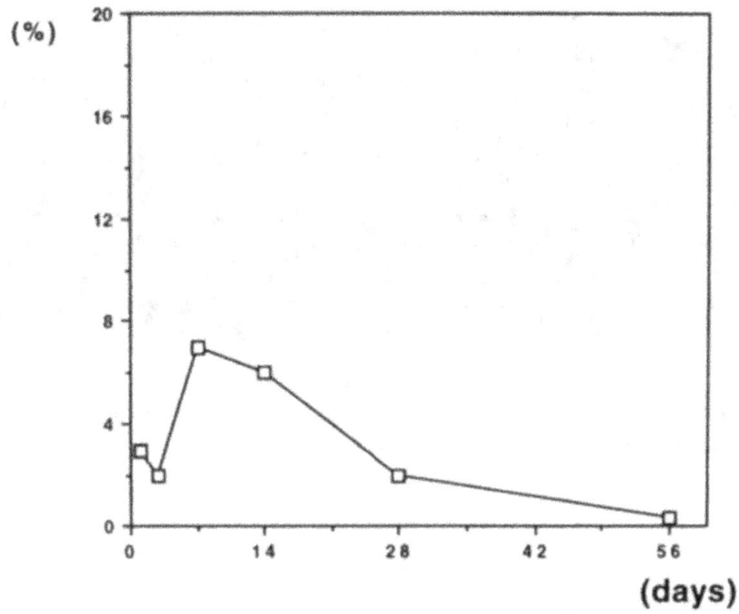

Fig. 4. LacZ-bearing cells present in the injured area up to 56 d after transfection, with the peak of expression at d 7.

in gene transfer compared to liposomes without HVJ, and the method has been successfully used for the introduction of foreign genes and antisense oligonucleotides (ODN) into several organs and tissues.

Gene Therapy in Ligament and Tendon Repair

Introduction of Marker Gene

Initial gene therapy studies focused on the introduction of a marker gene (β-galactosidase; LacZ) into normal and healing ligament and tendon tissues to evaluate the effectiveness of ex vivo or in vivo gene transfer. Nakamura et al. injected the lacZ plasmid DNA directly into rat patellar ligament scar using HVJ liposomes *(58)*. LacZ-bearing cells were present in the injured area up to 56 d after transfection, with the peak of expression at d 7 (7% of cells at the wound site; Fig. 4). With double labeling for marker antigens for monocyte/macrophage (ED-1) and for collagen I aminopropeptide (pN collagen I), it was revealed that fibroblastic (pN collagen I-positive) cells accounted for 63% and monocyte/macrophage lineage cells for 32% of the LacZ-labeled cells in the d-7 wound. On d 28, they formed 58% and 35% of the LacZ-labeled cells in the wound, respectively. Moreover, specific labeling of the transfected cells revealed a biological event, i.e., that the cells in and around the injured site infiltrate into the uninjured ligament substance and come to populate the whole length of the ligament substance as repair progresses. Although a potentially less invasive intraarterial delivery of lacZ gene in HVJ liposomes into the healing rat patellar ligament has been explored *(59)*, a comparable expression of the lacZ gene product was observed. This alternative delivery method could be advantageous for gene delivery to deeper tissues. With regard to viral vectors,

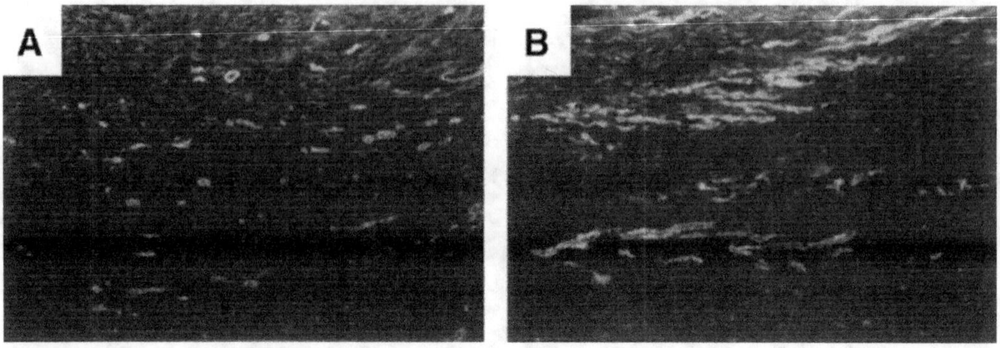

Fig. 5. (**A**) Using the HVJ-liposome method, the PDGF-B gene was introduced into healing rat patellar ligaments. (**B**) PDGF-B gene transfer resulted in the enhanced expression of PDGF in the healing ligament up to 4 wk after transfection, leading to an initial promotion of angiogenesis.

using the ex vivo and in vivo strategy, the lacZ gene has been introduced into normal rabbit patellar tendon retrovirally and adenovirally, respectively, and the duration of gene expression was at least 6 wk by both delivery methods *(60)*. The efficiency of transfection *in situ* by this delivery technique has not been clarified. The same research group also introduced the LacZ gene into normal and injured rabbit MCL and the anterior cruciate ligament (ACL) of the knee. They confirmed transgene expression for over 6 wk within normal and injured ligaments *(61)*. Adenoviral vector-mediated gene transfer of the lacZ gene to chicken tendon and tendon sheath has also been investigated. Descriptive analysis of lacZ gene expression has been performed, and expression persisted for over 75 d in both tissues *(62)*. Recently, to obtain longer-term gene expression in the joint, unique myoblast mediated ex vivo gene transfer has also been investigated. The transduced myoblasts were found in the ACL and in the synovial tissue surrounding the ACL at 4-, 7-, 14-, and 21-d postinjection. The myoblasts fused and formed myotubes in the ligament *(63)*. This unique gene transfer method may be applicable to the biological manipulation of ligament healing; further study is expected.

Gene Therapy to Accelerate Ligament/Tendon Repair

As described, recent studies have shown the positive effects of growth factors on wound healing and ligament/tendon repair. Therefore, initial gene transfer studies have focused on the overexpression of growth factors to accelerate healing. Using the HVJ-liposome method, the PDGF-B gene was introduced into healing rat patellar ligaments *(64)*. This PDGF-B gene transfer resulted in the enhanced expression of PDGF in the healing ligament up to 4 wk after transfection, leading to an initial promotion of angiogenesis (Fig. 5) and subsequent enhanced collagen I deposition in the wound (Fig. 6). There has been no in vitro study showing the direct effect of PDGF on the synthesis of collagen I; yet, it is known that PDGF stimulates macrophages to produce TGF-β1 which stimulates collagen formation *(65)*. Therefore, some stimulating factors of matrix synthesis (e.g., TGF-β1) could be simultaneously overexpressed in the PDGF gene–transferred healing ligament. No significant collagen I deposition was detected in the

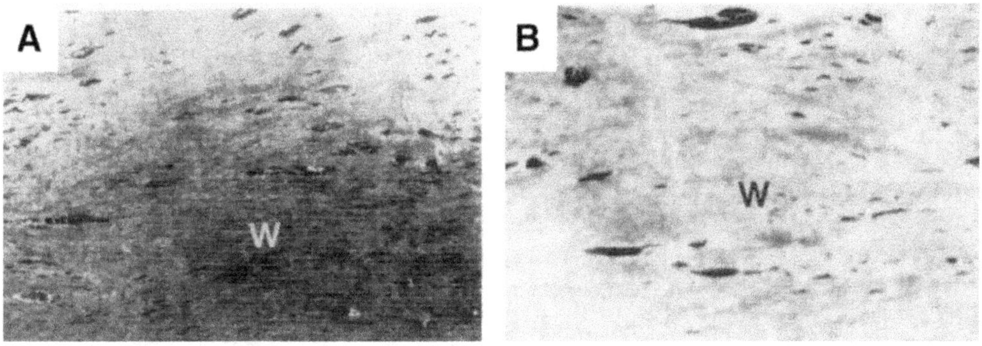

Fig. 6. **(A)** PDGF-B gene transfer resulted in the enhanced expression of PDGF in the healing ligament up to 4 wk after transfection, leading to an initial promotion of angiogenesis and **(B)** subsequent enhanced collagen I deposition in the wound.

gene-transferred wound at 8 wk by semiquantitative morphological analysis. However, it should be noted that the amount of collagen deposition in the gene-transferred wound was a comparable amount with that of the control wound 4 wk earlier. This could be interpreted as the acceleration of ligament healing by gene transfer. With focus on a strong in vivo angiogenic action, gene transfer of HGF into healing rat patellar ligament has been also investigated using the HVJ-liposome method *(66)*. Although the results were preliminary, in vivo introduction of HGF resulted in enhanced angiogenesis and collagen synthesis for the first 4 wk following gene transfer. Further analysis is pending.

As noted previously, the induction of neotendon/ligament-like tissue by BMP-12, -13, and -14 has been demonstrated *(31)*. Accordingly, to enhance neotendon tissue formation following injury, the effect of BMP-12 gene transfer on tendon cells and chicken tendon healing has been investigated. Adenoviral BMP-12 gene transfer into chicken tendon cells increased type I collagen synthesis and gene transfer into injured tendon resulted in a twofold increase of tensile strength and stiffness of repaired tendons, indicating improved tendon healing in vivo *(67)*. Adenoviral BMP-13 transfer into rat thigh muscle also resulted in the formation of collagenous matrix with the ultrastructural appearance of neotendon/neoligament. At the same time, small foci of bone and fibrocartilage were also seen within the treated tissue *(68)*. Thus, based on these results, gene transfer of BMP-12 and BMP-13 might be a promising procedure for improving the ligament/tendon repair. However, it should be emphasized that local administration of these BMPs into healing tissues, where a number of immature mesenchymal cells are recruited, has the potential risk of producing chondrogenic and bony tissue, because these BMPs are also known for their strong chondrogenic and bone morphogenic action *(69)*. More optimization studies would be required for appropriate tissue induction.

Gene Therapy to Prevent Tissue Adhesion

Adhesion is a critical complication in tendon healing. Lou et al. researched the effect of the local administration of focal adhesion kinase ($pp125^{FAK}$) in tendon adhesion *(70)*.

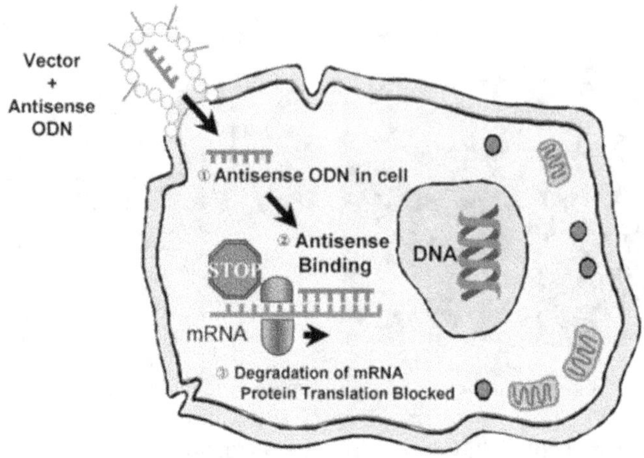

Fig. 7. Complementary ODN specifically bind to mRNA or pre-mRNA by base pairing, thus enhancing the degradation of target mRNA and also blocking the translation of the target gene.

The intracellular focal adhesion kinase (FAK)-related signaling pathway may be related to cell–cell and cell–ECM interactions via the cell surface adhesion receptors, including the integrins and cadherins *(71)*, and may be one of the mechanisms involved in the induction of tendon adhesions. Gene transfer of $pp125^{FAK}$ to the tendon sheath resulted in abnormal tendon adhesion. This finding suggested a possible relationship between cell–ECM interaction via the integrins and overproduction of the ECM leading to tissue adhesion.

Gene Therapy to Alter Collagen Ultrastructure

As mentioned, collagen fibril diameter may correlate with the mechanical properties of connective tissues *(36,37)*. Healing ligament contains mainly a homogenous population of small-diameter collagen fibrils as commonly observed in scar tissues *(5)* and is inferior to normal tissue biomechanically *(4,6,8)*. Therefore, the production of larger-diameter collagen fibrils could be used as a strategy to improve the mechanical properties of healing ligament. As shown in Table 3, several matrix molecules have been identified to regulate collagen fibril diameter. The results of in vitro binding experiments, molecular and biochemical analyses of tendon development, and knockout mouse studies, collectively indicate the involvement of decorin (a member of the SLRPs) in downregulating collagen fibril diameters *(43–45,72)*. Moreover, the presence of decorin mRNA *(73)* and protein *(74)* in the ligament scar has been observed. Based on these results, it could be hypothesized that decorin inhibition during early ligament healing would possibly enhance the lateral growth of newly synthesized collagen fibrils in the ligament scar. To suppress a specific molecule, antisense approaches have been investigated in a variety of studies. Antisense ODN inhibit gene expression in a sequence-specific manner. Complementary ODN specifically bind to mRNA or pre-mRNA by base pairing, thus enhancing the degradation of target mRNA and also blocking the translation of the target gene (Fig. 7). Therefore, in vivo antisense therapy could potentially suppress targeted gene expression in a specific tissue *(75)*. Studies

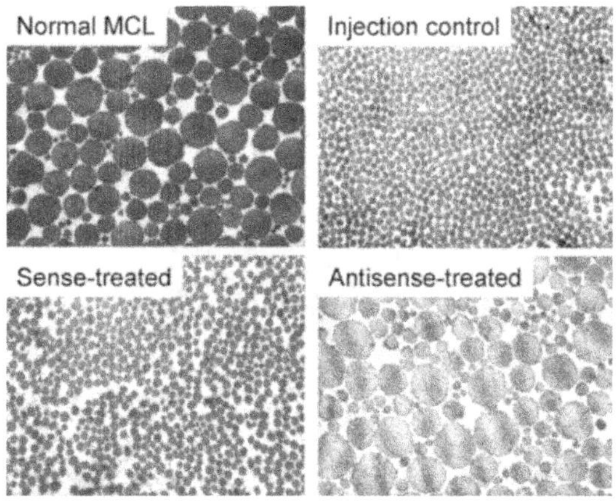

Fig. 8. Development of larger-diameter collagen fibrils within scars.

have shown that the in vivo introduction of fluorescence-labeled ODN into a healing rabbit MCL can be achieved using the HVJ-liposome-mediated gene transfer method *(74)*. With systematic direct injection into the ligament scars using a dispenser and a microgrid mesh system to distribute the liposomes, scar cells were effectively transfected when assessed 1 d after transfection. Furthermore, introduction of antisense ODN for the small proteoglycan decorin has resulted in decorin suppression at both the mRNA and protein levels over 4 wk following exposure to the HVJ liposomes. Such changes in decorin expression have led to the development of larger-diameter collagen fibrils within scars (Fig. 8; *76*) but results are somewhat variable among the animals with the same treatment. The degree of increase in collagen fibril size varied according to the location, implying that collagen fibril assembly was not improved in the whole area of each ligament scar by this single antisense treatment, but it had clearly altered the morphology of most scars in several locations. The average collagen fibril diameter in antisense treated scars was 104.7 ± 51.1 nm, whereas the control scars and normal MCL were 74.8 ± 11.0 nm and 189.1 ± 104.0 nm, respectively. In mechanical assessments, this antisense therapy caused enhanced resistance of the healing ligament scar tissue to elongation by creep (Fig. 9; *6,8*). Antisense-treated scars were significantly less suspectible to creep during low stress creep testing (at 2.2 Mpa) than control scars (by 18–22%), and they also revealed 33–48% less irrecoverable creep after the same recovery period than control scars (Table 4). Antisense-treated scars also failed at a higher stress than control scars (by 82–84%) (Fig. 10; *25,76,77*). This study is the first demonstration of in vivo manipulation of collagen fibrillogenesis during soft connective tissue repair processes, as well as the first report that shows such a treatment can improve the functional properties of ligament scarring. However, it is not likely that there is a simple, direct cause-and-effect relationship between downregulation of decorin expression and the increase in collagen fibril diameters, as well as the improvement in the biomechanical properties of the scar tissue. Although the ODNs were designed to be specific for decorin based on available evidence, it is possible that secondary regulation of other molecules could be involved

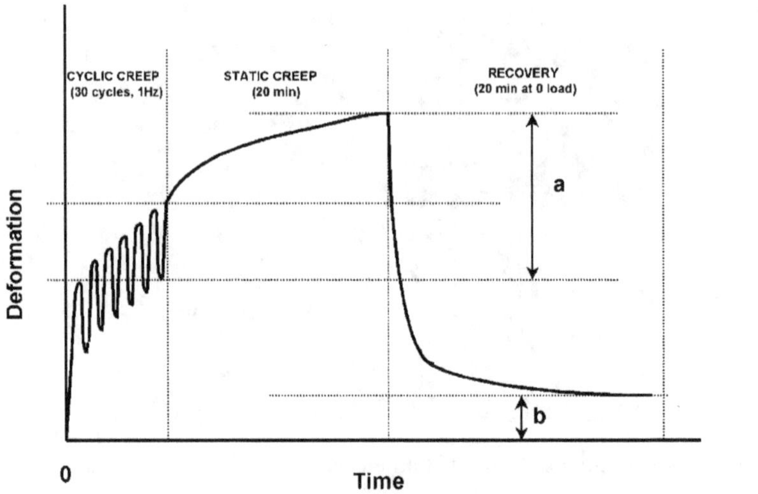

Fig. 9. The antisense therapy caused enhanced resistance of the healing ligament scar tissue to elongation by creep.

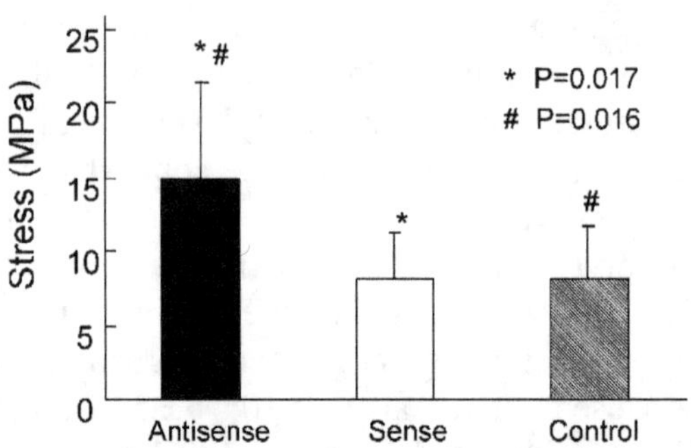

Fig. 10. Antisense-treated scars failed at a higher stress than the control scars.

in vivo. In fact, mRNA levels for collagens I, III, biglycan, and lumican were significantly suppressed in the antisense-treated samples when compared with the sense-treated *(25)*. As total RNA was not altered by the antisense treatment, decorin antisense treatment might have affected scar cell metabolism secondarily in a specific manner. Finally, it must be reinforced that this technique has not yet been fully optimized for this application, and there was only partial recovery of the biomechanical properties. Yet, a recent study has succeeded in suppressing $\alpha 1$ chain of collagen V, which is also shown to inhibit collagen fibrillogenesis in vitro and to be abundant in ligament scarring *(78)* in human patellar tendon fibroblasts by antisense treatment *(79)*. Administration of this treatment in vivo could also potentially alter collagen ultrastructure in

Table 4
Summary of Creep Testing (Average ± SD)

Treatment group	Antisense-treated	Sense-treated	Injection control
Scar cross-sectional area (mm^2)	7.64 ± 0.90	9.40 ± 1.69	7.98 ± 1.72
Total creep strain (%)	2.57 ± 0.35 [a,b]	3.18 ± 0.42 [a]	3.29 ± 0.74 [b]
Irrecoverable creep strain (%)	1.60 ± 0.32 [c,d]	2.40 ± 0.83 [c]	3.05 ± 1.44 [d]

SD, standard deviation.
[a] $p < 0.014$.
[b] $p < 0.045$.
[c] $p < 0.035$.
[d] $p < 0.030$.

healing ligament. With further optimization of the dosage, timing, and delivery techniques, antisense therapy strategy may not only help to improve the understanding of the structure–function relationships in connective tissue but may also significantly enhance the quality of soft-tissue healing in vivo.

CONCLUSIONS

The recent advances in gene therapy to improve ligament healing have been reviewed. Encouraging results have been reported that bode well for future clinical trials. However, optimal therapeutic strategies will not be obtained without a thorough understanding of the scientific basis of tissue repair. Further investigations in the mechanisms underlying tissue regeneration are required.

ACKNOWLEDGMENT

We thank Richard S. Boorman, MD, MSC, FRCS(C), University of Calgary, for substantial discussion and helpful editorial work.

REFERENCES

1. Frank CB, Bray RC, Hart DA, et al.. Soft tissue healing. In Fu F, Harner CD, Vince KG, eds. *Knee Surgery*, Williams & Wilkins, Baltimore, MD, 1994, pp. 189–230.
2. Hirshman HP, Daniel DM, Miyasaka K. The fate of unoperated knee ligament injuries. In Daniel DM, Akeson WH, O'Connor JJ, eds. *Knee Ligaments: Structure, Function, Injury, and Repair*, Raven Press, New York, NY, 1991, pp. 351–364.
3. Deuel TF, Kawahara RS, Mustoe TA, Pierce AF. Growth factors and wound healing: platelet derived growth factor as a model cytokine. *Ann Rev Med* 1991;42:567–584.
4. Frank CB, Woo SL-Y, Amiel D, Harwood F, Gomez M, Akeson W. Medial collateral ligament healing: a multidisciplinary assessment in rabbits. *Am J Sports Med* 1983;11:379–389.
5. Frank C, McDonald D, Shrive N. Collagen fibril diameters in the rabbit medial collateral ligament scar: a longer term assessment. *Connect Tissue Res* 1997;36:261–269.
6. Thornton GM, Leask GP, Shrive NG, Frank CB. Early medial collateral ligament scars have inferior creep behaviour. *J Orthop Res* 2000;18:238–246.
7. Holden JP, Grood ES, Korvick DL, Cummings JF, Butler DL, Bylski-Austrow DI. In vivo forces in the anterior cruciate ligament: Direct measurements during walking and trotting in a quadruped. *J Biomech* 1994;27:517–526.

8. Boorman RS, Shrive NG, Frank CB. Immobilization increases the vulnerability of rabbit medial collateral ligament autografts to creep. *J Orthop Res* 1998;16:682–689.
9. Toyoda M, Takayama H, Horiguchi N, et al. Overexpression of hepatocyte growth factor/scatter factor promotes vascularization and granulation tissue formation in vivo. *FEBS Lett* 2001;509:95–100.
10. Cowin AJ, Kallincos N, Hatzirodos N, et al. Hepatocyte growth factor and macrophage-stimulating protein are upregulated during excisional wound repair in rats. *Cell Tissue Res* 2001;306:239–250.
11. Mustoe TA, Pierce GF, Thomason A, Gramates P, Sporn MB, Deuel TF. Accelerated healing of incisional wounds in rats induced by transforming growth factor-beta. *Science* 1987;237:1333–1336.
12. Pierce GF, Mustoe TA, Lingelbach J, et al. Platelet-derived growth factor and transforming growth factor-beta enhance tissue repair activities by unique mechanisms. *J Cell Biol* 1989;109:429–440.
13. Yang L, Qiu CX, Ludlow A, Ferguson MW, Brunner G. Active transforming growth factor-beta in wound repair: determination using a new assay. *Am J Pathol* 1999;154:105–111.
14. Brown GL, Curtsinger LJ, White M, et al. Acceleration of tensile strength of incisions treated with EGF and TGF-beta. *Ann Surg* 1988;208:788–794.
15. Pierce GF, Mustoe TA, Senior RM, et al. In vivo incisional wound healing augmented by platelet-derived growth factor and recombinant c-sis gene homodimeric proteins. *J Exp Med* 1988;167:974–987.
16. Tsuboi R, Rifkin DB. Recombinant basic fibroblast growth factor stimulates wound healing in healing-impaired db/db mice. *J Exp Med* 1990;172:245–251.
17. Breitbart AS, Grande DA, Laser J, et al. Treatment of ischemic wounds using cultured dermal fibroblasts transduced retrovirally with PDGF-B and VEGF121 genes. *Ann Plast Surg* 2001;46:555–561.
18. Ozawa K, Kondo T, Hori O, et al. Expression of the oxygen-regulated protein ORP150 accelerates wound healing by modulating intracellular VEGF transport. *J Clin Invest* 2001;108:41–50.
19. Sciore P, Boykiw R, Hart DA. Semiquantitative reverse transcription-polymerase chain reaction analysis of mRNA for growth factors and growth factor receptors from normal and healing rabbit medial collateral ligament tissue. *J Orthop Res* 1998;16:429–437.
20. Natsu-ume T, Nakamura N, Shino K, Toritsuka Y, Horibe S, Ochi T. Temporal and spatial expression of transforming growth factor-beta in the healing patellar ligament of the rat. *J Orthop Res* 1997;15:837–843.
21. Lee J, Harwood FL, Akeson WH, Amiel D. Growth factor expression in healing rabbit medial collateral and anterior cruciate ligaments. *Iowa Orthop J* 1998;18:19–25.
22. Panossian V, Liu SH, Lane JM, Finerman GA. Fibroblast growth factor and epidermal growth factor receptors in ligament healing. *Clin Orthop* 1997;342:173–180.
23. Bidder M, Towler DA, Gelberman RH, Boyer MI. Expression of mRNA for vascular endothelial growth factor at the repair site of healing canine flexor tendon. *J Orthop Res* 2000;18:247–252.
24. Boyer MI, Watson JT, Lou J, Manske PR, Gelberman RH, Cai SR. Quantitative variation in vascular endothelial growth factor mRNA expression during early flexor tendon healing: an investigation in a canine model. *J Orthop Res* 2001;19:869–872.
25. Hart DA, Nakamura N, Marchuk L, et al. Complexity of determining cause and effect in vivo after antisense gene therapy. *Clin Orthop* 2000;379S:242–251.
26. Shah M, Foreman DM, Ferguson MW. Neutralisation of TGF-beta 1 and TGF-beta 2 or exogenous addition of TGF-beta 3 to cutaneous rat wounds reduces scarring. *J Cell Sci* 1995;108:985–1002.
27. Batten ML, Hansen JC, Dahners LE. Influence of dosage and timing of application of platelet-derived growth factor on early healing of the rat medial collateral ligament. *J Orthop Res* 1996;14:736–741.

28. Hildebrand KA, Woo SL, Smith DW, et al. The effects of platelet-derived growth factor-BB on healing of the rabbit medial collateral ligament. An in vivo study. *Am J Sports Med* 1998;26:549–554.
29. Kobayashi D, Kurosaka M, Yoshiya S, Mizuno K. Effect of basic fibroblast growth factor on the healing of defects in the canine anterior cruciate ligament. *Knee Surg Sports Traumatol Arthrosc* 1997;5:189–194.
30. Fukui N, Katsuragawa Y, Sakai H, Oda H, Nakamura K. Effect of local application of basic fibroblast growth factor on ligament healing in rabbits. *Rev Rhum Engl Ed* 1998;65: 406–414.
31. Wolfman NM, Hattersley G, Cox K, Celeste AJ, Nelson R, Yamaji N, et al. Ectopic induction of tendon and ligament in rats by growth and differentiation factors 5, 6, and 7, members of the TGF-beta gene family. *J Clin Invest* 1997;100:321–330.
32. Luyten FP. Cartilage-derived morphogenetic protein-1. *Int J Biochem Cell Biol* 1997;29: 1241–1244.
33. Houston P, Campbell CJ, Svaren J, Milbrandt J, Braddock M. The transcriptional corepressor NAB2 blocks Egr-1-mediated growth factor activation and angiogenesis. *Biochem Biophys Res Commun* 2001;283:480–486.
34. Bryant M, Drew GM, Houston P, Hissey P, Campbell CJ, Braddock M. Tissue repair with a therapeutic transcription factor. *Hum Gene Ther* 2000;11:2143–2158.
35. Bateman JF, Lamande SR, Ramshaw JAM. Collagen superfamily. In Comper, W.D. (ed). *Extracellular Matrix*, Vol. 2. Harwood Academic Publishers, Amsterdam, Netherlands, 1996, pp. 22–67.
36. Parry DAD, Barnes GRG, Craig AS. A comparison of the size distribution of collagen fibrils in connective tissues as a function of age and a possible relationship between fibril size distribution and mechanical properties. *Proc R Soc Lond B Biol Sci* 1978;203: 305–321.
37. Doillon C, Dunn MG, Bender E, Silver F. Collagen fiber formation in repair tissue: development of strength and toughness. *Collagen Rel Res* 1992;5:481–492.
38. Birk DE, Mayne R. Localization of collagen types I, III and V during tendon development. Changes in collagen types I and III are correlated with changes in fibril diameter. *Eur J Cell Biol* 1997;72:352–361.
39. Romanic AM, Adachi E, Kadler KE, Hojima Y, Prockop DJ. Copolymerization of pNcollagen III and collagen I. pNcollagen III decreases the rate of incorporation of collagen I into fibrils, the amount of collagen I incorporated, and the diameter of the fibrils formed. *J Biol Chem* 1991;266:12703–12709.
40. Birk DE, Fitch JM, Babiarz JP, Doane KJ, Linsenmayer TF. Collagen fibrillogenesis in vitro: interaction of types I and V collagen regulates fibril diameter. *J Cell Sci* 1990;95: 649–657.
41. Marchant JK, Hahn RA, Linsenmayer TF, Birk DE. Reduction of type V collagen using a dominant-negative strategy alters the regulation of fibrillogenesis and results in the loss of corneal-specific fibril morphology. *J Cell Biol* 1996;135:1415–1426.
42. Nurminskaya MV, Birk DE. Differential expression of genes associated with collagen fibril growth in the chicken tendon: identification of structural and regulatory genes by subtractive hybridization. *Arch Biochem Biophys* 1998;350:1–9.
43. Vogel KG, Trotter JA. The effect of proteoglycans on the morphology of collagen fibrils formed in vitro. *Coll Rel Res* 1987;7:105–114.
44. Birk DE, Nurminskaya MV, Zycband EI. Collagen fibrillogenesis in situ: fibril segments undergo post-depositional modifications resulting in linear and lateral growth during matrix development. *Dev Dyn* 1995;202:229–243.
45. Danielson KG, Baribault H, Holmes DF, Graham H, Kadler KE, Iozzo RV. Target disruption of decorin leads to abnormal collagen fibril morphology and skin fragility. *J Cell Biol* 1997;136:729–743.

46. Kuc IM, Scott PG. Increased diameters of collagen fibrils precipitated in vitro in the presence of decorin from various connective tissues. *Connect Tissue Res* 1997;36:287–296.
47. Hedbom E, Heinegard D. Interaction of a 59-kDa connective tissue matrix protein with collagen I and collagen II. *J Biol Chem* 1989;264:6898–6905.
48. Ezura Y, Chakravarti S, Oldberg A, Chervoneva I, Birk DE. Differential expression of lumican and fibromodulin regulate collagen fibrillogenesis in developing mouse tendons. *J Cell Biol* 2000;151:779–788.
49. Chakravarti S, Magnuson T, Lass JH, Jepsen KJ, LaMantia C, Carroll H. Lumican regulates collagen fibril assembly: skin fragility and corneal opacity in the absence of lumican. *J Cell Biol* 1998;141:1277–1286.
50. Kyriakides TR, Zhu YH, Smith LT, et al. Mice that lack thrombospondin 2 display connective tissue abnormalities that are associated with disordered collagen fibrillogenesis, an increased vascular density, and a bleeding diathesis. *J Cell Biol* 1998;140:419–430.
51. Liaw L, Birk DE, Ballas CB, Whitsitt JS, Davidson JM, Hogan BL. Altered wound healing in mice lacking a functional osteopontin gene (spp1). *J Clin Invest* 1998;101:1468–1478.
52. Evans CH, Robbins PD. Possible orthopaedic application of gene therapy. *J Bone Joint Surg* 1995;77A:1103–1114.
53. Eming SA, Morgan JR, Berger A. Gene therapy for tissue repair: approaches and prospects. *Brit J Plast Surg* 1997;50:491–500.
54. Oligino TJ, Yao Q, Ghivizzani SC, Robbins P. Vector systems for gene transfer to joints. *Clin Orthop* 2000;379:S17–S30.
55. Musgrave DS, Fu FH, Huard J. Gene therapy and tissue engineering in orthopaedic surgery. *J Am Acad Orthop Surg* 2002;10:6–15.
56. Kaneda Y, Morishita R, Tomita N. Increased expression of DNA cointroduced with nuclear protein in adult rat liver. *J Mol Med* 1995;73:289–297.
57. Kaneda Y. Improvements in gene therapy technologies. *Mol Urol* 2001;5:85–89.
58. Nakamura N, Horibe S, Matsumoto N, et al. Transient introduction of a foreign gene into healing rat patellar ligament. *J Clin Invest* 1996;97:226–231.
59. Ozkan I, Shino K, Nakamura N, et al. Direct in vivo gene transfer to healing rat patellar ligament by intra-arterial delivery of HVJ-liposomes. *Eur J Clin Invest* 1999;29:63–67.
60. Gerich TG, Kang R, Fu FH, Robbins PD, Evans CH. Gene transfer to the rabbit patellar tendon: potential for genetic enhancement of tendon and ligament healing. *Gene Ther* 1996; 3:1089–1093.
61. Hildebrand KA, Deie M, Allen CR, et al. Early expression of marker genes in the rabbit medial collateral and anterior cruciate ligaments: the use of different viral vectors and the effects of injury. *J Orthop Res* 1999;17:37–42.
62. Lou J, Manske PR, Aoki M, Joyce ME. Adenovirus-mediated gene transfer into tendon and tendon sheath. *J Orthop Res* 1996;14:513–517.
63. Menetrey J, Kasemkijwattana C, Day CS, et al. Direct-, fibroblast- and myoblast-mediated gene transfer to the anterior cruciate ligament. *Tissue Eng* 1999;5:435–442.
64. Nakamura N, Shino K, Natsuume T, et al. Early biological effect of in vivo gene transfer of platelet-derived growth factor (PDGF)-B into healing patellar ligament. *Gene Ther* 1998;5: 1165–1170.
65. Roberts AB, Sporn MB, Assoian RK, et al. Transforming growth factor type β: rapid induction of fibrosis and angiogenesis in vivo and stimulation of collagen formation in vitro. *Proc Natl Acad Sci USA* 1987;83:4167–4171.
66. Natsuume T, Nakamura N, Shino K, et al. *In Vivo Introduction of Hepatocyte Growth Factor/Scatter Factor (HGF/SF) in Healing Patellar Ligament*. Abstract 94, Proceedings of the 44th Meeting of the Orthopaedic Research Society, New Orleans, LA, 1998.
67. Lou J, Tu Y, Burns M, Silva MJ, Manske P. BMP-12 gene transfer augmentation of lacerated tendon repair. *J Orthop Res* 2001;19:1199–1202.

68. Helm GA, Li JZ, Alden TD, et al. A light and electron microscopic study of ectopic tendon and ligament formation induced by bone morphogenetic protein-13 adenoviral gene therapy. *J Neurosurg* 2001;95:298–307.
69. Buxton P, Edwards C, Archer CW, Francis-West P. Growth/differentiation factor-5 (GDF-5) and skeletal development. *J Bone Joint Surg* 83A Suppl 2001;1:S23–30.
70. Lou J, Kubota H, Hotokezaka S, Ludwig FJ, Manske PR. In vivo gene transfer and overexpression of focal adhesion kinase (pp125 FAK) mediated by recombinant adenovirus-induced tendon adhesion formation and epitenon cell change. *J Orthop Res* 1997;15: 911–918.
71. Parsons JT, Martin KH, Slack JK, Taylor JM, Weed SA. Focal adhesion kinase: a regulator of focal adhesion dynamics and cell movement. *Oncogene* 2000;19:5606–5613.
72. Weber IT, Harrison RW, Iozzo RV. Model structure of decorin and implications for collagen fibrillogenesis. *J Biol Chem* 1996;271:31767–31770.
73. Boykiw R, Sciore P, Reno C, Marchuk L, Frank CB, Hart DA. Altered levels of extracellular matrix molecules mRNA in healing rabbit ligaments. *Matrix Biol* 1998;17:371–378.
74. Nakamura N, Timmermann SA, Hart DA, et al. A comparison of in vivo gene delivery methods for antisense therapy in ligament healing. *Gene Ther* 1998;5:1455–1461.
75. Crooke ST, Bennett CF. Progress in antisense oligonucleotide therapeutics. *Ann Rev Pharmacol Toxicol* 1996;36:107–129.
76. Nakamura N, Hart DA, Kaneda Y, et al. Decorin antisense gene therapy improves functional healing of early rabbit ligament scar with enhanced collagen fibrillogenesis in vivo. *J Orthop Res* 2000;18:517–523.
77. Hart DA, Nakamura N, Boorman R, et al. Functional improvement in ligament scar tissue following antisense gene therapy: A model system for in vivo engineering of connective tissues. *Gene Ther Mol Biol* 1999;4:285–290.
78. Niyibizi C, Kavalkovich K, Yamaji T, Woo SL. Type V collagen is increased during rabbit medial collateral ligament healing. *Knee Surg Sports Traumatol Arthrosc* 2000;8: 281–285.
79. Shimomura T, Jia F, Niyibizi C, Woo SL. Antisense oligonucleotides reduce synthesis of procollagen alpha1 (V) chain in human patellar tendon fibroblasts: potential application in healing ligaments and tendons. *Connect Tissue Res* 2003;44:167–172.

Index

www.ingramcontent.com/pod-product-compliance
Lightning Source LLC
Chambersburg PA
CBHW081742030826
49219CB00006B/406
* 9 7 8 1 5 8 8 2 9 1 7 4 5 *